T0202203

Prevention, Policy, and Public Health

Prevention, Policy, and Public Health

Edited by
Amy A. Eyler
Jamie F. Chriqui
Sarah Moreland-Russell
and
Ross C. Brownson

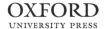

OXFORD
UNIVERSITY PRESS

OXFORD
UNIVERSITY PRESS

Oxford University Press is a department of the University of Oxford. It furthers
the University's objective of excellence in research, scholarship, and education
by publishing worldwide.Oxford is a registered trade mark of Oxford University
Press in the UK and certain other countries.

Published in the United States of America by Oxford University Press
198 Madison Avenue, New York, NY 10016, United States of America.

© Oxford University Press 2016

First Edition published in 2016

Cataloging-in-Publication data is on file at the Library of Congress
ISBN 978-0-19-022465-3

Contents

Preface

Policy impacts our health in many ways. Do you get a drink of water from the faucet? Do you wear a safety belt in your car? Do you find fresh produce options at your grocery store? We can do these things often without a second thought, because of the policies in place. In fact, policies had a role in every one of the 10 public health achievements of the last century. Sanitation of water, vaccination mandates, motor vehicle safety, and the recognition that tobacco is a public health threat were guided by policy action to influence practice and prioritize resources. One simple way of measuring policy-related impact is in life expectancy, which historically, increased very slowly. Since 1900, however, Americans have gained over 30 years of life due largely in part to health-related policy measures. Policies also play an important role globally. The World Health Organization has deemed "Health in all policies" the guiding principle for all global health activities. The goal of this principle is to improve population health, health equity, and the context in which health systems function by amending public policymaking across sectors in order to achieve the most favorable health impacts.

Although increasingly important to public health, understanding how public policy works can be challenging. An old quote attributed to Otto Van Bismark says something like, "Laws are like sausages and you should never watch either one being made." It is true that the policy process can be complicated, messy, and potentially unappetizing, but as the previous examples indicate, the results can be positive. Public health professionals can be instrumental in ensuring a beneficial policy outcome.

Stakeholders from many agencies and disciplines often come together to develop, implement, enforce, oppose, or support various policies. Public health representatives play an important role on these stakeholder teams by making sure that the principle of "health in all policies" is considered. They also can provide input on evidence, best practices, and effective evaluation strategies. Communicating research information, as well as advocating for the best possible policy option, are also important responsibilities of public health professionals.

Although policy plays a major role in health promotion and disease prevention, training public health students, researchers, and professionals to be effective in the policy arena remains a need. Information on public policy theoretical frameworks, analysis, and relevant policy applications are often lacking in public health professional preparation or development programs. Knowledge and skills related to policy are imperative in order to address the complex health challenges within today's society successfully. This book will provide the basis for understanding the dynamics of policies and politics for public health students, researchers, and professionals.

ORGANIZATION OF THE BOOK

This book presents policy information in three distinct yet related sections. Section 1 outlines fundamental policy concepts. This information lays the foundation for readers to gain a better understanding of the intricacies of policy. Chapter 1 sets the stage for the rest of the book and outlines the importance of policy in preventing disease and premature death. This chapter provides historical and current examples of policy impact on public health. Although the book is not about *healthcare* policy, this chapter describes how the Affordable Care Act is an important public policy that relates to health promotion and disease prevention. Chapter 2 explains the process and particulars of public policy, including governmental basics. Chapter 3 outlines and describes the most commonly used policy theories in public health. Tools that can help in ascertaining appropriate policy strategies through policy analysis, evidence-base, and measurement are presented in Chapter 4. The last chapter in this section describes policy implications of social and economic determinants of health.

Section 2 explores policies related to selected risk factors for premature death. Each chapter in this section describes a specific health topic, its implications, and public policy strategies used to address the problem. The chapters also include illustrative "real world" case studies of specific policy examples related to each topic. These topics include tobacco, nutrition and obesity policy, physical activity, alcohol, infectious disease, injury, violence against women, sexual behavior, and illicit drug use.

Section 3 provides next steps for improving public health through policy. Chapter 15 describes policy tracking and surveillance for assessing policy adoption and content for advocacy and evaluation purposes. In Chapter 16, effective strategies on communicating research to policy and practice are outlined, with relevant examples provided. Chapter 17 describes the importance of advocacy and identifies several advocacy approaches for prevention policy. Lastly, the book ends with a chapter on future directions for professionals seeking to better facilitate public health improvement through policy. Together, these sections can be considered a primer to truly understanding the connections between prevention, policy, and public health.

About the Editors

Amy A. Eyler, PhD, is an Assistant Professor and Assistant Dean of Public Health at the Brown School, Washington University in St. Louis. Her main research interests are health promotion through community policy and environmental interventions, with a focus on physical activity and obesity prevention. For over a decade, she served as Principal Investigator for the Physical Activity Policy Research Network (PAPRN), a national network of researchers who study the influence of policy on population physical activity. She is the Past Chair of the physical activity section of the American Public Health Association, a member of the American College of Sports Medicine, and a Certified Health Education Specialist.

Jamie F. Chriqui, PhD, MHS, is a Professor of Health Policy and Administration and a Fellow in the Institute for Health Research and Policy in the School of Public Health at the University of Illinois at Chicago. She is considered a nationwide expert on public health policy surveillance and evaluation and has led or is involved with numerous nationwide studies examining public health policies and their impacts, particularly on chronic disease risk factors such as tobacco use, physical activity, diet and nutrition, obesity, and substance use. Her research is supported by the National Institutes of Health, the Centers for Disease Control and Prevention, the U.S. Department of Agriculture, and the Robert Wood Johnson Foundation. She holds a BA in political science from Barnard College, Columbia University, an MHS in Health Policy from the Johns Hopkins University School of Hygiene and Public Health, and a PhD in policy sciences (health policy concentration) from the University of Maryland, Baltimore County.

Sarah Moreland-Russell, PhD, is an Assistant Research Professor at Washington University in St. Louis. Sarah is involved in several studies, including some with national, state, and local-level focus that assess public health policy implementation. Specifically, her research focuses on health policy analysis and evaluation, specifically regarding tobacco control and obesity prevention initiatives, organizational and systems science and evaluation, and dissemination and implementation of public health policies. Her work has been supported by the Centers for Disease Control and Prevention and the National Institutes of Health and has contributed toward the need for local level public health policy adoption, strategies for disseminating results for more effective implementation of evidence-based policy, and the evaluation of public health programs.

Ross C. Brownson, PhD, is the Bernard Becker Professor of Public Health at Washington University in St. Louis. He is involved in numerous community-level studies designed to understand and reduce modifiable risk factors such as physical inactivity, obesity, and tobacco use. In particular, he is interested in the impacts of environmental and policy interventions on health behaviors, and he conducts research on disseminating evidence-based interventions. His research is supported by the National Institutes of Health, the Centers for Disease Control and Prevention, and the Robert Wood Johnson Foundation.

Contributors

Gabriela J. Camberos
Brown School
Washington University in St. Louis
St. Louis, Missouri

Tonya Edmond
Brown School
Washington University in St. Louis
St. Louis, Missouri

Robert Fields
Brown School
Washington University in St. Louis
St. Louis, Missouri

Roberta R. Friedman
Rudd Center for Food
    Policy & Obesity
University of Connecticut
Hartford, Connecticut

James Gilsinan
Professor of Political Science
Saint Louis University
St. Louis, Missouri

Shelley D. Golden
University of North Carolina Gillings
    School of Global Public Health
Chapel Hill, North Carolina

Richard A. Grucza
Department of Psychiatry
Washington University School of
    Medicine
St. Louis, Missouri

Melissa Jonson-Reid
Brown School
Washington University in St. Louis
St. Louis, Missouri

Harry T. Kwon
Division of Research Education
Office of Extramural Research,
    Education, and Priority Populations
Agency for Healthcare Research
    and Quality
Rockville, Maryland

Janet L. Lauritsen
University of Missouri, St. Louis
St. Louis, Missouri

Duane C. McBride
Behavioral Sciences
Institute for Prevention of Addictions
Andrews University
Berrien Springs, Michigan

David E. Nelson
Cancer Prevention Fellowship Program
Division of Cancer Prevention
National Cancer Institute
Bethesda, Maryland

Andrew D. Plunk
Department of Pediatrics
Eastern Virginia Medical School
Norfolk, Virginia

William G. Powderly
Institute for Public Health
Washington University School of Medicine
St. Louis, Missouri

Jason Q. Purnell
Brown School
Washington University in St. Louis
St. Louis, Missouri

Christina N. Sansone
School of Public Health
University of Illinois at Chicago
Chicago, Illinois

F. David Schneider
Saint Louis University
St. Louis, Missouri

Marlene B. Schwartz
Rudd Center for Food Policy & Obesity
Department of Human Development &
    Family Studies
University of Connecticut
Hartford, Connecticut

Frederic E. Shaw
Centers for Disease Control and
    Prevention
Atlanta, Georgia

Sarah Simon
Center on Society and Health Virginia
    Commonwealth University
Richmond, Virginia

David A. Sleet
Division of Unintentional Injury
National Center for Injury Prevention
Centers for Disease Control
    and Prevention
Atlanta, Georgia

Bradley Stoner
Department of Anthropology
Washington University in St. Louis
St. Louis, Missouri

Yvonne M. Terry-McElrath
Institute for Social Research
University of Michigan
Ann Arbor, Michigan

Curtis J. VanderWaal
Department of Social Work
Andrews University
Berrien Springs, Michigan

Sabrina K. Young
Institute for Health Research and Policy
School of Public Health
University of Illinois at Chicago
Chicago, Illinois

Emily B. Zimmerman
Center on Society and Health Virginia
    Commonwealth University
Richmond, Virginia

Marissa Zwald
Brown School
Washington University in St. Louis
St. Louis, Missouri

Part 1
Fundamental Policy Concepts

1

The Power of Policy to Improve Health

Amy A. Eyler and Ross C. Brownson

"Public policy can be one of the most effective approaches to protecting and improving the health of the population."[1]
Institute of Medicine, 2012

LEARNING OBJECTIVES

1. Provide historical examples of policy success in public health.
2. Explain rationale for policy as a strategy to improve health.
3. Describe examples of various levels of policy related to disease prevention.

INTRODUCTION

Policies are fundamentally linked to health promotion and disease prevention. They create opportunities for broad and sustainable improvements in population health, and currently, there is a definite need for improvement. The societal burden of *preventable* chronic disease is staggering. Roughly 80% of deaths in the United States are now caused by chronic diseases such as heart disease, cancer, hypertension, stroke, and diabetes.[2] Mortality is not the only concern, because these diseases are also the biggest drivers of healthcare expenditures in the United States, accounting for more than 75% of annual spending on medical care. Costs of lost productivity due to illness add to the economic burden. For example, the total estimated cost of diabetes in the United States for 2012 was $176 billion in direct medical costs and an additional $69 billion in reduced productivity.[3] The amount for cardiovascular disease is even greater, with costs reported as $273 billion for direct medical care and $172 in lost productivity.[4] These totals are estimated to grow exponentially as costs rise and the population ages.[2-4] This problem, although dire, is not insurmountable. These diseases are linked to many modifiable lifestyle or behavioral risk factors that can be addressed through interventions that include policy changes. The power of policy is exemplified by the fact that every one of the top 10 public health achievements in the last century was facilitated by some sort of policy action to influence practice and prioritize resources (see Table 1.1).[5]

Historically, policies that focused on prevention greatly affected disease rates, increased life expectancy, and improved quality of life. In 1900, there were approximately 100 cases of typhoid fever for every 100,000 persons living in the United States.[6] In 2006, the rate had declined to 0.1 cases for every 100,000 persons (only 353 cases of illness in total) and approximately 75% of these—or 265 cases—occurred among international travelers.[7] This dramatic decrease is linked to policies related to improving water quality through disinfection and sanitation, the first of which was

Table 1.1 Ten Public Health Achievements of the Last Century and Examples of Related Policy Strategies

Public Health Achievement	Related Policy Strategies
Vaccination	• Requiring vaccination for school children • Requiring vaccination for healthcare workers • Improvements in access to vaccines for elderly
Motor-vehicle safety	• Requiring safety belts and child restraints • Requiring motorcycle helmets • Programs for decreased drinking and driving
Safer workplaces	• Requirements on reduced exposure to hazards • Improvements in workplace safety monitoring
Control of infectious diseases	• Sanitation requirements • Required testing for water safety • Improvements in development and distribution of antimicrobial therapy
Decline in deaths from coronary heart disease and stroke	• Requirements related to risk reduction (e.g., smoking) • Improvements in access to early detection and better treatment
Safer and healthier foods	• Requirements for testing for microbial contamination • Increased surveillance • Improvements in food labeling
Healthier mothers and babies	• Improvements in access to prenatal care • Improvements in nutrition for mothers and children
Family planning	• Increased access to contraception • Promotion of barrier contraceptives to prevent pregnancy and sexually transmitted diseases
Fluoridation of drinking water	• Requirements for fluoridation
Recognition of tobacco as a health hazard	• Decreased access to tobacco for youth • Clean indoor air regulations • Advertisement restrictions

Source: Centers for Disease Control and Prevention. 1999. Ten great public health achievements—United States, 1900–1999. *MMWR.* 48(12):241–243.

implemented in 1908 in Jersey City, New Jersey.[7] Many U.S. cities followed suit with similar policies, and this movement resulted in the dramatic decrease of disease. Policies to ensure a safe and reliable water supply continue to emerge. The Clean Water Act, passed in 1972, addressed environmental contaminants and sources of water pollution, such as sewage.[8] Policies related to treating water to remove or kill disease-causing contaminants or to monitoring water quality remain a health priority.

Immunization or vaccine policies also improved population health by preventing outbreaks of disease. The late 1770s saw an emerging acceptance of Dr. Edward Jenner's cowpox inoculation to prevent smallpox. As a result, governments became aware of the potential and widespread impact of preventing this devastating disease. The science of developing successful vaccinations for infectious diseases advanced and lawmaking agencies realized their value in protecting population health, productivity, and societal security.[9] In 1855, Massachusetts passed the first state law requiring vaccinations for school children,[10] which was soon followed by many other state, organizational, and school district policies requiring vaccines. After 1949, there were no endemic cases of smallpox in the United States.[11] Vaccination policies have had global impact, too. In the 1960s and 1970s, the World Health Organization (WHO) launched a large-scale smallpox vaccination campaign. This successful effort culminated in the last naturally occurring case of smallpox in Somalia in 1977.[12] (See Chapter 10 for more information on policies related to vaccines.)

Another example of a public health issue addressed through past regulation and policy is tobacco control. Laws regulating taxes, access, advertising, and use contributed to the substantial reduction in smoking- and tobacco-related morbidity and mortality.[13-15] Figure 1.1 depicts a timeline of historical events and policy-related strategies plotted with the per capita use of cigarettes. Policies such as broadcast advertisement bans, increased taxes, and others increasing the availability of nicotine replacement contributed to the declining rates of smoking over time. (See Chapter 6 for more details on policies related to tobacco.)

Recognizing the influence of policy on health, many international, federal, state, and local efforts to improve health now emphasize *policy change* as a way to make health promotion strategies more impactful and sustainable. WHO recommends effective and up-to-date policies for successful impact on many health issues. For example, the 2014 Ebola outbreak prompted WHO to facilitate the development and implementation of new policies across many different sectors.[16] Policies related to strengthening health systems, vaccination trials, and emergency preparedness expedited reduced prevalence of this deadly disease.[16] The Patient Protection and Affordable Care Act (ACA) is a U.S. federal policy that includes many provisions for health promotion and disease prevention. (See Box 1.1.)

In 2009, The Centers for Disease Control and Prevention (CDC) published *Recommended Community Strategies and Measurements to Prevent Obesity in the United States*.[23] This document outlined ways in which local governments can promote healthy eating and active living through policy and environmental changes. Many of the recommendations require formal public policy. In order to implement recommendations such as "enhance infrastructure for walking and bicycling" or "restrict access to less healthy foods at public venues" most effectively, policies need to be developed,

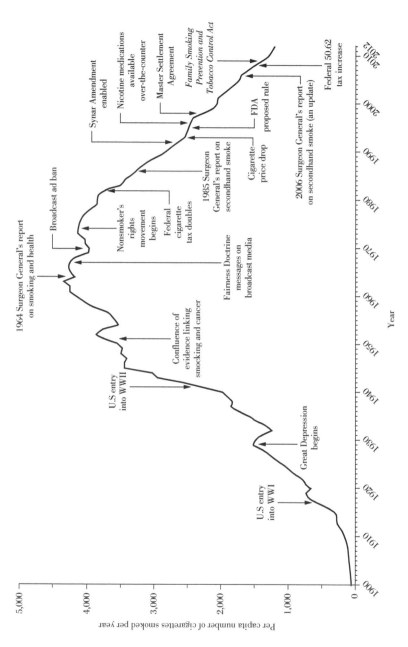

Figure 1.1 Adult per capita cigarette consumption and major historical and policy events. (Adults ≥ 18 years of age as reported annually by the Census Bureau.)

Sources: Adapted from Warner 1985 with permission from Massachusetts Medical Society; U.S. Department of Health and Human Services, 1989; Creek et al, 1994; U.S. Department of Agriculture, 2000; U.S. Census Bureau, 2013; U.S. Department of the Treasury 2013.

Box 1.1 Federal Prevention Policy: Prevention and Public Health within the Affordable Care Act

The Affordable Care Act (ACA) established the Prevention and Public Health Fund (PPHF) to provide expanded and sustained national investments in prevention and public health, to improve health outcomes, and to enhance health care quality. The U.S. Congress authorized $18.75 billion for this fund between 2010 and 2022 and $2 billion per year after that.[17] PPHF is the first mandatory funding stream dedicated to providing resources for public health programs to reduce the leading causes of death and disability through a broad range of evidence-based activities. Funds are being used to support a variety of community and clinical prevention programs, to enhance the public health infrastructure and workforce, and to expand public health research and tracking efforts. In spite of being a landmark fund allocation for public health, the amount initially funded was reduced when Congress passed legislation that cut the fund by $6.25 billion over a 9-year period (2013–2021), in order to offset a scheduled cut to Medicare physician payments. In 2014, $1 billion was allocated to the fund through the Consolidated Appropriations Act of 2014, but sequestration cut $72 million, leaving $928 million for prevention and wellness activities as of fiscal year 2014.[18]

The ACA also expands access to preventive services for women. Through the ACA, women's preventive healthcare services are already covered and with no cost sharing under some health plans. The eight prevention services for women are: well-woman visits; gestational diabetes screening; Human Papilloma Virus DNA testing; Sexually Transmitted Infections counseling; HIV screening and testing; contraception and contraception counseling; breast-feeding support, supplies, and counseling; and interpersonal and domestic violence screening and counseling.[19]

Another way ACA has promoted prevention is through the formation of the National Prevention, Health Promotion, and Public Health Council (National Prevention Council), which provides leadership and coordination related to health and prevention at the federal level. Chaired by the U.S. Surgeon General, this council is made up of heads of 20 federal departments and agencies to emphasize that health is a transdisciplinary cross-sector effort. The council was tasked with the development of the first National Prevention Strategy (NPS) and has provided a platform for making the federal government a leader in prevention, with a particular focus on reducing tobacco use and increasing access to health food.[17,20]

Another important aspect of prevention within ACA is the provision for menu labeling. In 2011, the Food and Drug Administration (FDA) published two proposed rules in the *Federal Register* on nutritional labeling for vending machines and chain restaurants.[21] These rules require restaurants and similar retail food establishments that are part of a chain with 20 or more locations to provide calorie and other nutrition information for standard menu items, including food on display and self-service food. In 2014, a detailed calorie-labeling component was added to the *Federal Register*.[22] (See Chapter 7 for more information on nutrition and obesity policies.)

Box 1.2 Communities Putting Prevention to Work

As a result of the growing burden of preventable chronic disease, the U.S. Department of Health and Human Services created the Communities Putting Prevention to Work (CPPW) program, which is led by the Centers for Disease Control and Prevention (CDC). Fifty communities around the country were funded in 2010 to implement policy, systems, and environmental interventions geared toward reducing obesity, tobacco use, and second-hand smoke exposure.[25] These interventions were developed locally by community leadership teams comprising representatives from public health, education, planning, health care, transportation, agriculture, business, local government, and other sectors. Within 12 months, 790 policy, systems, and environmental outcome objectives were planned.[24] Examples of policies to improve food access within CPPW communities included wellness policies, partnering with food assistance programs, and pricing strategies. To increase physical activity, these communities worked on policies that support the creation of sidewalks and bike lanes, urban design and land use policies that encourage physical activity, and policies to require daily physical activity in childcare and afterschool settings. For tobacco use prevention, CPPW communities worked to develop comprehensive smoke-free policies and pricing strategies.[24] Overall, the program has a potential to reach 55 million people, or 1 out of 6 Americans who live within the funded jurisdictions.[24,25]

implemented, and enforced.[23] In a recent grant program, CDC relied on sustainable, high-impact policy, system, and environmental changes for sustained success in the Communities Putting Prevention to Work (CPPW) projects.[24,25] (See Box 1.2.)

The Institute of Medicine's reports, *Accelerating Progress on Obesity Prevention*[26] and *Childhood Obesity Prevention Actions for Local Governments*[27] also called for policy-related interventions. National reports outline policy action for other public health topics. Recent Institute of Medicine reports called for a policy to increase the minimum age to purchase tobacco products[28] and outlined policies to impact alcohol access to reduce underage drinking.[29]

National advocacy agencies also rely on public policies to enhance their efforts. For example, the American Heart Association (AHA) recognizes the importance of policies in fighting cardiovascular disease. The *Guide to Improving Cardiovascular Health at the Community Level*[30] outlines ways that local programs and policies can complement clinical guidelines in the prevention of heart disease and stroke. Ensuring clean indoor air is one of the community strategies in the AHA guide that is promoted through policy. State and local laws that restrict smoking in public areas reduce the exposure to the whole population in that jurisdiction which, in turn, reduces the population disease risk.

PUBLIC POLICY AND PUBLIC HEALTH WITHIN A SOCIO-ECOLOGICAL FRAMEWORK

For the purposes of this book, we will focus on *public policy*, which is defined as laws, regulatory measures, courses of action, and funding priorities concerning a given topic by a governmental entity or its representatives.[31,32] To understand the role and impact of public policy, it is also important to understand the various policy systems and players. Governmental policy systems vary widely in their structure and scope, ranging from totalitarian to democratic governments. In this book, the descriptions of public policy are focused primarily on multicentric (democratic) governments, which are more common in middle and upper income countries. Whether at a local, state, or federal level, the purpose of a representative body is to enact rules, laws, or ordinances that are, in turn, implemented by executive or administrative agents.

Public policies can be described in the context of a broader framework related to population health. McLeroy and colleagues outlined a socio-ecological framework that emphasizes the linkages and relationships among multiple factors affecting health.[33] The framework is most often drawn using concentric circles, with policy as the outermost layer that encompasses individual, organizational, and community characteristics. The outer circle depicts *public policy* at the federal, state, and local levels that regulates or promotes healthy behaviors or actions. This framework is not intended to be one-directional and each level contributes to health in unique and interrelated ways. Individual level characteristics can influence a behavioral outcome. These characteristics can be compounded by the influence of the organizational and community factors that can interact to facilitate or hinder the behavior. For example, eating a healthy diet may depend on individual characteristics such a motivation to eat healthy or taste preferences, but also on interpersonal factors such as social support from family. Additionally, organizational factors such as adequate break time for eating at work, community factors such as nearby places to buy healthy foods, and public policy such as tax incentives for stores to be located in communities, can all play a role in an individual's healthy eating behaviors. (See Chapter 3 for more information on policies and the socio-ecological framework.)

WHY USE POLICY TO PREVENT DISEASE AND IMPROVE POPULATION HEALTH?

The greatest public health challenges today are complex and require broad, multi-faceted solutions. Policies are beneficial in that they have the potential to affect *both* the environment and behavior to reduce health risks. Policies that result in systemic improvements in economic, physical, and social environments can provide opportunities, support, and cues for healthy behaviors.[34] Policies enforcing fines for the sale of alcoholic beverages to minors, for example, create less access to alcohol for minors and may reduce underage drinking. Requiring that healthy food be served in schools can promote an increase in fruit and vegetable consumption in children. Policies can alter social norms by influencing environments, too. As stricter bans on smoking in public places increased, the expectation of smoke-free air became the norm.[35] In numerous cities across Europe, local policies support active travel, making commuting by foot or bicycle the norm.[36,37]

Another benefit of using policies to promote health is that they have a broad scope. Unlike clinical or individual-level approaches, policies have the potential to reach a large population. Policy changes can benefit *all* people exposed to the environment rather than focusing on changing behaviors one person at a time.[38] If a school district implements a policy change, it has the potential to influence every student within that district. If a state mandates a curricular policy change, all public school students in the state will be affected. The CPPW program (Box 1.2) is another good example of the broad reach of policy. One in six Americans were exposed to policy, system, and environmental changes made through this program to prevent obesity and reduce tobacco use.[24,25] At a time when funding and resources for public health interventions are not abundant, broad population reach is vital.

Policy interventions also are more sustainable than individually focused efforts.[24,34] Influence exerted on individual factors such as knowledge or perception may not last over time because people may continue to be exposed to an environment that inhibits healthy behavior. Additionally, public policies are more permanent strategies for chronic disease prevention because they are formally embedded into local, state, or federal government. Enacted policies that are implemented and enforced can be sustained over time and can potentially affect the health of generations. The Public Health Cigarette Smoking Act of 1969 banned advertising of cigarettes on television and radio and remains enforced today.[39] Generations of children will not have been exposed to this type of advertising because of this law.

INTEGRATING POLICY WITH PUBLIC HEALTH RESEARCH AND PRACTICE

There is a growing body of research on the development, implementation, and outcome of policies related to public health. A content analysis of articles published in 16 top peer-reviewed public health journals from 1998 to 2008 revealed a marked increase in the number of articles related to tobacco policy, school policy, and healthcare policy over this 10-year period.[40] A growing number of research networks aim to study policies related to various health topics. Table 1.2 lists a selection of these networks and describes their purpose or mission.

Many of these networks emphasize the transdisciplinary or multidisciplinary nature of their work. Because stakeholders from a wide range of sectors are needed to develop and implement effective policy, a diverse network is essential. Think about a policy to reduce access to methamphetamines. Who is needed for input? The list includes representatives from the public health sector to help outline the extent of the problem, academics to help provide evidence base, businesses (e.g., drug stores) for information on implementation, public safety for enforcement, advocates to represent the public, and of course, policymakers. This breadth of expertise and input is needed if policies are to be successful in affecting complex health outcomes. The chapters in the second section of this book highlight examples of groups of stakeholders appropriate for specific public health policy topics.

Policies are an important aspect of international health research and practice. "Health in All Policies" (HiAP) is a phrase coined in the late 1990s and now is a

Table 1.2 Examples of Policy Research Networks

Network	Purpose or Mission
Active Living Research http://activelivingresearch.org	To work with governments, the private sector, and advocacy groups to apply the lessons of research to building great communities.
Alcohol Research Network http://www.dmu.ac.uk/research/research-faculties-and-institutes/health-and-life-sciences/health-policy-research-unit/alcohol-research-group.aspx	To pool expertise in alcohol research, build networks and partnerships, strengthen external funding capacity, and ensure that alcohol research is transferred into teaching, research, and practice.
Center for a Livable Future (Food Policy Network) http://www.jhsph.edu/research/centers-and-institutes/johns-hopkins-center-for-a-livable-future/about/index.html	To promote research and to develop and communicate about the complex interrelationships among diet, food production, environment and human health; to advance the ecological perspective in reducing threats to the health of the public; and to promote policies that protect health, the global environment, and the ability to sustain life for future generations.
Center for Infectious Disease Research and Policy http://www.cidrap.umn.edu/about-us/mission	To prevent illness and death from targeted infectious disease threats through research and translation of scientific information into real-world, practical application, polices, and solutions.
Global Health Policy Research Network http://www.cgdev.org/initiative/global-health-policy-research-network	To develop original research focused on high-priority global health policy issues.
Healthy Eating Research Network http://healthyeatingresearch.org/who-we-are/about-us/	Supports research on environmental and policy strategies that have strong potential to promote healthy eating among children.
Injury and Violence Prevention Network http://www.safestates.org/?IVPN	Supports injury and violence prevention policies at the national level and advocates for federal funding for injury and violence prevention.
Physical Activity Policy Research Network + http://www.globalobesity.org/gopc-news/paprn.html	To conduct and communicate policy research so it can be used by stakeholders in multiple sectors to support more physical activity for all Americans.
Research Network on Mental Health Policy Research http://www.macfound.org/press/info-sheets/research-network-mental-health-policy-research-information-sheet/	Develop a knowledge base linking mental health policies, financing, and organization to their effects on access to quality care.

cornerstone of global WHO activities. The goal of HiAP is to improve population health, health equity, and the context in which health systems function by amending public policymaking across sectors in order to achieve the most favorable impacts. This concept encompasses public policies within and outside of the public health sector.[41] HiAP also includes factors such as unintended health consequences as part of understanding the holistic effect of policy on health. Good examples of HiAP are zoning and land use laws that could effectuate changes to the built environment to enable healthy food access and physical activity opportunities within communities.

Policies also are fundamentally integrated with public health practice in the United States. In a document outlining a framework for the National Public Health Performance Standards program, 10 essential public health services are identified. Two of these services are explicitly related to policy: 1) develop policies and plans that support individual and community health efforts and 2) enforce laws and regulations that protect and ensure safety. Other essential services such as disease surveillance are implicitly related to public policy because programs and monitoring systems are guided by regulations and laws. In spite of the broad emphasis on using policy to improve health, many public health researchers and professionals are not adequately prepared to understand the policy process or effectively advocate for policy change.[42] Recognizing this deficit and the importance of policy as a public health strategy, The Association of Schools and Programs of Public Health (ASPPH) outlines the significance of policy within its "Critical Content of the Core for a 21st Century Master of Public Health Degree." They describe one of the foundational areas as:

> *legal, ethical, economic, and regulatory dimensions of health care and public health policy, the roles, influences, and responsibilities of the different agencies and branches of government, and approaches to developing, evaluating, and advocating for public health policies.*[43] *(p.5)*

Developing and engaging in policy is imperative to successfully addressing the complex health challenges within today's society. In order to do so, knowledge of the basic dynamics of the policy process, political theories, key terms, and policy analysis skills is needed.

SUMMARY

From both historical and current examples, it is clear that policies play a major role in health promotion and disease prevention. *Public policies* in particular, are broad in scope, have the potential to impact large populations, and will likely be more sustainable than individual-level efforts. Policies are not developed or implemented solely by policymakers. The process usually involves a transdisciplinary team of stakeholders with a vested interest in the issue. There is an important place for public health researchers and practitioners within these teams to provide input on evidence, best practices, and effective evaluation strategies.

REFERENCES

1. Institute of Medicine. *For the Public's Health: Revitalizing Law and Policy to Meet New Challenges.* Washington, DC: The National Academies Press; 2011.

2. Freudenberg N, Olden K. Getting serious about the prevention of chronic diseases. *Prev Chron Dis.* Jul 2011;8(4):A90.

3. American Diabetes Association. Economic costs of diabetes in the U.S. in 2012. *Diabetes Care.* Apr 2013;36(4):1033–1046.

4. Heidenreich PA, Trogdon JG, Khavjou OA, et al. Forecasting the future of cardiovascular disease in the United States: a policy statement from the American Heart Association. *Circulation.* Mar 1 2011;123(8):933–944.

5. Centers for Disease Control and Prevention. Ten great public health achievements—United States, 1900–1999. *MMWR.* 1999;48(12):241–243.

6. Centers for Disease Control and Prevention. Achievements in public health, 1900–1999: Safer and healthier foods. *MMWR.* 1999;48(40):905–932.

7. Abellera J, Adams D, Anderson W, et al. Summary of notifiable diseases—United States, 2009. *MMWR.* 2011;58(53):1–100.

8. United States Environmental Protection Agency. Clean Water Act (CWA). 2014; http://www.epa.gov/agriculture/lcwa.html#National%20Pollutant. Accessed April 10, 2015.

9. Stern AM, Markel H. The history of vaccines and immunization: familiar patterns, new challenges. *Health Affairs.* May–Jun 2005;24(3):611–621.

10. College of Physicians of Philadelphia. History of Vaccines: Government Regulation. 2015; http://www.historyofvaccines.org/content/articles/government-regulation. Accessed May 4, 2015.

11. Belongia EA, Naleway AL. Smallpox vaccine: the good, the bad, and the ugly. *Clinl Med Res.* Apr 2003;1(2):87–92.

12. Henderson DA. Edward Jenner's vaccine. *Public Health Reports.* Mar–Apr 1997; 112(2):116–121.

13. Instituteof Medicine BR, Stratton K, Wallace RB, Richard Bonnie Robert Wallace KS. *Ending the Tobacco Problem: A Blueprint for the Nation.* Washington, DC: The National Academies Press; 2007.

14. Levy DT, Chaloupka F, Gitchell J. The effects of tobacco control policies on smoking rates: a tobacco control scorecard. *J Pub Health Manag Pract.* Jul–Aug 2004;10(4):338–353.

15. U. S. Department of Health and Human Services. *The health consequences of smoking—50 years of progress: a report of the Surgeon General.* Washington, DC: U.S. Department of Health and Human Services; 2014.

16. World Health Organization. *The role of WHO within the United Nations Mission for Ebola Emergency Response: Report of the Secretariat.* Geneva, Switzerland: World Health Organization; 2015.

17. U.S. Department of Health and Human Services. Prevention and Public Health Fund. 2015; http://www.hhs.gov/open/prevention/index.html.

18. Association. APH. *Prevention and Public Health Fund: Dedicated to improving our nation's public health.* Washington, DC: APHA; 2014.

19. U.S. Department of Health and Human Services. Affordable Care Act rules on expanding access to preventive services for women. 2011; http://www.hhs.gov/healthcare/facts/factsheets/2011/08/womensprevention08012011a.html. Accessed April 3, 2015.

20. Shearer G. *Prevention provisions in the Affordable Care Act.* Washington, DC: American Public Health Association; 2010.

21. Henry J. Kaiser Family Foundation. Health reform implementation timeline. 2015; http://kff.org/interactive/implementation-timeline/. Accessed May 22, 2015.

22. Kux L. Food labeling; Nutrition labeling of standard menu items in restaurants and similar retail food establishments. *Federal Register: The Daily Journal of the United States Government.* 2014; https://www.federalregister.gov/articles/2014/12/01/2014-27833/food-labeling-nutrition-labeling-of-standard-menu-items-in-restaurants-and-similar-retail-food#h-4. Accessed May 22, 2015.

23. Keener D, Goodman K, Lowry A, Zaro S, Kettel Khan L. *Recommended community strategies and measurements to prevent obesity in the United States: Implementation and measurement guide.* Atlanta, GA: U.S. Department of Health and Human Services, Centers for Disease Control and Prevention; 2009.

24. Bunnell R, O'Neil D, Soler R, et al. Fifty communities putting prevention to work: accelerating chronic disease prevention through policy, systems and environmental change. *J Comm Health.* Oct 2012;37(5):1081–1090.

25. Centers for Disease Control and Prevention. Communities putting prevention to work. 2013; http://www.cdc.gov/nccdphp/dch/programs/communitiesputtingpreventiontowork/.

26. Institute of Medicine. *Accelerating progress in obesity prevention: solving the weight of the nation.* Washington DC: The National Academies Press; 2012.

27. Institute of Medicine. *Childhood obesity prevention actions for local governments.* Washington, DC: The National Academies Press; 2009.

28. Institute of Medicine. *Public health implications of raising the minimum age of legal access to tobacco products.* Washington, DC: The National Academies Press; 2015.

29. Institute of Medicine. *Reducing underage drinking: A collective responsibility.* Washington, DC: The National Academies Press; 2004.

30. Pearson TA, Palaniappan LP, Artinian NT, et al. American Heart Association Guide for Improving Cardiovascular Health at the Community Level, 2013 Update: a scientific statement for public health practitioners, healthcare providers, and health policy makers. *Circulation.* Apr 23 2013;127(16):1730–1753.

31. Evans S. *Public policy issues: research trends.* Nova Science Pub, Inc; 2008.

32. Centers for Disease Control and Prevention. Public health policy. 2013; http://www.cdc.gov/stltpublichealth/policy/index.html. Accessed May 1, 2015.

33. McLeroy K, Bibeau D, Steckler A, K. G. An ecological perspective on health promotion programs. *Health Educ Q.* 1998;15(4):351.

34. Brownson RC, Haire-Joshu D, Luke DA. Shaping the context of health: a review of environmental and policy approaches in the prevention of chronic diseases. *Ann Rev Pub Health.* 2006;27:341–370.

35. Hyland A, Barnoya J, Corral JE. Smoke-free air policies: past, present and future. *Tob Control.* 2012;21(2):154–161.

36. de Geus B, De Bourdeaudhuij I, Jannes C, Meeusen R. Psychosocial and environmental factors associated with cycling for transport among a working population. *Health Educ Res.* Aug 2008;23(4):697–708.

37. Goetzke F, Rave T. Bicycle use in Germany: explaining differences between municipalities with social network effects. *Urban Studies.* 2011;48(2):427–437.

38. Brownson RC, Baker EA, Housemann RA, Brennan LK, Bacak SJ. Environmental and policy determinants of physical activity in the United States. *Am J Public Health.* Dec 2001;91(12):1995–2003.

39. Centersfor Disease Control and Prevention. Smoking and tobacco use: legislation. 2012; http://www.cdc.gov/tobacco/data_statistics/by_topic/policy/legislation/index.htm. Accessed April 4, 2015.
40. Eyler AA, Dreisinger M. Publishing on policy: trends in public health. *Prev Chron Dis*. Jan 2011;8(1):A22.
41. World Health Organization. Health in all policies. 2013; http://www.healthpromotion2013.org/health-promotion/health-in-all-policies. Accessed May 5, 2015.
42. Institute of Medicine. *Who will keep the public healthy? Educating public health professionals for the 21st century*. Washington, DC: The National Academies Press; 2003.
43. Association of Schools & Programs of Public Health. *A Master of Public Health degree for the 21st Century*. Washington, DC: ASPPH; 2014.

2

Public Policy Explained

Shelley D. Golden and Sarah Moreland-Russell

LEARNING OBJECTIVES

1. Describe the difference between policy types.
2. Explain when government intervention is appropriate in relation to prevention.
3. Provide prevention policy examples for each branch of government.
4. Identify the stakeholders who help shape public policy.

WHAT IS PUBLIC POLICY?

What exactly is meant by *policy*? When many people think of public policy they might think of formal laws, rules, or regulations enacted by elected officials intended to direct or influence the actions, behaviors, and decisions of others.[1] Most of this book focuses on these "*big P Policies.*" But the term policy also is used to refer to "*little p policies,*" or organizational rules and practices, and sometimes normative behaviors in a specific setting. The development, implementation, and evaluation of "big P" and "little p" policies can differ but also can share some key tenets. Furthermore, the two can interact. Formal laws can make specific requirements of organizations, such as mandating physical education time in schools or setting guidelines for what constitutes sexual harassment in the workplace, but the ways in which schools and workplaces put those into day-to-day practice depend on more local, sometimes less formal, rules and systems of organization. Similarly, organizations can be breeding grounds for new policy ideas. For example, the smoke-free movement was born out of voluntary adoption of smoke-free workplace policies that spread and were developed into formal mandatory county, city, and/or state level smoke-free laws.[2]

Governments, and to some extent other organizations, do a variety of things through policymaking and other rulemaking. They collect money from individuals and businesses, usually in the form of taxes or fees, and then spend it on programs, services, subsidies, and grants. They outline the source and amounts of tax income, as well as the details of expenditures, in written budgets. Governments also regulate behaviors and practices of groups and individuals, outline private rights to which citizens are entitled, and help ensure those rights are not violated. They use the tools at their disposal to foster economic activity, as well as an informed and educated populace.

WHEN IS GOVERNMENT INTERVENTION CONSIDERED APPROPRIATE?

Public policy is a tool used by societies to allocate communal resources, solve social problems, and improve conditions. Public policies are particularly useful when individuals are unable to resolve specific conflicts on their own, but do agree on a political process for collective decision-making. By their nature, public policies usually allocate community resources in identified ways and/or place restrictions on the behavior or choices of individuals or groups. Yet democracies also value the freedom of people to live as they choose. As a result, policymakers and citizens themselves often design government structures to limit the scope of government action. Beliefs about when and why governments should intervene vary among individuals, due to their own life experiences, personal interests, and affinity for different ideologies.[3] Common rationales for government action that have been applied to public health policies, described in the next sections, include: (1) provision of public goods; (2) ensuring access to accurate information; (3) accounting for costs or benefits incurred by third parties (i.e., positive and negative externalities); (4) protection of vulnerable populations; and (5) ameliorating prior government failure.

Provision of Public Goods

Public goods are resources that are both available to everyone and inexhaustible. In other words, use of a public good by one person does not reduce the availability of that good for another. Examples of public goods include fresh air, national security, and street lighting. Other resources, like community parks or public roads, may have limits on consumption at extreme levels, but fit the definition on most occasions. Because people can benefit from public goods without paying for them, they will often choose not to, and government intervention, sometimes in partnership with other organizations, is required to produce them. The Global Polio Eradication Initiative, a public–private partnership to eliminate polio through worldwide vaccination and surveillance, is an example of a public health effort, supported in part by national governments, to provide a public good—a world free of polio.[4]

Ensuring Access to Accurate Information

In order for individual members of a society to make informed choices about their health, they must have access to available information about the costs, quality, and consequences of various goods and options. Governments often take action to ensure that health-related information is available to the public by dedicating resources to educational efforts. In some cases, other entities intentionally or unintentionally provide limited or misleading information to individuals or groups, prompting policy intervention. For example, evidence that the tobacco industry hid from its consumers health and addiction risks related to the products they sold has been used to advocate for restrictions on product marketing and availability.[5]

Accounting for Costs or Benefits Incurred by Third Parties

Sometimes the production or consumption of a good leads to unintended outcomes—positive and negative—for others. These indirect consequences are called *externalities*. Pollution from production facilities is a traditional example of negative externalities, but the concept applies elsewhere in public health as well. Alcohol use, for example, is associated with motor vehicle crashes and interpersonal violence, each of which can produce injuries for nondrinkers, as well as healthcare costs sometimes born by society at large.[6] Policies designed to raise the price of alcohol or limit outlet density could be justified, in part, as measures to recoup or prevent these externalities.[7]

Protection of Vulnerable Populations

Whether through Constitutional protection, other legislative means, or simply public opinion, societies often deem certain groups of people as deserving of extra protection from governments. Some groups, like children, may warrant special attention because they are less capable of self-protection or rational decision-making. Others, like racial minorities in the United States, may not have fair or equal access to information, power, and social resources due to longstanding prejudice. As a result, governments may implement specific policies to ensure that groups with limited decision-making authority are not manipulated by others, to prevent health risks from both historical and current discriminatory practices, and to extend health resources to underserved groups. Laws prohibiting the sale of sugar-sweetened beverages in schools[8] or to provide funding for targeted cancer screening programs[9] are two examples of policy efforts to improve health outcomes for vulnerable groups.

Ameliorating Prior Government Failure

Governments are run by individual people, and as such are imperfect organizations. Politicians are rarely experts in every topic they address, and may, therefore, make choices they might make differently with more information and input. In addition, politicians, as well as government staff, may adopt short-term views on problems and solutions, especially if pressured to document short-term returns to maintain their positions or political viability. Proliferation of the bureaucracy that characterizes modern political systems also creates interagency competition and redundancy, sometimes leading to inefficiency in addressing problems. Agencies within government can jockey for position and power in the larger political structure, leading to poor collaboration or inefficient use of resources. Finally, policies can be adopted using language that is confusing or in ways that contradict other policies. Some policies, in fact, cannot be financially or practically implemented by the agencies tasked with doing so. As a consequence, a number of policies are adopted to provide redress for previous mistakes, often after those mistakes have been brought into the spotlight.[10] In 2006, for example, a coal mine explosion in Sago, West Virginia that killed 12 miners triggered state and national investigations into not only the causes of the explosion, but also the reasons the mine remained open despite hundreds of reports of regulation violations.[11] Several months later, after a second explosion killed five miners in Kentucky, the Mine Improvement and New Emergency Response (Miner) Act of 2006, which modified previous federal mine safety legislation to enhance safety training, improve communication systems, and increase penalties for violations, was signed into law.[12]

OVERVIEW OF THE U.S. POLITICAL SYSTEM

The United States is a federal constitutional republic. This means that a system of governance, in which powers and responsibilities are divided between federal and state entities, and the representation of the citizenry by elected individuals, is described in a written Constitution that serves as the supreme law of the country. The U.S. Constitution specifically delineates a separation of powers among three branches of federal government: a legislative branch responsible for passing laws, an executive branch that carries out laws and commands the Armed Forces, and a judicial branch, which interprets the Constitution to evaluate whether laws are consistent with it (Figure 2.1). In the federal government, the legislative branch consists of the U.S. House of Representatives and the U.S. Senate, which together form the U.S. Congress. The executive branch is led by the President, who, in turn, appoints the heads of federal agencies that are responsible for day-to-day administration of federal laws. Finally, the judicial branch consists of regional district and appeals courts, as well as the Supreme Court of the United States, which reviews selected decisions of lower federal or state courts. Each state also has a constitution. Most are modeled off the U.S. Constitution, creating a legislative branch led by one or two lawmaking bodies, an executive branch headed by a governor, and a system of state courts. Federal and state systems were designed to include a system of "checks and balances," in which each branch of government can amend or veto actions of another branch of government. For example, the executive branch usually appoints judges to fill vacancies in courts, which the legislative branch must approve, while courts interpret laws and presidential actions. Similarly, while legislative branches are tasked with making laws, presidents and governors can veto them. With enough support in the legislative body, however, an executive veto can be overridden, preventing governors and presidents from complete control over law enactment. The various branches of government can employ a variety of policymaking instruments, including (1) legislative law, which is executed by the legislative branch; (2) executive orders, which are executed through the executive branch; and (3) common and administrative law, which is executed by the judicial branch.

Certain governing powers are solely in the purview of the federal government, whereas others belong to the state. Foreign affairs, including declarations of war, are conducted at the federal level. The federal government also regulates currency and interstate commerce and is in charge of ensuring certain individual rights (e.g., voting rights) are protected. In general, powers not specifically delegated to the federal government in the Constitution belong to the states, including the ability to issue licenses,

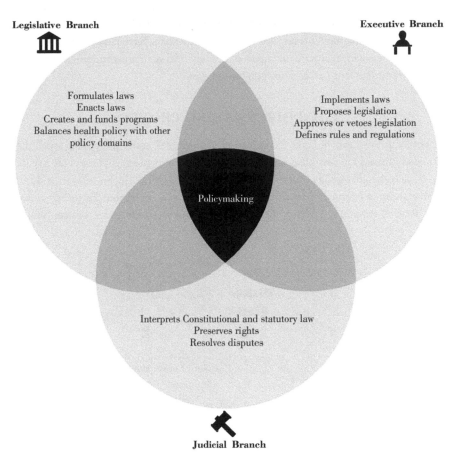

Legislative Branch

Formulates laws
Enacts laws
Creates and funds programs
Balances health policy with other
policy domains

Executive Branch

Implements laws
Proposes legislation
Approves or vetoes legislation
Defines rules and regulations

Policymaking

Interprets Constitutional and statutory law
Preserves rights
Resolves disputes

Judicial Branch

Figure 2.1 Branches of government in the United States.

regulate intrastate commerce, conduct elections, and provide for public health and safety. An additional power of the state is to establish local governments and grant them authority in certain areas. Local governments, usually established at the county and municipal levels, often are tasked with maintaining public services, like police and fire departments, housing services, parks and recreation departments, public transportation, and public works, and with establishing rules for zoning, planning, and local economic development.

The federal, state, and sometimes the local government share responsibility for other tasks, such as paying for and providing public education and maintaining roads and highways. Each level of government also can levy and collect taxes, set up court systems, and make laws or spend money to improve the general welfare of people living in the jurisdiction. Shared authority, however, can lead to problems if laws implemented at different levels of government contradict each other. In most cases of clear conflict, when it is difficult or impossible to comply with two laws at the same time, laws passed at the higher jurisdiction displace, or preempt, those passed at a lower jurisdiction. In some cases, federal or state laws will specifically restrict lower-level governments from enacting laws that do not necessarily conflict with, but instead are more stringent than, those passed at the higher level. For example, some states have laws prohibiting retail alcohol outlets within certain distances of schools, and state preemption can prevent a local government from extending such boundaries.[13]

THE POLICYMAKING PROCESS

Whether prevention policies are adopted at the local, state, or federal level, they are made through a complex, interactive, and cyclical process that involves five distinct, yet related steps, as illustrated in Figure 2.2: (1) *Problem Prioritization* during which an issue becomes part of the public agenda and is targeted for policy action; (2) *Policy Formulation* during which various policy solutions are conceptualized

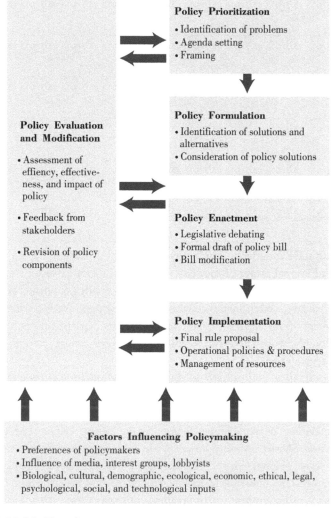

Figure 2.2 Model of the policy process.

and considered; (3) *Policy Enactment* during which a specific policy solution is formally adopted; (4) *Policy Implementation* during which the policy solution is implemented and enforced; and (5) *Policy Evaluation* during which the intended and unintended effects of the policy are analyzed, in order to inform policy modification. Although the notion of policymaking steps as distinct, linear components offers a useful heuristic device,[14] policymaking is usually less efficient or straightforward than the illustration depicts. Because the policymaking process is an open system in which processes interact and events and circumstances can change at any given stage, it can be hard to dissect. In addition, policymaking in public health (as in other areas) largely evolves through incremental steps and utilizes the constant feedback generated as the process moves forward.[15,16] As a result, existing policies often serve as the foundation for new policy efforts; rather than focusing on radical shifts or new policy instruments, change is often made through small, progressive modifications. For example, tobacco control advocates have long sought comprehensive restrictions on tobacco use, access, and secondhand smoke exposure. However, public policies regarding these concerns were developed over decades and continue to evolve with the advent of new problems (tobacco product expansion) and identification of solutions. Much of this evolution resulted from the evaluation of policies and through the "feedback loop" where information flows back into the process system and is used to inform modification and development for new policies (Chapter 4 discusses the feedback loop more extensively). Therefore, we present this model for the purposes of understanding the various stages, including the constant feedback loop, and components of policymaking. In the next section, we elaborate on the inherent politics that operate within the policymaking process by discussing the wide range of factors and considerations that influence the process[15] and that often result in chaotic and irrational decision-making.

Problem Prioritization

Prevention policymaking ultimately involves the matching of public health problems with policy solutions. However, simply identifying a public health problem is not usually sufficient to generate a policy response. There are many issues potentially deserving of public attention and these compete for prioritization on the policy agenda. Policymakers must be convinced of the importance of the problem, as well as its relevance to their constituency and sometimes even to themselves as policymakers. Furthermore, the issue must be perceived as more important than other public issues vying for attention. *Agenda setting* is the process by which a particular problem emerges, gains sufficient public and political interest, and advances to the next stage,[17] in which solutions are identified. Several factors influence whether a particular public health issue will rise on the policy agenda, including the strength, resources, and connectedness of advocacy networks interested in the issue; skills and resources of groups with opposing interests or alternative agenda priorities; scientific or technical information about the problem; and public attention to the issue, as well as perceived urgency of the need to address it.[18,19]

The way in which an issue is framed and defined also can impact public and political support. Theories of framing indicate that perceptions of a topic are influenced by the manner in which the topic is presented. A variety of factors, including changes in technology, perceived risks and fears, economic conditions, and perceived institutional capacity can all impact the ways in which health problems and potential solutions are presented.[20] Following the 2014 outbreak of Ebola in western Africa, for example, high rates of perceived risk prompted quarantining of individuals from many regions of Africa (including regions not impacted by the epidemic), and stories of how hospitals responded to infected individuals drove calls for improvements to public health infrastructure and training.[21] Public health professionals often can articulate the health ramifications of a particular concern, but health impacts are not necessarily enough to warrant public action. Public and policymaker support may grow if health-related problems can be tied to one or more of the rationales for government action listed in the previous section. For example, an issue could be framed in terms of deficits and excesses (e.g., "Too many children live in food-insecure households."); quantifying a problem (e.g., "Smoking is associated with one in five deaths annually in the United States."); describing the conditions that cause the problem (e.g., "Women cannot leave violent relationships if they have no safe place to go."); or incorporating the role of personal and social responsibility (e.g., "Working together, we can prevent the spread of flu."). Chapter 4 further defines how analysis and evaluation of policy is critical in identifying the range of possible policy solutions that might be proposed for consideration by the authoritative body.

Policy Formulation

Even when a problem is considered important, and political factors support action to address the problem, policy action cannot proceed until one or more viable policy solutions have been identified.[17] Policy professionals often develop several alternative courses of action and outline the advantages and disadvantages of each. Although public health professionals may favor a particular policy option, it may be useful to have a good understanding of less preferred policy choices as well in order to engage in productive discussions regarding the efficiency, equity, and effectiveness of the proposed policy. Policy alternatives to address public health issues can derive from creative brainstorming about how various tasks of government (e.g., taxing, public services, public education, and licensing or regulating behavior) could be applied, from investigating parallel policies adopted to address other health—and nonhealth—issues, or from creating multisectoral policies that address multiple needs. For example, many public health professionals are interested in policies to promote active transportation (i.e., walking and biking) in order to increase physical activity and decrease obesity, but these initiatives also are supported by city and road planners interested in reducing traffic congestion and by environmental advocates focused on lowering greenhouse gas emissions.[22,23] Chapter 4 provides more detailed information on the specific criteria used to evaluate various alternatives.

Policy Enactment

Once problems are matched with potential solutions or alternatives, political circumstances are surmounted, and priority is achieved on the policy agenda for a particular policy solution, the next stage of the policy process ensues: *policy enactment.* The policy enactment stage involves a series of steps that occur via a variety of policymaking instruments, including the legislative process, executive orders, common and administrative law, and ballot measures. The details of a policy solution often evolve during this process, so that the final enacted policy may differ in some ways from the initial proposed idea.

Legislative Process

The legislative process involves a complex series of steps and interactions among legislative decision-making bodies, as shown in Figure 2.3. The first step in the legislative process is for the policy solution to be drafted as a bill. Most legislative bodies have staff who draft bills at the request of legislators, but in many cases, any competent person can draft a bill. Once drafted, the bill must be introduced to one of the legislative bodies (i.e., the House of Representatives or Senate at the federal level, or the parallel bodies at the state level) by a member of that body. All states with the exception of Nebraska have two legislative bodies, usually coined the House and the Senate. The bill is assigned a number and referred to the relevant committee for study, discussion, amendment, and recommendation. Standing committees are made up of a subgroup of legislators who examine bills focused on particular topics, such as agriculture, the environment, education, public utilities, and health. In addition, one or more committees specifically focus on appropriations, or legislation related to government operations and other budget relevance. If the committee votes in favor of the bill, it is considered by the full membership of the legislative body to which it was introduced. The bill is once again debated, and potentially amended, before the full body votes. If approved, the bill is sent to the other legislative body, where it goes through the same process (except in the case of Nebraska). In some cases, a bill is instead introduced into both legislative houses at close to the same time, and each proceeds through committee and floor votes concurrently.

Because amendments can be made by both legislative bodies, at the committee and full-body stages, different versions of the same bill could be approved by each legislative body. When this happens, a committee consisting of representatives from both bodies is usually appointed to reconcile the differences and recommend new language. The bill moves to the next stage if both houses approve the revised version, or returns to earlier stages of the process if they do not. Bills approved by both houses, and signed by their presiding officers are considered ratified, and usually go to the executive branch head (the President or Governor) for approval or veto. If approved, the bill becomes a law. If vetoed, the bill returns to the legislative branch, where a specified majority (e.g., 2/3 at the federal level) of votes are needed in support of the bill to override the veto and have the bill become a law. Policies at the local

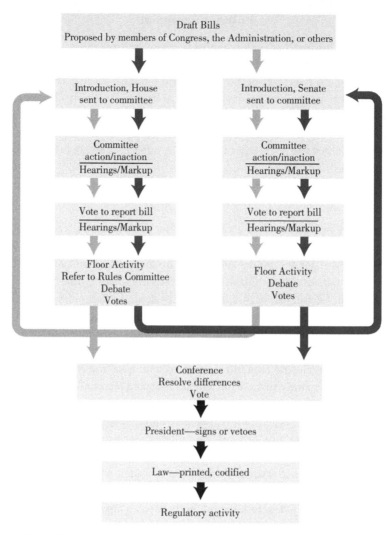

Figure 2.3 Legislative process.

level are usually called ordinances, rather than laws, and follow a similar adoption process. Although processes vary by municipality, ordinances are generally passed by a legislative body (e.g., city council) and signed by a city or county executive (e.g., mayor). Regardless of the level of government, passage and signage result in official policy adoption. As described in the section on administrative law below, however, additional rulemaking often is needed to direct the implementation and enforcement of a new policy.

The majority of preventive health-related policies are established through this process. Improvements to public health have resulted from legislative laws that require vaccination before entry into school, ban smoking in restaurants or workplaces, require use of child safety seats, and criminalize violations of violence-related protective orders.

Executive Orders

Executive orders are directives with the full force of law if their subject matter is within the explicit purview of the executive branch, as detailed in the federal or state constitution. Executive orders are issued by presidents or governors, often to manage the operations of government or handle emergencies, and can have implications for public health. In 2005, for example, New Jersey's acting governor used an executive order to create a new program to address the abuse of anabolic steroids, which increases the risk of cancer and other diseases.[24]

Administrative Law

Administrative law, also called regulatory law, is created by administrative agencies that make rules, issue regulations, or establish procedures to support legislatively enacted policy goals. This can include the executive branch's roles in designing regulations for implementation of a policy, adjudication, or the enforcement of a specific policy. In the judicial branch, administrative law judges are appointed at the local, state, and federal levels and hear the appeal of people or organizations concerned about provisions in new laws or dissatisfied with the way a law is implemented.

In public health administrative law, rulemaking plays a critical role in ensuring that policy is implemented appropriately. Developed legislation is often vague and non-specific, requiring the regulatory agency to further define the rules that will allow for the implementation of the laws passed. In other words, the legislation provides the "skeleton" for the law, and the regulations provide the "meat" or details. For example, the Healthy, Hunger-Free Kids Act was enacted by Congress (federal legislative branch), which then granted the U.S. Department of Agriculture the authority to regulate the sale of all foods sold in schools outside of the school meal programs. The U.S. Department of Agriculture then went through the rulemaking process to promulgate the Smart Snacks standards, which provide very detailed minimum nationwide standards for the sale of foods and beverages outside of school meals, with specific restrictions on fats, sugars, sodium, portion sizes, calories, etc. In another example, state and local legislatures have responsibility for taxation of goods and services. The tax codes are written by the local or state legislature, which often specifies what is or is not taxable. The state or local Department of Revenue further clarifies these tax codes by defining rules and regulations for what is "counted" as a taxable product and subject to taxation.

Common Law

Most lawmaking processes reviewed so far reside primarily in the legislative or executive domain, but the judicial branch also can establish policy. Common law, also called case law or precedent, are established through decisions of the judicial branch of government, rather than the legislative or executive. Generally, courts rely upon previous reasoning in similar court decisions to adjudicate disputes, but on occasion they can create new precedent, especially when considering new kinds of cases, or when social shifts warrant review of previous reasoning. Public nuisance laws that prohibit the use of property in a way that harms others, for example, have generally been established through common law, and used by public health advocates to limit environmental hazards, and as the basis for zoning laws that facilitate active living.[25]

Ballot Measures

There is a final means of policymaking driven more by citizen action than branches of government. Ballot measures are proposed statutes or amendments to state constitutions that are approved by popular vote, rather than by members of a legislative body. In some situations (and depending on the jurisdiction), laws created through ballot measures may bypass the legislative process entirely, originating in an initiative, in which individuals or groups gather signatures in support of placing the policy idea on the ballot for vote. In other circumstances, however, legislative bodies refer the legislation for popular vote (i.e., ballot referendum), either voluntarily or as part of a constitutional amendment procedure. One important difference between initiatives and referendums is that referendums can merely repeal laws, while direct ballot initiatives can both repeal old laws and replace them with new ones. Ballot initiatives and referendums have become increasingly important in public health policy, particularly in the chronic disease areas focused on tobacco, illicit drug control and regulation, and obesity prevention. In the 2014 elections, citizens cast votes on a host of health-related ballot initiatives, including personhood amendments with implications for abortion policy, "right to try" measures that allow drug makers to provide not-yet-approved drugs to people with terminal illnesses, and requirements for drug and alcohol testing for physicians.[26] One important distinction between ballot measures and general legislative policymaking is the process in which a law is determined for consideration. In a legislature, many interested parties contribute to the drafting of a proposed law and there is an extensive vetting process. Interested parties can identify drafting flaws, argue for more optimal solutions, and suggest modifications. In contrast, direct ballot initiatives are drafted by a sponsor, and the text is finalized prior to beginning signature collection. In most cases, there is no informed deliberation, no consensus-building, and no compromise. It is, therefore, extremely important for public health lawyers, scientists, and advocates to play a role in the drafting of initiatives put forth for a vote.

Policy Implementation

Regardless of how laws are enacted, they remain to be implemented. The implementation phase involves taking the actions approved through the policy development phase and assigning formal actions necessary to operationalize and implement the policies. An implemented policy can affect the many levels explained by the socioecological model (refer to Chapter 3) of health, including the physical environment and social culture in which people work and live. Therefore, prevention policies must be implemented comprehensively and effectively to affect these many determinants of health. For instance, the impact of a law may be severely reduced if resources are inadequately allocated for the enforcement of it.

Once legislation has reached this point in the process, whether it has been enacted at the federal, state, or local level, policymaking shifts from the legislative branch to the executive branch. However, the legislative and judicial branches continue to play a role as checks and balances across the continuum of implementation. The policy implementation responsibilities incurred within each branch are described below, and the unique responsibilities and processes for budget bills are described in Box 2.1.

Executive Branch Responsibilities

In the case of public health or prevention policies, executive bodies that focus on health and justice (and the agencies within them) are the main organizations responsible for implementation and operationalization of the policy. Implementing organizations within the executive branch are established and maintained to carry out the intent of the policies as enacted. At the federal level, the Department of Health and Human Services, the Department of Agriculture, the Department of Transportation, and the Department of Justice are just some of the agencies responsible for overseeing the implementation of prevention policies. Executive bodies and agencies at the state and local levels are tasked with and undergo a similar process of policy implementation.

Box 2.1 The Special Case of Budget Bills

The development and approval of federal and state budgets follows a unique process that incorporates aspects of legislative, executive, and administrative lawmaking. First, administrative agencies request funding for specific resource needs. These are reviewed by state or federal budget offices, which provide recommendations to governors or the president. The head of the executive branch then presents a proposed budget to the legislative branch. Appropriations committees in each legislative house consider the proposed budget, and recommend their own budgets for consideration. Proposed budgets in each house then follow the same process as other bills, with separate consideration in each branch, and processes of reconciliation. The final budget is then returned to the governor or president, for full or partial veto, which the legislatures can overturn with significant majorities. The final budget gives agencies the authority to spend certain amounts of money for specific things, but the specific ways in which those monies are spent may rest with the agency head. One example is the creation of the Prevention and Public Health Fund under the Affordable Care Act. This fund was created to expand and sustain national investments in prevention and public health, to improve health outcomes, and to enhance the quality of care. The U.S. Department of Health and Human Services has been granted the authority to spend monies allocated through this fund; determination on how funds can be spent, however, is defined by Congress.

Operationalization of a policy includes outlining the formal regulations or rules necessary to fully affect the intent of the law, the responsibilities for the management of financial and human resources, and processes for monitoring, enforcing, and evaluating the law. Depending on the scale of the newly enacted law, the operationalization and management can be simple and straightforward or can require massive effort. The process of outlining formal regulations or rules for implementation begins with the promulgation of the proposed new regulations. A proposed regulation is essentially a draft of the set of rules that will guide the implementation of the law while the rules are being finalized. At this time in the implementation process, regulations can be added, modified, or deleted, based on the input of the public or stakeholders. For instance, as part of the 2010 Healthy Hunger-Free Kids Act, the USDA was granted authority to regulate foods sold in schools. Even though the Healthy Hunger-Free Kids Act was enacted on December 13, 2010, it took until June 28, 2013 for the USDA to promulgate an interim final rule. Over the course of time between enactment and implementation, the USDA published a proposed rule to obtain public comment and engaged in a lengthy feedback process. The current rule is only an interim final rule, as the USDA continues to seek feedback from local education agencies and school food authorities regarding implementation. The timeline for the implementation of this law continues to be revised as implementation challenges have been identified.

Concurrent with the development and refinement of the rules and regulations of the law is the process for outlining how its implementation will be managed. As noted above, the delegation of human, financial, and other resources and persons responsible for oversight, enforcement, and evaluation according to the objectives defined in the legislation are outlined as part of the management component of implementation. Government staff, employed by departments under the auspices of the executive branch (i.e., civil servants or appointees), are the main persons responsible for overseeing the management of implementation. These staff members outline the organizational structure, allocate budgets for the effective operation of programs and processes outlined within the policy, and define policies and procedures to support overall management, operation, and maintenance of the policy.

Legislative Branch Responsibilities

Although the organizations within the executive branch bear most of the implementation responsibilities, the legislative branch maintains responsibility for oversight of the implementation process. Specifically, legislative oversight is designed to ensure that the implementing organizations are adhering to the intent of the law, implementing the law effectively and efficiently according to the economy of the government, and implementing the law ethically and in a manner that reflects the public interest. Legislative bodies use their authoritative power through the approval of funding appropriations to continue the implementation of law and can slash departmental budgets in the case of inefficient implementation or abhorrent management.

Judicial Branch Responsibilities

The judicial branch offers a place for legislation and the regulations outlined for implementation to be challenged. The judiciary sets policy through common and administrative law. Common law (described above) is the body of law established by court decisions. There are a number of examples in which common law has decided the course of public health policy. One of the most important examples is a Supreme Court case involving the Food and Drug Administration (FDA) and the tobacco industry. In *FDA v. Brown & Williamson Tobacco Corp*, the tobacco industry challenged the 1996 "FDA Rule," which asserted FDA authority to regulate tobacco products. In this case, the Supreme Court ruled that the FDA did not possess the statutory authority (granted by Congress) to regulate tobacco products. It took until 2009, a decade later, for Congress to enact the Family Smoking Prevention and Tobacco Control Act to grant the FDA the authority it needed to regulate tobacco. Another example is the consideration of the constitutionality of the individual mandate portion of the Affordable Care Act in the 2010 U.S. District Court Case *Thomas More Law Center v. President Barack H. Obama*. In this case, the U.S. District Court ruled that the minimum coverage portion of the Affordable Care Act was Constitutionally sound, a ruling that was confirmed by the U.S. Court of Appeals for the Sixth Circuit in June 2011. In July 2011, the Thomas More Law Center petitioned the Supreme Court to review the case, but that petition was denied in July 2012.

Policy Evaluation

The final step in the policymaking process involves the evaluation of the implementation of the policy. Policymakers and the public want to understand the ramifications of policy actions, in part to determine whether to maintain or alter policy actions in the future. Policy implementation evaluation examines the inputs, activities, and outputs involved in the implementation of a policy. Policy evaluation is a key component of the policymaking process in that it ensures that the policy is implemented as intended and that the policy is meeting the criteria outlined above (i.e., efficient, equitable, compatible, etc.). This results in a feedback loop in which policy can be modified and improved. It also can provide important information about stakeholder perceptions and awareness, as well as barriers to and facilitators of implementation. Policy evaluation can have multiple aims or purposes, including (1) understanding how a policy was implemented; (2) identifying critical differences between planned and actual implementation; (3) identifying barriers to and facilitators of implementation; (4) measuring intended and unintended changes in health and other outcomes resulting from the policy; (5) documenting and comparing the implementation and effectiveness of different intensities or variations of policy; and (6) informing future policy development.

Policy evaluation has played a critical role in the development, implementation, revision, and diffusion of a host of policy issues across public health topic areas. We can illustrate the importance of policy evaluation as a part of the policy process with this example from injury prevention policy. In May 2009, the State of Washington passed the "Zackery Lystedt Law," which later became known as the "Return to Play" law, to address concussion management in youth athletics. The Washington law was the first state law to require a "removal and clearance for Return to Play" among youth athletes. To demonstrate the importance of measuring the influence of implementation on the impact of a violence and injury prevention policy, the National Center for Injury Prevention and Control (NCIPC) conducted an evaluation on the "Return to Play" implementation efforts. Through interviews with a variety of stakeholders at different levels, including state health departments, interscholastic athletic associations, regional athletic directors, and school personnel, the evaluation examined stakeholder perceptions, barriers to implementation, and implementation successes. The evaluation provided an understanding of key implementation factors within the state, compared barriers and facilitators to implementation, identified best practices for implementation, and identified any unintended consequences of "Return to Play" laws. Although this information was essential for evaluating the law in Washington, it was also important for informing the efforts of other states considering similar laws.[27] Chapter 4 further describes the important components of policy analyses and evaluation.

SHAPING PUBLIC POLICY

In the previous section, we outlined the central components of the policymaking process. There are several players in the game of policymaking, both within and outside the government, who help shape public policy throughout the process. This section highlights the many actors who can play a role in influencing policymaking. Although many in and around public policy believe policymakers "reign supreme," a fair body of research has challenged the view that elected officials completely control the policymaking process.[17] Many scholars have noted that elected policymakers often have trouble using their authority to effectively develop and enact policy in the manner intended.[28,29] Replacing this view is the idea of public policy as a also a product of nongovernmental actors and nongovernmental processes. Therefore, we provide an overview of both policymakers and the actors external to the government who can shape the policy process, including lobbyists, interest groups, the media, and citizens. We conclude by reflecting on the roles public health scientists and practitioners can and have played in shaping prevention policy.

Policymakers

The politics surrounding the policymaking process can be one of the most significant factors that influence policy consideration and enactment. A policymaker's ideology, ability to influence various groups and bargain with them, and individual position among key policymakers often contribute to the "backroom" politics that make the process so interesting yet inherently challenging to rationalize. A policymaker's political party can also drive the policy agenda through the content of their platforms, the impact of their leadership in Congress, and the ideologies they represent. Democrats are often portrayed as more "public health friendly" because they are viewed as more willing to support government regulation of the private sector and more willing to spend on social programs that define public health policy than are Republicans.[17] Bipartisan support, however, often has been necessary to achieve public health policy change. Changes in administration also can result in a reset of the policy agenda, changes in the conceptions of problems and possible solutions, and designation of priorities. For example, former New York City mayor Michael Bloomberg established policies to make the city more health-enabling, by making smoking illegal in public places, instituting calorie counts in restaurants, and implementing bicycle sharing programs. His successor, Mayor Bill de Blasio has echoed his predecessor's emphasis on public health, but appears poised to address it in different ways, instead prioritizing affordable housing, income inequality, and infrastructure repairs.

Lobbyists

Lobbying has deep roots in public policymaking and has been proven to be an important factor in federal and state policymaking.[30] This widely used and influential tactic is employed across many areas of public health policymaking. According to the Center for Responsive Policymaking, between the years 2006 and 2014, 614 clients reported lobbying on specific issues containing the word "public health," as revealed in filings related to a variety of topics, including general public health, tobacco, injury prevention, cancer prevention, and use of nuclear energy to name just a few.[31] The term "lobbying" often conjures a negative response for many public health stakeholders, mainly because of its association with the large amount of monies funneled through the tobacco, food, and pharmaceutical industries into the hands of policymakers in exchange for deleterious votes. Although this often occurs at the federal level, it also can occur at state and local levels. For instance, a study conducted by Morley et al. showed that in the 1990s, when tobacco control policymaking was active, the tobacco industry lobby spent more money in states and localities considering raising cigarette taxes and/or implementing smoke-free legislation.[32] However, pro-public health agencies (e.g., American Public Health Association, American Medical Association, Campaign for Tobacco Free Kids, etc.), play an important role in lobbying for public health policy efforts. In the summer of 2014, for example, a coalition of public health agencies, including the American College of Preventive Medicine, the National Association of County and City Health Officials, and the Public Health Advocacy Institute wrote a joint letter to the U.S. Food and Drug Administration (FDA) in reaction to proposals to revise food and beverage labels. Among other recommendations, they encouraged the FDA to align their "daily value" level with health guidelines for sodium content and develop daily value levels for calories.

Interest Groups

Interest groups can be defined as individuals or organizations who present a unified position regarding a specific problem or policy solution. Studies of the policy process indicate that interest groups often play a central role in setting the government agenda, defining policy solutions, influencing decisions, and directing implementation.[30,33–35] Interest groups have successfully influenced policy by expressing general support or disdain for a proposed policy, mobilizing constituents, and providing reports that outline research regarding a specific policy.[30] In the realm of public health and prevention policy, examples of interest groups that weigh in on public health policy include informal groups of like-minded citizens, state and national volunteer organizations and advocacy groups, community organizations, health-related professional organizations, business associations, employer unions, and consumer groups.

Media

The mass media are a powerful force in our society and becoming even more influential with the emergence of social media. Research has shown that the public's attention to governmental issues tracks rather closely with media coverage of the same issues.[36,37] All policy stakeholders including community groups, businesses, and institutions compete for time and attention within the media agenda. The problems that are identified in the media agenda are constructed by society and reflect this competition between varying stakeholders.

Mass media can be implemented as paid or earned. Paid media refers to publicity gained through paid advertising. Paid media comprises any mass media outlet including television, radio, print, and social sites on the Internet and may include a variety of formats including commercials, promotional articles, and billboards. Earned media (or free media) refers to publicity gained through promotional efforts other than advertising. Earned media may include any mass media outlets, such as newspaper, television, radio, and the social sites on the Internet, and may include a variety of formats, such as news articles or shows, letters to the editor, editorials, and polls on television and the Internet. Earned media cannot be bought or owned; it can only be gained when media editorial staff or others who control media messages deem it important, hence the term "earned." Studies have found earned media to be the most trusted source of information. Earned media also is considered the most cost-effective method of communicating an idea and, therefore, is replacing traditional paid media strategies.

Both paid and earned media have played important roles in public health policy by raising awareness of a problem, stimulating coverage of issues, generating support for proposed policy solutions, and communicating information regarding the implementation of a policy. Media advocacy, in the public health context, is the "strategic use of mass media to apply pressure to advance healthy public policy."[38] The most effective media advocates amplify authentic voices of concerned citizens to ensure they are "heard" by the public and by policymakers who have the power to make change. Through media advocacy, community members and other concerned stakeholders take ownership of a policy issue in the media, and generate change, ultimately resulting in an empowered population with better health outcomes.[38] For example, in the case of seat belt laws, a national "Click it or Ticket" media campaign assisted in helping the public understand the importance of seat belts in saving lives and the potential consequences of breaking the law. Tobacco control advocates also have used mass media to broadcast personal stories from former smokers regarding the harms and consequences of tobacco use. Intended to raise awareness around the issue, these also helped garner support for tobacco control policies such as smoke-free laws and taxation laws.

Citizens

Individual citizens play several important roles during the policymaking process, including electing policymakers, advocating for policies, and proposing policy solutions for consideration. The most fundamental form of citizen participation in policymaking is in the selection of policymakers, including the President, members of Congress, and state and local officials. But participation does not stop there. Citizens share their opinions on policy matters through correspondence with public officials, testimony at public hearings, and personal contact[39] with policymakers. In addition, citizens have the ability to advocate directly for a proposed law. Advocacy involves voicing public support for, or recommendation of, a particular cause or policy. Advocacy also can involve educating policymakers regarding the potential positive impacts of a policy solution. Often, citizens get engaged in larger, community-based organizations or interest groups that advocate for specific policy efforts. Finally, citizens have the authority to propose a potential policy solution for consideration.

Public Health Scientists and Practitioners

Public health and prevention scientists conduct "research designed to yield results directly applicable to identifying and assessing risk, and to developing interventions for preventing or ameliorating high-risk behaviors and exposures, the occurrence of a disease, disorder, or injury, or the progression of detectable but asymptomatic disease. Prevention research also includes research studies to develop and evaluate disease prevention and health promotion recommendations and public health programs."[40] This definition, provided by the National Institutes of Health, communicates the breadth and depth of prevention research and its potential value in public health policymaking. Public health and prevention scientists, as well as practitioners, communicate research and real-world public health stories to policymakers and the public. This communication can contribute to many stages of the policymaking process. Research plays an important role in documenting and establishing evidence related to health problems and issues, and, therefore, can be an essential part of agenda setting. There are many examples of the use of prevention science in policymaking. For example, public health researchers conducted studies of early seat belt laws, demonstrating greater effectiveness in states with primary laws, which allow police officers to stop a car expressly on suspicion of a seat belt violation, compared to states with secondary laws, which only allow a seat belt violation to be issued when a car has been stopped for other reasons.[41] The National Highway Traffic Safety Administration now cites these effects as the basis of its argument that states should transition to primary laws.[42] Credible prevention scientists who present evidence-based and well-conducted research provide policymakers with facts that potentially influence their consideration of a policy or decision to enact a policy.[43]

The second way in which public health and prevention scientists inform the policymaking process is through the analysis of proposed policy solutions and/or the evaluation of policy after it is implemented. This type of research, which is the focus of the next chapter, can present the potential effectiveness, efficiency, and equity of a proposed policy solution and also identify the possible unintended consequences of implementation. For example, public health research, as well as input from antiviolence advocates and individuals who work with survivors of intimate partner violence, played a large role in the original development of the 1994 Violence Against Women Act, as well as in the fight to reauthorize it with increased protections for certain groups in 2013.

CONCLUSION

If public health professionals want to engage in efforts to use policy as a population health strategy, they need to understand the priorities and foundations of policymaking. This chapter was designed to provide an overview of policymaking in the United States, outlining when government intervention may be considered appropriate, how the political system operates, and the role of various actors in the system. Many public health professionals have been active participants in these processes over time, and there continue to be opportunities for them to make policy solution suggestions, work in partnership with others to support policies that enable healthier populations, and evaluate the intended and unintended consequences of these efforts.

ACKNOWLEDGMENT

The authors would like to acknowledge Ms. Kimberly Prewitt, Project Coordinator at the Center for Public Health Systems Science, for assistance with graphic development for this chapter.

REFERENCES

1. Longest BB. *Health Policymaking in the United States*. 5th ed. Chicago, IL: Health Administration Press; 2010.
2. United States Department of Health and Human Services. *The Health Consequences of Involuntary Exposure to Tobacco Smoke: A Report of the Surgeon General*. Atlanta, GA: U.S.

Department of Health and Human Services, Centers for Disease Control and Prevention, National Center for Chronic Disease Prevention and Health Promotion, Office on Smoking and Health; 2006.

3. Blekesaune M, Quadagno J. Public attitudes toward welfare state policies: A comparative analysis of 24 nations. *Eur Sociol Rev.* 2003;19(5):415–427. doi:10.1093/esr/19.5.415.

4. Global Polio Eradication Initiative. Polio Eradication. http://www.polioeradication.org/. Accessed February 12, 2015.

5. Bero L. Implications of the tobacco industry documents for public health and policy. *Annu Rev Public Health.* 2003;24:267–288. doi:10.1146/annurev.publhealth.24.100901.140813.

6. World Health Organization. *Global Status Report on Alcohol and Health 2014.* Geneva, Switzerland;2014:1–392. doi:/entity/substance_abuse/publications/global_alcohol_report/en/index.html.

7. Greenfield TK, Ye Y, Kerr W, Bond J, Rehm J, Giesbrecht N. Externalities from alcohol consumption in the 2005 U.S. National Alcohol Survey: Implications for policy. *Int J Environ Res Public Health.* 2009;6(12):3205–3224. doi:10.3390/ijerph6123205.

8. Mello MM, Pomeranz J, Moran P. The interplay of public health law and industry self-regulation: The case of sugar-sweetened beverage sales in schools. *Am J Public Health.* 2008;98(4):595–604. doi:10.2105/AJPH.2006.107680.

9. Henson RM, Wyatt SW, Lee NC. The National Breast and Cervical Cancer Early Detection Program: A comprehensive public health response to two major health issues for women. *J Public Heal Manag Pract.* 1996;2(2):36–47. http://journals.lww.com/jphmp/Fulltext/1996/00220/The_National_Breast_and_Cervical_Cancer_Early.7.aspx.

10. Le Grand J. The theory of government failure. *Br J Polit Sci.* 1991;21(04):423–442. href="http://dx.doi.org/10.1017/S0007123400006244.

11. U.S. Department of Labor. Sago Mine Information Single Source Page. 2007. http://www.msha.gov/sagomine/sagomine.asp. Accessed May 2, 2015.

12. United States Public Laws. 109th Second Congress. *Mine Improvement and New Emergency Response Act of 2006 (MINER ACT).* 2006.

13. Mosher JF, Treffers RD. State pre-emption, local control, and alcohol retail outlet density regulation. *Am J Prev Med.* 2013;44(4):399–405.

14. Sabatier PA. *Theories of the Policy Process.* 2nd ed. Cambridge, MA: Westview Press; 2007.

15. Lindblom CE. The science of "muddling through." *Public Adm Rev.* 1959;19(2):79–88.

16. Brownson RC, Chriqui JF, Stamatakis K a. Understanding evidence-based public health policy. *Am J Public Health.* 2009;99(9):1576–1583. doi:10.2105/ajph.2008.156224.

17. Kingdon JW. *Agendas, Alternatives, and Public Policies.* New York: Longman; 2003. http://books.google.com/books?id=hSolAQAAIAAJ.

18. Sabatier PA. The advocacy coalition framework : revisions and relevance for Europe. *J Eur Public Policy.* 1998;5(1):98–130.

19. Laumann EO, Knoke D, Kim Y-H. An organizational approach to state policy formation: a comparative study of energy and health domains. *Am Sociol Rev.* 1985;50(1):1–19.

20. Aronowitz R. Framing disease: an underappreciated mechanism for the social patterning of health. *Soc Sci Med.* 2008;67(1):1–9.

21. Gronke P. The politics and policy of Ebola. *PS Polit Sci Polit.* 2015;48(01):3–18.

22. Giles-Corti B, Foster S, Shilton T, Falconer R. The co-benefits for health of investing in active transportation. *N S W Public Health Bull.* 2010;21(6):122–127. http://dx.doi.org/10.1071/NB10027.

23. Milner J, Davies M, Wilkinson P. Urban energy, carbon management (low carbon cities) and co-benefits for human health. *Curr Opin Environ Sustain.* 2012;4(4):398–404. doi:http://dx.doi.org/10.1016/j.cosust.2012.09.011.

24. Gakh M, Vernick JS, Rutkow L. Using gubernatorial executive orders to advance public health. *Public Health Rep.* 2013;128(2):127–130. http://www.ncbi.nlm.nih.gov/pmc/articles/PMC3560871/.

25. Schilling J, Linton LS. The public health roots of zoning: in search of active living's legal genealogy. *Am J Prev Med.* 2005;28(2 Suppl 2):96–104. doi:10.1016/j.amepre.2004.10.028.

26. Rovner J. Voters provide mixed messages on health ballot measures. *Kaiser Health News.* 2014. http://kaiserhealthnews.org/news/voters-provide-mixed-messages-on-health-ballot-measures/. Accessed February 12, 2015.

27. National Center for Injury Prevention and Control. *Brief 4: Evaluating Policy Implementation.*; 2010:1–4.

28. Nakamura F, Smallwood R. The politics of policy implementation. *Natl Civ Rev.* 1981;70(10):553–556. doi:10.1002/ncr.4100701010.

29. Pressman JL, Wildavsky A. *Implementation.* Oakland, CA: University of California Press; 1984.

30. Grossmann M. Interest group influence on U.S. policy change: An assessment based on policy history. *Interes Groups Advocacy.* 2012;1(2):171–192. doi:10.1057/iga.2012.9.

31. Center for Responsive Policymaking. Public Health Lobbiest List 2006–2014. https://www.opensecrets.org/lobby/clientissues.php?id=D000054075&year=2014&spec=public health. Accessed February 2, 2015.

32. Morley CP, Cummings KM, Hyland A, Giovino GA, Horan JK. Tobacco Institute lobbying at the state and local levels of government in the 1990s. *Tob Control.* 2002;11(Suppl 1):i102–i109. doi:10.1136/tc.11.suppl_1.i102.

33. Baumgartner FR, Jones BD, Mortensen PB. Punctuated equilibrium theory: Explaining stability and change in public policymaking. In Sabatier PA & Weible CM (Eds.), *Theor Policy Process, Edition 3.* Boulder, CO: Westview Press; 2014:59–103.

34. Patashnik E. After the public interest prevails: The political sustainability of policy reform. *Governance.* 2003;16(2):203–234.

35. Berry FS, Berry WD. Innovation and diffusion models in policy research. *Theory of Policy Process.* 2014;169:307–349.

36. Miller AH, Goldenberg EN, Erbring L. Type-set politics: Impact of newspapers on public confidence. *Am Polit Sci Rev.* 1979;73(01):67–84.

37. Erbring L, Goldenberg EN, Miller AH. Front-page news and real-world cues: A new look at agenda-setting by the media. *Am J Pol Sci.* 1980;24:16–49.

38. Wallack L, Dorfman L. Media advocacy: a strategy for advancing policy and promoting health. *Health Educ Q.* 1996;23(3):293–317.

39. Crooks GM. Shaping public policy. *Public Health Rep.* 1987;102(4 Suppl):85–90.

40. National Institutes of Health Office of Disease Prevention. Prevention research at NIH. https://prevention.nih.gov/prevention-research.

41. Wagenaar AC, Maybee RG, Sullivan KP. Mandatory seat belt laws in eight states: A time-series evaluation. *J Safety Res.* 1988;19(2):51–70.

42. National Highway Traffic Safety Administration. The nation's top strategies to stop impaired driving. http://www.nhtsa.gov/people/injury/alcohol/StrategiesStopID/pages/Primary SBL.html. Accessed January 1, 2015.

43. Moreland-Russell S, Barbero C, Andersen S, Geary N, Dodson EA, Brownson RC. "Hearing from all sides." How legislative testimony influences state level policy-makers in the United States. *Int J Health Policy Manag.* 2015;4(2):91–98. doi:10.15171/ijhpm.2015.13.

3

Use of Policy Theory
in Prevention Policymaking

Sarah Moreland-Russell, Marissa Zwald, and James Gilsinan

LEARNING OBJECTIVES

1. Explain how policy fits in to the socio-ecological framework.
2. Describe the key theories in the public policymaking process.
3. Provide examples of theory application in public health.
4. Describe the role of networks in the policy process.

POLICY THEORY IN PUBLIC HEALTH

Theories, as described by F. N. Kerlinger, are a "set of interrelated constructs, definitions, and propositions that present a systematic view of phenomena by specifying relations among variables, with the purpose of explaining and predicting."[1] Theories can be useful in public health research and practice for a number of reasons. They can be used to develop and test hypotheses, identify factors that influence certain health behaviors, determine program or policy activities to address specific health behaviors, implement programs or policies, and measure and evaluate program or policy effectiveness.[2] The domain of theories currently and most frequently applied in public health research and practice are health behavior theories. This includes such theories as the Health Belief Model, the Theory of Planned Behavior, or the Social Cognitive Theory. Although these health behavior theories are often used in public health, health behavior theories have been criticized for their emphasis on individual-level behaviors and their limited consideration of broader contextual factors that influence health behaviors, such as socioeconomic, environmental, and policy factors.[2-4]

These critiques align with a shift in public health from understanding and addressing health behaviors at an individual level to embracing frameworks and strategies that involve policy, environmental, and systems approaches. This is represented in the uptake of ecological models and frameworks like the Socio-Ecological Model (Figure 3.1) and the Health Impact Pyramid (Figure 3.2).[5,6] The Socio-Ecological Model is a leading framework among public health researchers and practitioners and the foundation of the model is that behavior is influenced by factors across the following

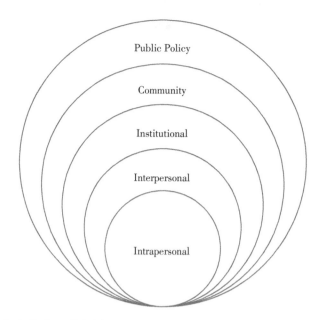

Figure 3.1 Socio-Ecological Model.

levels: intrapersonal (biological and psychological), interpersonal (social and cultural), organizational or institutional, community, and public policy.[7] Developed by Dr. Thomas Frieden, the Health Impact Pyramid describes how different types of public interventions impact population health. In ascending order, the framework

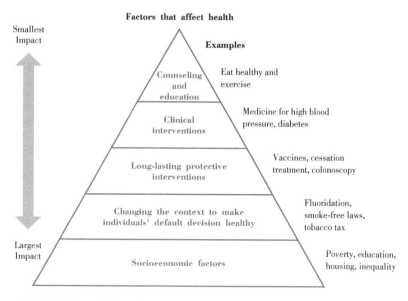

Figure 3.2 Health Impact Pyramid.
Source: Frieden T. A framework for public health action: The health impact pyramid. *Am J Public Health.* 2010;100(4):590–595.

posits that interventions with the greatest potential public health impact include (1) addressing socioeconomic factors, (2) changing the context to make individuals' default decisions healthy, (3) implementing long-lasting protective interventions, (4) employing clinical interventions, and (5) providing counseling or health education.[6] The foundation for these ecological models and approaches posits that factors at multiple, interacting, and interconnected levels impact health behaviors; and that addressing factors at broader levels instead of the individual level may have greater impacts on population health.[2,6] As such, there is a growing trend in public health practice to implement policies and interventions that change the contextual features of environments to establish healthier defaults and these shifts necessitate more useful theoretical approaches.[2,6,8–10]

Drawing from theoretical approaches used in other disciplines, particularly from public policy, may have important implications for a better understanding and implementation of the policy mechanisms that can influence environments and health behaviors. This chapter will provide an introduction to various policy theories (mostly drawn from the discipline of political science) that are relevant to understanding how the policy process can bring about change in society's perception of health-related issues. For example, because of success in tobacco control policy and adoption, the culture of tobacco use has changed from one in which society believed smoking to be an attractive and necessary habit with doctors promoting its use to societal recognition of tobacco use as a grotesque and deadly habit (Figure 3.3).

In Chapter 2, "Public Policy Explained," we describe the policymaking process as a complex, interactive, and cyclical process that involves five distinct yet

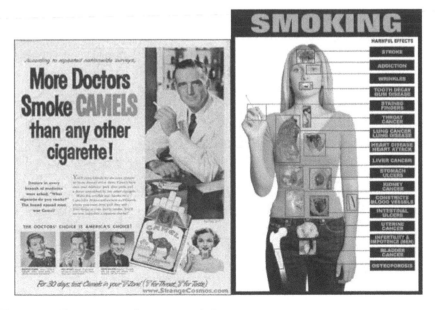

Figure 3.3 Changes in societal perceptions of tobacco use.

related steps, including (1) problem prioritization (including agenda setting); (2) policy formulation; (3) policy enactment; (4) policy implementation; and (5) policy evaluation. In this chapter, we present the theoretical frameworks that can improve our understanding of the interactions, events, and circumstances that are not explicitly represented in these steps, but that implicitly drive this five-step policymaking process. Specifically, we organize this chapter by theories that describe the various facets of the policymaking process moving from agenda setting (getting legislative attention) to theories of how the process actually works, specifically highlighting the frameworks of Institutional Rational Choice, Kingdon's Multiple Streams, and Social Construction. We also discuss theories that focus specifically on the importance of policy communities and networks in moving the process forward, including the Advocacy Coalition Theory and Policy Network Theory. Finally, we present the Diffusion of Innovation Theory to describe the characteristics of policies that allow for broad adoption. The list of theories chosen for inclusion in this chapter is certainly not exhaustive; however, we feel those presented are representative of concepts useful for understanding public health policy processes and for designing public health policy research. For each of the theories discussed, we provide applications across public health topics and levels of policymaking (federal, state, local, organization) for specific public health policy phenomena (Table 3.1).

THE POLICY COMMUNITY

Before diving into a presentation of the central theoretical tenets of the policymaking process and applications to public health policy, it is important to define the "policy community" and understand the environment in which this community operates. There are many definitions outlining the boundaries of the policy community. Policy communities can be comprised of any conglomeration of groups of people inside and outside of government who work collectively; these could include groups of people having cultural, religious, ethnic, or other characteristics or interests in common. These groups can be focused on community, state, or national priorities and can use a continuum of rationality in policymaking from value-based or normative to rational or evidence-based. Policy communities can include participants both inside and outside government, such as representatives of interest groups, advocacy organizations, academics, media, and the general public.[30]

For the purposes of this chapter, we define the policy community as a group of people trying to achieve a common policy goal. The theories highlighted in the next section not only provide frameworks for understanding policy progression and institutionalization, but also provide insight for understanding the setting in which the various actors interact to form policy communities. The policy goal being considered by the policy community is centered on public health and prevention policy and thereby recognizes both the altruistic nature of the discipline and the importance of evidence-based policy to achieve health for all peoples as a common good.

Table 3.1 Selected Publications Applying Policy Theory to Public Health Topics

Theory	Author (Year)	Public Health Area
Agenda setting	Holder and Treno (1997)[51]	Substance abuse
Institutional Analysis and Development Framework	• Fallin, Goodin, Rayens, et al. (2015)*[11]	Tobacco control
	• Martinez (2009)[12]	Tobacco control
Multiple Streams Framework	• Abiola, Colgrove, & Mello (2013)[13]	HPV vaccination
	• Craig, Felix, Walker, et al. (2010)*[14]	Childhood obesity prevention
	• Greathouse, Hahn, Chizmuzo, et al. (2005)[15]	Tobacco control
	• McHugh, Perry, Bradley, et al. (2014)[16]	Diabetes care
Social Construction Framework	• Blakely (2003)[17]	Influenza
	• Ludwig, Cox, & Ellahi (2011)[18]	Obesity
	• Nicholson-Crotty, & Nicholson-Crotty (2005)*[19]	Inmate health related to HIV & tuberculosis
Advocacy Coalition Framework	• Breton, Richard, Gagnon, et al. (2008)*[20]	Tobacco control
	• Larsen, Vrangbaek, & Traulsen (2006)[21]	Deregulation of distribution of medicine
	• Schorn (2005)[22]	Emergency contraception
	• Swigger & Heinmiller (2014)[23]	Mental health policy
Policy Network Theory	• Moreland-Russell et al. (2011)*[24]	Tobacco control
Diffusion of Innovation	• Dingfelder & Mandell (2011)[25]	Autism
	• Hall, Escoffery, Nehl, et al., (2010)	Skin cancer prevention
	• Moreland-Russell et al. (2015)*[26]	Active transportation
	• Nanney, Haire-Joshu, Brownson, et al. (2007)[27]	Nutrition education
	• Olstad, Campbell, Raine, et al. (2015)[28]	Physical activity in schools
	• Storms & Wallace (2003)[29]	Mammography screening

*Study described further within chapter text.

KEY THEORIES OF THE POLICYMAKING PROCESS

The policymaking process is an open system in which processes and components interact and events and circumstances can change at any given stage. This complexity can make the process difficult to dissect. In this section, we present several theories with varying explanations on how to understand and study this complex process. This section presents four theoretical frameworks: Agenda Setting, Institutional Rational Choice, Kingdon's Multiple Streams, and the Social Construction Theory. These theories describe the policy process as well as the importance of interaction among the various components that impact the process, and the influence of these components on policy outcomes.

Agenda Setting

Agenda setting is an important first step in the policymaking process. Agenda setting involves prioritization of an issue or a process by which a particular problem emerges, gains enough public and political interest, and advances to the next stage in which solutions are identified.[30] The agenda setting theory originally was developed by communication scholars, Drs. Max McCombs and Donald Shaw, in a study on the 1968 presidential election, where McCombs and Shaw outlined the importance of the national mass media in guiding public perceptions and determining public opinion.[31] McCombs and Shaw's work has been adapted to explain how the many issues potentially deserving of public attention compete for prioritization on the policy agenda. So how does a problem gain recognition and salience for policy action? First, the policy must be prioritized on the policy agenda. Policymakers must be convinced of the significance of the problem, as well as its relevance to their constituency (i.e., prioritized on the public agenda), and sometimes to themselves as policymakers. Furthermore, the issue must be perceived as more important than other public issues vying for attention.

Several factors play a role in the agenda-setting process, including gatekeepers, focusing events, interpersonal communications, and real-world indicators. Gatekeepers represent media leadership, advocates, policy staff, and others, each with unique values, routines, and cultures that allow or disallow and shape news content.[32] It is important to note that within the agenda-setting process, people (including those inside and outside government, the media, the policy community, and the general public) are not passive consumers of information but rather active seekers and users of information.

Focusing events also influence the agenda: these are rare events that reveal harms or potential harms to society and may be especially problematic for specific population groups or geographic areas.[33] Further, focusing events prompt changes in the issues presented by the media, influence public and policy agendas, and mobilize interest groups to either expand or contain the issue.[33] For example, the release of the 2006 Surgeon General Report, *Health Consequence of Involuntary Exposure to Tobacco Smoke,*[34] concluded that there was "no risk-free level of secondhand smoke exposure." This spurred action on media, public, and policy agendas, resulting in smoke-free policy actions across the nation. Next, interpersonal communication (e.g., communication between media staff, advocates, or policymakers) can dictate the salience of issues and events throughout the agenda-setting process. Interpersonal communication among decision makers can facilitate the inclusion of topics into the public and policy agendas.[35,36] A variety of factors, including the media agenda, the public agenda, changes in the environment such as technological advances, perceived risks and fears, economic conditions, and perceived institutional capacity can all impact the ways in which health problems and potential solutions are communicated to decision makers.[37]

Finally, real-world indicators play a role in the development of media, public, and policy agendas. Real-world indicators are objective measures of the severity or risk of an agenda issue, event, or social problem.[38] In tobacco control, results of population-based studies indicating high rates of lung cancer and billions of dollars spent annually on tobacco-related healthcare costs are examples of real-world indicators of a public health problem.

Public Health Policy Application: Use of News as a Means to Advance Policy Action

The use of the agenda setting theory in public health research is extensive and documents the various factors that impact the rise of a particular public health issue on media, public, and policy agendas, as well as the social and political change (or stability) that results from the agenda-setting process. Specifically, research has identified: (1) how media advocacy can determine salience of an issue and also affect policy outcomes[39-43]; (2) how the public and policymakers rank the importance of various issues, as well as the perceived urgency of the need to address a particular problem[41,44]; (3) characteristics of media content (use of stories vs. data, use of rhetoric, etc.)[45-49] and the use of framing to allow for problem recognition[39,50]; and (4) the power of groups, including those with opposing interests or alternative priorities, in setting public health policy agendas.[44]

One specific example of the use of the agenda setting theory in public health is highlighted in a study by Holder and Treno. This study examined the strategic use of news media to advance a public policy focused on drinking and driving within the Community Trials Project, a community-based intervention designed to alter alcohol use patterns and reduce high-risk drinking among people of all ages. Within the Community Trials Project, mass communication was used to re-establish a public agenda related to alcohol-involved trauma, to increase public concern about risk of arrest for driving under the influence (DUI), and to increase support of DUI enforcement. The investigators specifically examined how the news media was used in defining the problem of drunk driving, gaining recognition around the problem, and advancing policy action and adherence among the public. The study also documented increases in alcohol-related and DUI news coverage and compared this increased coverage to changes in public perception regarding the risk of arrest after drinking and driving. Results of their study indicated that as news coverage (both electronic [TV] and print [newspaper]) increased, the media did increase public awareness of alcohol issues, and public attention and support of alcohol prevention policy increased.[51]

Institutional Rational Choice and Institutional Analysis and Development

Institutional Rational Choice represents a group of frameworks that seeks to explain the influence of institutions on policy outcomes.[52,53] Institutions can refer to many different types of entities and can be broadly conceptualized as "shared concepts used by individuals in repetitive situations organized by rules, norms, and strategies."[52] Frameworks within Institutional Rational Choice assume that policy actors are "intendedly rational."[54] This means that institutional actors seek to realize goals or solutions in an efficient and effective manner while recognizing that they may not able to completely ascertain the probable consequences of their chosen solutions.

Within the Institutional Rational Choice family of frameworks, the Institutional Analysis and Development (IAD) Framework is commonly used to understand the formal and informal institutions whose established rules influence the behavior of rational individuals. To note, according to the IAD Framework, institutional rules can vary from mutually shared norms to explicitly enforced guidelines. In public policy studies, the independent variable of interest is often the institution or institutional rule and the dependent variable is usually the policy outcome.[52]

To understand the factors that influence the processes and outcomes of institutional policies, the IAD Framework takes a multitier approach, considering three tiers of action: constitutional, collective choice, and operational. The *constitutional tier* represents where decisions are made about who is eligible to participate in the policy process and which rules will be used throughout the policy process. An example of this tier could be federal- or state-level policymaking. The *collective choice* tier represents where decision-makers have to make policy decisions within the constraints of a set of collective-choice rules. An example of this tier could be local policymaking, where actors repeatedly make policy decisions within the limitations set by the constitutional tier. Finally, the *operational tier* represents the "street-level" actors and activities necessary to develop, adopt, or implement a policy.

Within these tiers of action, the first step of analyzing a policy problem is to identify the "action arena," which represents where interactions between policy actors and decision-making processes occur. Several variables are used to describe the policy situations and actors that make up the action arena: (1) the set of participants (individuals or groups); (2) positions that exist (e.g., within an organization); (3) potential outcomes; (4) allowable actions; (5) the control the participants exercise; (6) available information; and (7) costs and benefits of actions and outcomes. In addition, broader contextual attributes such as the physical setting, attributes of the community, and governing rules can impact the action arena. It is also important to note that the IAD Framework demands that a wide range of issues are considered in any policy analysis. The more complete the analysis, the better the policy solution and potential to eliminate possible unintended consequences of the policy. Figure 3.4 represents the components and interactions of the IAD Framework.[52]

Public Health Application: Institutional Analysis and Development Framework and Tobacco Control Policies

Although the IAD Framework has limitations in its practical application, in that many of its concepts are broad and unspecific, making it challenging to operationalize

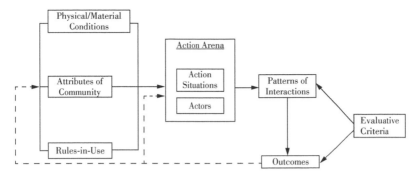

Figure 3.4 Institutional Analysis and Development Framework.
Source: Ostrom E. (2007). Institutional rational choice: An assessment of the Institutional Analysis and Development Framework. In: *Theories of the Policy Process.* Sabatier P (Ed.). Boulder, CO: Westview Press.

certain components of the framework,[55] it nonetheless has been applied in public health prevention, particularly within the realm of tobacco control policies.[11,12] One specific example includes a study by Fallin and colleagues that applied the IAD Framework to examine smoke-free policy implementation effectiveness at the collective-choice and operational levels in three counties in Kentucky. Using mixed methods, the investigators described the collective-choice tier as encompassing adoption of the smoke-free policies in workplaces, restaurants, and bars. In this phase, the action arena was considered the presence, strength, and length of time of a local smoke-free policy enacted by local government officials. The rules in use represented the voluntary smoke-free policies adopted by schools and large manufacturing employers in the counties.

Within the operational tier, or street-level policy implementation, the researchers conceptualized the action arena as community adherence and the enforcement capacity of the smoke-free policies. This included level of compliance with the smoke-free policies in selected businesses. The rules in use were operationalized as the availability of tobacco cessation programs.[11]

In comparing the three Kentucky communities in this exploratory case study, findings demonstrated that a comprehensive smoke-free policy adopted at the collective-choice level and positive policy implementation indicators at the operational level (i.e., high community adherence and enforcement capacity) may have contributed to positive population health outcomes, including lower exposure to secondhand smoke and demand for tobacco cessation services. Although this study included only selected variables from the IAD Framework to examine policy adoption and implementation effectiveness in a small sample of communities, the investigators' operationalization of constructs provide a guide for examining factors that impact processes and outcomes of institutional policies. Furthermore, this study represents only one application of the IAD Framework to one public health prevention area.[11] The IAD Framework has been used to understand a wide array of questions, including how institutions influence primary health care, urban policing, education, natural resources, and many other public policy areas that impact health.[54]

Multiple Streams Framework

Drawing from concepts of the "Garbage Can" model by Cohen and colleagues,[56] John Kingdon developed the Multiple Streams Framework, which uses an analogy of three streams converging to illustrate how policy change occurs.[30] These streams include the problem, policy, and politics (Figure 3.5). The *problem stream* represents the problems that policymakers and citizens want addressed. Problems often change according to systematic indicators that demonstrate the existence of the problem, focusing events that call attention to the problem, or feedback that typically takes the form of public opinion or existing programs. The *policy stream* represents the many possible solutions to policy problems. The *politics stream* consists of the national mood, campaigns, and administrative or legislative changes. Kingdon suggests that these streams typically function independently of one another, without any stream preceding others chronologically, except when a "window of opportunity" opens. A window of opportunity, usually prompted or opened because of a focusing event, represents a critical juncture, which allows for the separate streams to become coupled. Critical junctures are major events that disrupt the existing political and economic balance in one or many societies and can occur at the international, national, state, and local levels of policymaking. An example of a critical juncture in the realm of public health includes the 1964 release of the Surgeon General Report that declared "cigarette smoking is

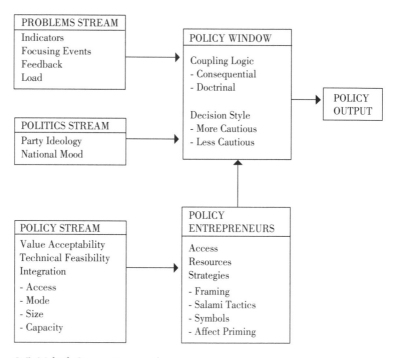

Figure 3.5 Multiple Streams Framework.

Source: Zahariadis N. (2007). The Multiple Streams Framework: structure, limitations, and prospects. In: *Theories of the Policy Process*. Sabatier P (Eds). Boulder, CO: Westview Press.

a health hazard of sufficient importance in the US to warrant appropriate remedial action" and outlined the harmful effects of tobacco use. This landmark definition of the problem allowed for the problem and politics and even the policy streams to align in the development of smoke-free policies around the world. A "policy entrepreneur" represents a key player in the policy process who is willing to devote resources, such as time, energy, reputation, or funding, in hope of a future benefit and is often credited with helping align the three streams.[30,57]

Public Health Application: Multiple Streams in Childhood Obesity Prevention Policies

The Multiple Streams Framework has been widely applied across a variety of public health prevention areas, from the enactment of smoke-free laws to the development of diabetes management programs.[15,58] Craig and colleagues used the Multiple Streams Framework to provide insight on the what, when, and how of policymaking related to the passage of Arkansas Act 1220 of 2003, a comprehensive childhood obesity prevention bill. Act 1220 included the following short-term and long-term actions at state, local, and school levels: (1) the development of a statewide Child Health Advisory Committee to create recommendations regarding physical activity and nutrition standards in school; (2) the requirement of school districts to establish a Nutrition and Physical Activity Advisory Committee to develop and implement local policies and programmatic activities; (3) the statewide enactment of school-based body mass index (BMI) screening, including reports to parents of all K–12 public school children; (4) the restriction of vending machines in public elementary schools and full and public disclosure of vending contracts into which public schools enter; and (5) the requirement of the state department of health to hire community health promotion specialists to support public schools developing, implementing, and evaluating the rules and regulations included in the Act.

Through a historical review of documents and key informant interviews, Craig and colleagues sought to understand the policy process that led to this window of opportunity and the passage of Arkansas Act 1220. Their findings demonstrated that the problem stream was comprised of systematic indicators and focusing events that drew attention to the childhood obesity problem. Public health leaders from a state university and the department of health provided annual updates to legislators on the burden of obesity, which included important health indicators on childhood obesity rates in the state and related chronic disease prevention rates. Additionally, personal health problems associated with obesity that both the state Speaker of the House and the Governor at the time experienced served as focusing events that brought visibility to the obesity epidemic.

The politics stream that supported the enactment of Arkansas Act 1220 included several meetings that brought together various legislative and administrative actors to discuss challenges and opportunities related to childhood obesity in Arkansas. First, the state legislature commissioned the state department of health to establish a statewide obesity task force to examine the problem of obesity in children and adults and recommend actions to reduce obesity rates. The taskforce presented findings to the state legislature and made recommendations that focused on improvements to school nutrition and physical activity policies and practices. Additionally, a number of Arkansas legislators, policymakers, and public health leaders had opportunities to discuss the childhood obesity epidemic in their state and devise practical policy strategies to promote improved nutrition and physical activity in schools. This included a National Foundation for Women Legislators Conference; an additional conference sponsored by the National Council of State Legislators, the National Governors Association, and the Association of State and Territorial Health Officials; and a third summit on Preventive Nutrition and Physical Activity. The aforementioned opportunities for public health leaders, policymakers, and additional stakeholders to engage with one another around childhood obesity-related policy issues and discuss solutions promoted changes in the political environment.

The policy stream for the enactment of Arkansas Act 1220 comprised feasible and acceptable policy solutions to reversing the childhood obesity problem within the state. In particular, one Arkansas policymaker was concerned about the caffeine and sugar in foods and beverages available to children in school vending machines. As a result, this policymaker led several legislative hearings to generate policy solutions to the problem of unhealthy foods and beverages served in schools. In addition, Arkansas legislators were becoming more aware of school-based childhood obesity initiatives from efforts going on in other states. Pilot studies in other states, such as California and Massachusetts, included statewide efforts to collect BMI data from public school students and notify parents of results. Thus, the policy stream generated several possible solutions to address the rising childhood obesity rates in Arkansas.

After mapping the policy process, Craig and colleagues determined that because of changes in the political and problem streams, a temporary policy window of opportunity opened, which allowed comprehensive school-based childhood obesity prevention legislation to be considered an acceptable policy solution. The Arkansas Speaker of the House, who brought attention to the obesity epidemic through the obesity-related personal health problems he experienced, was credited as the policy entrepreneur. The Speaker asked the state department of health to draft the potential bill and advocated for the bill's passage. Public health professionals who were engaged in the events described in the problem and political stream also were considered policy entrepreneurs. Their preparation of policy solutions that were introduced and discussed at the various taskforce meetings, conferences, and summits where other public health leaders, legislators, and policymakers were present allowed the window of opportunity to be seized and Arkansas Act 1220 of 2003 was passed.[14]

Social Construction Framework

One limitation of the aforementioned policy theories is that they do not examine the question of who benefits from and who is burdened by policy changes. To address this gap in policy theories, the concept of social construction was introduced in the 1980s.

The Social Construction Framework posits that when policy actors (generally policy-makers) are designing policies, their perceptions of reality are strongly influenced by negative and positive "social constructions" of target populations.[59] More specifically, social constructions represent cultural characterizations or popular images such as power or worthiness of a target population, or individuals or groups that are impacted by policy. As such, benefits and burdens of policies often are distributed in such a way as to maintain these underlying social constructions.

As depicted in Figure 3.6, both previous and current policy designs can influence institutions and culture, target populations, and society. The bottom of Figure 3.6 demonstrates that the dynamics of policymaking, such as the dynamics of special interest groups, government agencies, or elected officials, can influence future policy designs. When power and social constructions converge, four types of target populations typically emerge: advantaged, contenders, dependents, and deviants. Advantaged groups are both powerful and positively constructed; contenders are powerful but negatively constructed; dependents are considered politically weak but positively constructed; and deviants lack power and are negatively constructed.[59]

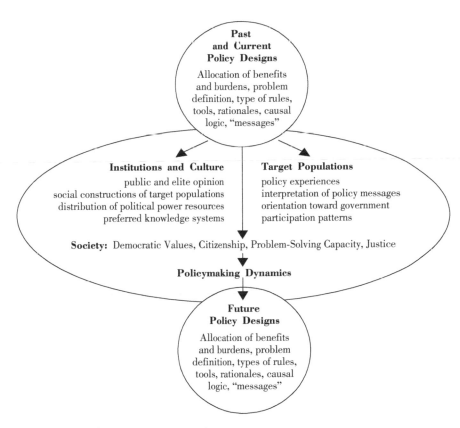

Figure 3.6 Social Construction Framework.
Source: Ingram H, Schneider A, de Leon P. (2007). Social construction and policy design. In: *Theories of the Policy Process.* Sabatier P (Ed.). Boulder, CO: Westview Press.

The Social Construction Framework was applied to understand how the social construction of inmates impacted funding and implementation of policies and programs to prevent the spread of HIV/AIDS and tuberculosis in state correctional systems across the United States. In assessing the relationship between social construction of the target group and policies for HIV/AIDS and tuberculosis prevention in correctional facilities, the investigators conceptualized social construction of the target group as the perceptions policymakers have of inmates and the perceived political power experienced by inmates. Using this definition of social construction of the target population, investigators found that policymakers' perceptions of inmates was, in fact, associated with funding and policy decisions of state legislators. Among a target population that lacks political power and is negatively constructed, the study found that inmates received few benefits related to HIV/AIDS and tuberculosis prevention.[19] As demonstrated in this section and from this case study, social constructions of specific groups may ultimately lead to how policies are developed, adopted, and implemented.

ROLE OF NETWORKS IN POLICY PROCESSES

The networks that form out of relationships among actors within policy communities also have been found to be important to advancing policy process. A term that is widely used (with varied uses in mathematics and ecology as well as economics, sociology, and political science), "networks" is inherently difficult to define. For the purposes of this section, we provide an overarching definition of networks as formal or informal structures that link actors (individuals or organizations) who share a common interest on a specific issue or who share a general set of values.[60-63] Within the contexts of policy, a "policy network" is often used as an umbrella term to describe any network that relates to the policy process comprised of actors from both inside and outside government, highly integrated with the policymaking process.[64] These networks could include coalitions, iron triangles, policy subsystems or subgovernments,[65] and policy communities. A considerable body of evidence suggests that networks can help improve policy processes. For instance, Young and Quinn (2002) found networks important in introducing a problem to the policy agenda—or "turning the problem into an issue."[66] In addition, actors within policy networks and subsystems can influence diffusion of policy ideas across larger policy systems.

This section presents two frameworks that explain the characteristics and roles of policy networks within policy communities that advance policy change. Specifically, we introduce the Advocacy Coalition Framework and the Policy Network Theory.

Advocacy Coalition Framework

The Advocacy Coalition Framework suggests that advocacy coalitions, or actors from a variety of institutions with shared policy beliefs, coordinate as a policy network around issue-specific policy activities, such as tobacco control or obesity prevention. Members of advocacy coalitions are vast and include intergovernmental and nongovernmental actors, such as government officials, and special interest groups, as well as researchers and journalists invested in the policy issue.

A core element of the Advocacy Coalition Framework is the difference between policy subsystems and the broader political environment. A policy subsystem would be considered the basic unit of analysis. It represents a network focused on a specific policy topic and can be comprised of multiple advocacy coalitions that may compete with one another. Policy change within a policy subsystem can occur by deviations in policy beliefs or fluctuations in resources.

As shown in Figure 3.7, policy change that occurs within a subsystem also can be impacted by the factors associated with the broader political environment. This could include factors that are relatively stable, such as fundamental sociocultural values; external system events, such as socioeconomic conditions; and long-term coalition opportunity structures, such as the degree of consensus needed for major policy change.[67]

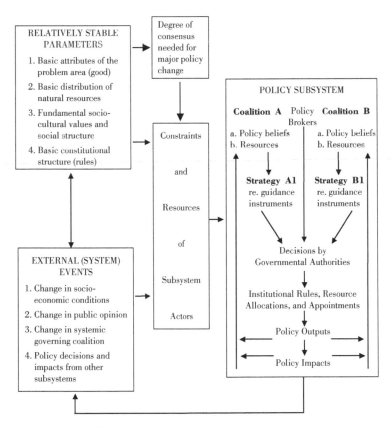

Figure 3.7 Advocacy Coalition Framework.
Source: Sabatier PA, Weible CM. (2007). The Advocacy Coalition Framework: innovations and clarifications. In: *Theories of the Policy Process.* Sabatier P (Ed.). Boulder, CO: Westview Press.

The Advocacy Coalition Framework demonstrates why it can be difficult to stimulate major policy change. Typically, policy subsystems are highly stable over time and for a significant policy change to occur, the Advocacy Coalition Framework suggests that there must first be change to the external environment of a policy subsystem.[68] The framework also emphasizes the importance of advocacy coalitions that can form to support or oppose a specific issue.

Public Health Application: Advocacy Coalition Framework and Tobacco Control Policies

The Advocacy Coalition Framework has been most frequently applied to understand the policy change process of tobacco policy subsystems.[4,20] One such example is the application of this Framework to understand the factors underlying the adoption of Quebec's Tobacco Act of 1998, which was the first statute to govern tobacco use. Through a content analysis of articles from daily newspapers in Quebec, government documents, and transcripts of parliamentary debates, as well as a qualitative analysis of semistructured interviews with stakeholders involved in promoting the Tobacco Act, the investigators identified relatively stable parameters and external events that contributed to the "tobacco policy subsystem."[20] Within this study, the tobacco policy subsystem comprised coalitions advocating in favor of the Tobacco Act (e.g., healthcare professionals and institutions within the governmental public health system, nongovernmental organizations working in tobacco control, including the Quebec coalition for tobacco control and the Quebec Division of the Canadian Cancer Society) and against the Tobacco Act (e.g., tobacco manufacturers and other opponents).

As previously stated and shown in Figure 3.7, the construct of relatively stable parameters within the Framework consists of attributes of the policy problem, the distribution of natural resources, sociocultural values and social structures, and constitutional structures or rules. The investigators identified the following stable parameters and their influence on stakeholders making up the tobacco policy subsystem: the lethality and addictive properties of smoking; the legitimacy of government to intervene in tobacco use, particularly to protect the majority of the population, who do not smoke; and the belief that any legislation considered cannot impede the Quebec economy.[20]

External events that impacted the tobacco policy subsystem also were identified. According to the Framework, such events can include changes in socioeconomic conditions, public opinion, or systematic governing coalitions, as well as policy decisions and impacts from other subsystems. The external events that impacted the tobacco policy subsystem in this case study included the 1986 enactment of an Act to respect the protection of nonsmokers in certain public places; a surge in youth smoking following legislation enacted in 1994 that reduced cigarette taxes to curb smuggled cigarettes from the United States; a 1995 government election that led to changes in elected officials and political parties; a 1995 Supreme Court ruling that allowed the freedom of expression in tobacco advertising; and finally, constant negative publicity toward the tobacco industry, including coverage of tobacco control interventions from the U.S. Food and Drug Administration and tactics used by tobacco manufacturers to attract new smokers.[20]

Ultimately, the relatively stable parameters and external events detailed above allowed advocates of tobacco control, including governmental public health agencies, nongovernmental organizations working in tobacco control, healthcare professionals, journalists, and the Minister of Health, to promote their vision of the tobacco problem within the tobacco policy subsystem and pass the Tobacco Act of 1998.[20]

Policy Network Theory

A policy network represents a group of actors with a shared interest in a specific policy topic, wherein the actors are linked directly or indirectly to one another.[69] The foundation of studying policy networks is based on the concept that regular and frequent communication and exchange of information and ideas among actors can result in stronger relationships and improved coordination of policy activities. Still in its infancy, the concept of policy networks can be used for three different approaches: (1) to designate a distinct, new governing structure; (2) to understand various patterns of interaction among public and private actors as they relate to a specific policy topic; and (3) to conduct social network analysis. The latter approach uses tools of social network analysis to identify actors (or nodes) within a network and the relationships (or ties) among actors. Network analysis allows for the development of visualizations of network structures and quantitative results that can characterize aspects of a network, such as attributes of the degree of centralization, connectedness, and density of a network.[70]

The policy network theory is still developing; in fact, a frequent critique of taking a policy network perspective is that rather than result in any predictive power, it is explanatory.[69] Others, however, have proposed that characteristics of networks and network participants can yield important information on policy outcomes.[71]

Public Health Application: Policy Networks and Local and Regional Adoption of Secondhand Smoke Policy

Though not explicitly documented, there is broad application of the concepts outlined in the Policy Network Theory across public health research. One specific application is in Moreland-Russell's study of policy network formation and influence in advancing smoke-free policy adoption across many communities within the Greater Metropolitan Area of Kansas City, Missouri. In this study, Moreland-Russell used social network analyses and qualitative interviewing to define the policy network involved in the policy process and document the influence of the network in defining the problem and setting the media, public, and policy agendas around smoke-free policy action. In this study, cities that were successful in adopting smoke-free policies had community-based policy networks comprising actors representing a variety of interests (e.g., public health experts, parents, doctors, business owners) who had strong ties and who communicated and collaborated often. Some actors within these successful community-based policy networks, specifically those highly central actors deemed policy entrepreneurs, were not only important in their connection to many actors within their own community, but also in creating links with other community-based networks in the region who also were working on smoke-free policy. The connections among these policy entrepreneurs and other community-based smoke-free policy networks inadvertently created a regional policy network that bridged governmental boundaries and catalyzed a greater regional coordination around the issue. Results from this study highlight four key ways in which smoke-free policy networks (both regional and community-based) influenced the policy process: (1) increasing visibility around the problem and solution throughout the policy process; (2) building consensus among a diverse set of actors; (3) providing resources and expertise to the policy process; and, (4) broadening and sustaining the reach of policy efforts.[24]

POLICY DIFFUSION

In the previous sections, we have presented frameworks that explain the policy process and the role of networks in policy change. The last framework that we introduce describes the specific characteristics of policy innovations that allow for diffusion across a large system.

Diffusion of Innovation

Although not technically a public policy theory, given that it derived from the sociology and anthropology disciplines, the Diffusion of Innovation theory increasingly has been used to examine policy diffusion.[72–74] Four elements characterize the theory of Diffusion of Innovation: (1) an innovation, (2) communication channels, (3) time, and (4) a social system.[72] The innovation refers to an idea, practice, or object that is perceived as new to an individual or institution. Communication represents a "process in which participants create and share information with one another to reach a mutual understanding" and a channel reflects the means by which communication occurs. Examples of communication channels include mass media or interpersonal communication. While time accounts for the time dimension in the diffusion process, the social system refers to the individuals who engage in aligned problem-solving to accomplish a common goal.[72,75]

Important factors that influence the diffusion process include characteristics of the innovation (shown in Table 3.2), characteristics of the communication channels, and characteristics of the change agents promoting diffusion. Characteristics of the adopters are also important when promoting an innovation, whereas adopters are often categorized into the following groups: innovators, early adopters, early majority, late majority, and laggards.[72,75]

Lastly, in considering the decision to adopt an innovation, Rogers suggests that an individual passes through several stages, including knowledge, persuasion, decision, implementation, or confirmation.[72] A description of each of these stages is provided in Table 3.3. Many factors can affect the passage from one decision-making step to

Table 3.2 Characteristics of Innovations that Affect Policy Diffusion

Attribute	Description
Relative advantage	Degree to which the innovation is perceived as better than the idea it supersedes
Compatibility	Degree to which the innovation fits with the values, past experiences, and needs of intended audience
Complexity	Degree to which the innovation is perceived as easy to understand and use
Trialability	Degree to which an innovation can be experimented with before making a decision to adopt
Observability	Degree to which the results of the innovation are visible and easily measurable
Reinvention	Degree to which the innovation can be altered or reinvented to meet the needs of the intended audience

the next. Specifically, the time and manner in which decision makers are exposed to or learn about specific policies, may affect their decision on whether or not to actively pursue the policy innovation. For instance, at the state level, policy innovations may diffuse through policymaker networks (e.g., National Council of State Legislatures) where information and lessons are shared and policy alternatives are suggested.

Public Health Application: Diffusion of Innovation Theory and Diffusion of Complete Streets Policies across the United States

Rogers's Diffusion of Innovation Theory has been applied to a variety of disciplines including public health, agriculture, education, social services, sociology, and communication science and spans various political levels including international, national, state, and local.[76] Examples within the field of public health of how the Diffusion of Innovation Theory is applied include a study that explored the adoption and diffusion of Complete

Table 3.3 Stages in the Innovation–Decision Process

Stage	Description
Knowledge	Individual is exposed to the innovation and gains an understanding of how it works
Persuasion	Individual develops a favorable or unfavorable attitude toward the innovation
Decision	Individual accepts or rejects an innovation at this stage
Implementation	Individual puts the new innovation to use
Confirmation	Individual finalizes his or her decision to continue using the innovation

Streets policies across communities in the United States.[26] Complete Streets policies represent a set of policies and planning practices that consider the diverse needs of all users, including pedestrians, bicyclists, motorists, and public transit riders, of all ages and abilities.[77] Guided by the Diffusion of Innovation Theory, Moreland-Russell and colleagues examined community- and state-level factors associated with the widespread diffusion of these types of built environment policies. Factors that were hypothesized to influence the adoption of a Complete Streets policy within a city, county, or a region included state-level funding dedicated to obesity prevention efforts; the state-level obesity rate; the state-level rate of active transportation among commuters; the presence of a state-level Complete Streets policy; the rural or urban status of the community; and the presence of an adjacent community with a Complete Streets policy.[26]

Using a method called Event History Analysis, the researchers found that Complete Streets policies were more likely to be adopted in communities where the state obesity rate was higher, where the percentage of people who walked or biked to work in the state was greater, and where there was an adjacent community with a Complete Streets policy in place. The associations between a higher state-level obesity rate, in addition to a higher state-level active commuting rate, and an increased likelihood of Complete Streets policy adoption demonstrates the importance of norms within a social system.[26] Rogers suggests that norms can serve as a guide or a standard for members within a social system.[72] Thus, if opinion leaders within a social system are concerned by the obesity epidemic or if active transportation is increasingly valued or accepted by community members within a social system, it can be expected that support for policies that address these issues would increase.

The study finding related to the presence of a bordering community with a Complete Streets policy being associated with increased odds of Complete Streets policy adoption corresponds with the Diffusion of Innovation Theory constructs of compatibility and observability of the innovation. As outlined in Table 3.2, compatibility is the degree to which an innovation is considered consistent with current values, previous experiences, and the needs of potential adopters, whereas observability is the degree to which the results of an innovation are observable to potential adopters. Therefore, the geographic proximity to successful Complete Streets policy adopters demonstrates how important it is for communities that have not yet adopted such policies to perceive these policy innovations as consistent with their values, experiences, and needs, and to also believe the policy innovation will produce tangible results.[26]

As one of the first studies to apply the Diffusion of Innovation framework to understand factors associated with adoption and diffusion of policies related to the built environment, the theoretical perspective and methodological approaches used by the investigators in this case could potentially be replicated to examine the diffusion of many other public health policy interventions.[26]

CONCLUSION

There is a shift occurring in public health prevention from individual-level approaches to policy and environmental strategies to support healthy behaviors. However, limited research exists in public health prevention that identifies or draws connections to theoretical underpinnings that can help understand policy interventions. Thus, opportunities exist to draw from the theoretical frameworks found in various disciplines, especially public policy. The policy change theories discussed in this chapter can improve our understanding of why some policy and environmental approaches in public health may gain traction and move forward while others do not, and can provide lessons learned for future policy development, adoption, and implementation in various public health prevention areas.[20]

REFERENCES

1. Kerlinger FN. *Foundations of Behavioral Research*. 3rd ed. New York, NY: Holt, Rinehart, & Winston; 1986.

2. Glanz K, Rimer BK, Viswanath K. Theory, research, and practice in health behavior and health education. In: Glanz K, Rimer BK, Viswanath K, eds. *Health Behavior and Health Education: Theory, Research, and Practice*. 4th ed. San Francisco, CA: Jossey-Bass; 2008.

3. Bernier NF, Clavier C. Public health policy research: making the case for a political science approach. *Health Promot Int*. 2011;26(1):109–116. doi:10.1093/heapro/daq079.

4. Breton E, De Leeuw E. Theories of the policy process in health promotion research: a review. *Health Promot Int*. 2011;26(1):82–90. doi:10.1093/heapro/daq051.

5. Sallis JF, Owen N, Fisher EB. Ecological models of health behavior. In: Glanz K, Rimer BK, Viswanath K, eds. *Health Behavior and Health Education: Theory, Research, and Practice*. 4th ed. San Francisco, CA: Jossey-Bass; 2008.

6. Frieden TR. A framework for public health action: the health impact pyramid. *Am J Public Health*. 2010;100(4):590–595. doi:10.2105/AJPH.2009.185652.

7. McLeroy K, Bibeau D, Steckler A, Glanz K. An ecological perspective on health promotion programs. *Health Educ Q*. 1998;15(4):351.

8. Leeman J, Sommers J, Vu M, et al. An Evaluation Framework for Obesity Prevention Policy Interventions Center TRT's Approach to Policy Evaluation. *Preventing Chronic Disease*. 2012;9(6):1–9.

9. Huang TT, Drewnoski A, Kumanyika S, Glass T a. A systems-oriented multilevel framework for addressing obesity in the 21st century. *Prev Chronic Dis*. 2009;6(3):A82. PMID: 19527584.

10. Committee on Accelerating Progress in Obesity Prevention Food and Nutrition Board. *Accelerating Progress in Obesity Prevention: Solving the Weight of the Nation*. Washington, DC; 2012. http://www.iom.edu/Reports/2012/Accelerating-Progress-in-Obesity-Prevention.aspx.

11. Fallin A, Goodin A, Rayens MK, Morris S, Hahn EJ. Smoke-free policy implementation: theoretical and practical considerations. *Policy Polit Nurs Pract*. 2015;15(3-4):81–92. doi:10.1177/1527154414562301.

12. Martinez C. Barriers and challenges of implementing tobacco control policies in hospitals: applying the institutional analysis and development framework to the Catalan Network of Smoke-Free Hospitals. *Policy Polit Nurs Pract*. 2009;10(3):224–232.

13. Abiola SE, Colgrove J, Mello MM. The politics of HPV vaccination policy formation in the United States. *J Health Polit Policy Law*. 2013;38(4):645–681. doi:10.1215/03616878-2208567.

14. Craig RL, Felix HC, Walker JF, Phillips MM. Public health professionals as policy entrepreneurs: Arkansas's childhood obesity policy experience. *Am J Public Health.* 2010;100(11):2047–2052. doi:10.2105/AJPH.2009.183939.

15. Greathouse LW, Hahn EJ, Okoli CTC, Warnick T a, Riker C a. Passing a smoke-free law in a pro-tobacco culture: a multiple streams approach. *Policy Polit Nurs Pract.* 2005;6(3):211–220. doi:10.1177/1527154405278775.

16. McHugh SM, Perry IJ, Bradley C, Brugha R. Developing recommendations to improve the quality of diabetes care in Ireland: a policy analysis. *Health Res Policy Syst.* 2014;12:53. doi:10.1186/1478-4505-12-53.

17. Blakely BDE. Social construction of three influenza pandemics in the New York Times. *Journal Mass Commun Q.* 2003;80(4):884–902.

18. Ludwig AF, Cox P, Ellahi B. Social and cultural construction of obesity among Pakistani Muslim women in North West England. *Public Health Nutr.* 2009;14(10):1842–1850.

19. Nicholson-crotty J, Texas A. Social construction and policy implementation : Inmate Health as a Public Health Issue. *Social Science Quarterly.* 2004;85(2):240–256.

20. Breton E, Richard L, Gagnon F, Jacques M, Bergeron P. Health promotion research and practice require sound policy analysis models: the case of Quebec's Tobacco Act. *Soc Sci Med.* 2008;67(11):1679–1689. doi:10.1016/j.socscimed.2008.07.028.

21. Larsen JB, Vrangbaek K, Traulsen JM. Advocacy coalitions and pharmacy policy in Denmark—solid cores with fuzzy edges. *Soc Sci Med.* 2006;63(1):212–224. doi:10.1016/j.socscimed.2005.11.045.

22. Schorn MN. Emergency contraception for sexual assault victims: an advocacy coalition framework. *Policy Polit Nurs Pract.* 2005;6(4):343–353. doi:10.1177/1527154405283410.

23. Swigger A, Heinmiller BT. Advocacy coalitions and mental health policy : The adoption of community treatment orders in Ontario. *Polit Policy.* 2014;42(2):246–270. doi:10.1111/j.1747-1346.2009.00174.x/abstract.

24. Moreland-Russell S. *Policy Processes and Networks: An Examination of the Diffusion of Smokefree Policies throughout the Kansas City Area;* 2011.

25. Dingfelder HE, Mandell DS. Bridging the research-to-practice gap in autism intervention: an application of diffusion of innovation theory. *J Autism Dev Disord.* 2011;41(5):597–609. doi:10.1007/s10803-010-1081-0.

26. Moreland-Russell S, Carothers BJ. (2015) An Examination of Two Policy Networks Involved in Advancing Smokefree Policy Initiatives. *Int. J. Environ. Res. Public Health.* 2015; 12, 11117–11131.

27. Nanney MS, Haire-joshu D, Brownson RC, Kostelc J, Stephen M, Elliott M. *Disseminated Dietary Curriculum.* 2000:64–73.

28. Olstad DL, Campbell EJ, Raine KD, Nykiforuk CI. A multiple case history and systematic review of adoption, diffusion, implementation and impact of provincial daily physical activity policies in Canadian schools. *BMC Public Health.* 2015;15(1). doi:10.1186/s12889-015-1669-6.

29. Levy-Storms L, Wallace SP. Use of mammography screening among older Samoan women in Los Angeles County: a diffusion network approach. *Soc Sci Med.* 2003;57(6):987–1000. doi:10.1016/S0277-9536(02)00474-4.

30. Kingdon JW. *Agendas, Alternatives, and Public Policies.* 2nd ed. Glenview, IL: Longman; 2011.

31. McCombs ME, Shaw DL. The agenda setting function of mass media. *Public Opin Q.* 1972;36(2):176–187.

32. Mccombs ME, Donald L. The evolution of agenda-setting research: Twenty-five years in the marketplace of ideas. *J Commun*. 1992;3:58–67.

33. Birkland TA. Focusing events, mobilization, and agenda setting. *J Public Policy*. 1998;18(1):53–74.

34. United States Department of Health and Human Services. *The Health Consequences of Involuntary Exposure to Tobacco Smoke A Report of the Surgeon General.*; 2006. http://www.surgeongeneral.gov/library/reports/secondhandsmoke/fullreport.pdf.

35. Wanta W, Wu Y-C. Interpersonal communication and the agenda setting process. *Journal Mass Commun Q*. 1992;69:847–855.

36. Yang J, Stone G. The powerful role of interpersonal communication in agenda setting. *Mass Commun Soc*. 2003;6(1):57–74.

37. Aronowitz R. Framing disease: an underappreciated mechanism for the social patterning of health. *Soc Sci Med*. 2008;67(1):1–9.

38. Dearing JW, Rogers EM. *Communication Concepts and Agenda-Setting*. Thousand Oaks, CA: Sage Publications; 1996.

39. Harris JK, Shelton SC, Moreland-Russell S, Luke D a. Tobacco coverage in print media: the use of timing and themes by tobacco control supporters and opposition before a failed tobacco tax initiative. *Tob Control*. 2010;19(1):37–43. doi:10.1136/tc.2009.032516.

40. Holder HD, Andrew J. Media advocacy in community prevention : news as a means to advance policy change. 1997;92(November 1996).

41. Jernigan DH, Wright PA. Media advocacy: Lessons from community experiences. *J Public Health Policy*. 1996;17:306–311.

42. Niederdeppe J, Farrelly MC, Hayiland ML. Confirming "truth": More evidence of a successful tobacco countermarketing campaign in Florida. *Am J Public Health*. 2004;94:255–257.

43. Niederdeppe J, Farrelly MC, Wenter D. Media advocacy, tobacco control policy change and teen smoking in Florida. *Tob Control*. 2007;16(1):47–52.

44. Laumann EO, Knoke D, Kim YH. An organizational approach to state policy formation: A comparative study of energy and health domains. *Am Sociological Rev*. 1985;50(1):1–19.

45. Moreland-Russell S, Harris JK, Israel K, Schelle S, Mohr A. Anti-smoking data is exaggerated vs. The data are clear and indisputable: examining Letters to the Editor about Tobacco. *J Health Commun*. 2012;17(4):443–459.

46. Demers DK. Structural pluralism, corporate newspaper structure, and news source perceptions: Another test of the editorial vigor hypothesis. *Journal Mass Commun Q*. 1998;75:572–592.

47. Dorfman L. Studying the news on public health: How content analysis supports media advocacy. *Am J Health Behav*. 2003;27:S217–S226.

48. Hinyard LJ, Kreuter MW. Using narrative communication as a tool for health behavior change: A conceptual, theoretical, and empirical overview. *Heal Educ Behav*. 2007;34:777–792.

49. Smith KC, McLeod K, Wakefield M. Australian letters to the editor on tobacco: Triggers, rhetoric, and claims of legitimate voice. *Qual Health Res*. 2005;15:1180–1198.

50. Wakefield M, Smith KC, Chapman S. Framing of Australian newspaper coverage of a secondhand smoke injury claim: Lessons for media advocacy. *Crit Public Health*. 2005;15(1):53–63.

51. Holder HD, Treno AJ. Media advocacy in community prevention: news as a means to advance policy change. *Addiction*. 1997;92(Suppl 2):S189–S199.

52. Ostrom E. Institutional rational choice: An assessmentof the Institutional Analysis and Development Framework. In: Sabatier P, ed. *Theories of the Policy Process*. 2nd ed. Cambridge, MA: Westview Press; 2007.

53. Ostrom E. Background on the Institutional Analysis and Development Framework. *Policy Stud J.* 2011;39(1):7–28.

54. Sabatier P. The need for better theories. In: Sabatier P, ed. *Theories of the Policy Process*. 2nd ed. Cambridge, MA: Westview Press; 2007.

55. Rutten A, Gelius P, Abu-Omar K. Action theory and policy analysis: The ADEPT model. In: Clavier C, de Leeuw E, eds. *Health Promotion and the Policy Process*. Oxford, UK: Oxford University Press; 2013.

56. Cohen MD, March JG, Olsen JP. A Garbage Can Model of Organizational Choice. *Adm Sci Q.* 1972;17(1):1–25.

57. Zahariadis N. The Multiple Streams Framework: structure, limitations, prospects. In: Sabatier P, ed. *Theories of the Policy Process*. 2nd ed. Cambridge, MA: Westview Press; 2007.

58. Mamudu HM, Dadkar S, Veeranki SP, He Y, Barnes R, Glantz S a. Multiple streams approach to tobacco control policymaking in a tobacco-growing state. *J Community Health.* 2014;39(4):633–645. doi:10.1007/s10900-013-9814-6.

59. Ingram H, Schneider AL, de Leon P. Social construction and policy design. In: Sabatier P, ed. *Theories of the Policy Process*. 2nd ed. Cambridge, MA: Westview Press; 2007.

60. Borkan J. Mixed methods studies: A foundation for primary care research. *Ann Fam Med.* 2004;2(1):4–6.

61. Steinberger PJ. Typologies of public policy: Meaning construction and the policy process. *Soc Sci Q.* 1980;63:185–187.

62. Tennyson R. *The Partnering Toolbook.* (International Business Leaders' Forum, ed.).; 2003.

63. Perkin E, Court J. *Networks and Policy Processes in International Development: A Literature Review.* London, UK; 2005. Published by Overseas Development Institute. Whitepaper found at http://www.odi.org/sites/odi.org.uk/files/odi-assets/publications-opinion-files/160.pdf

64. Stone D, Denham A. *Think Tank Traditions: Policy Research and the Politics of Ideas.* Manchester: Manchester University Press; 2004. http://publicpolicy.ceu.edu/node/14543

65. Leiper FJ, Stevens JP. A theoretical and conceptual reexamination of subsystem politics. *Public Policy Adm.* 1987;2(1):9–24.

66. Young E, Quinn L. *Writing Effective Public Policy Papers: A Guide for Policy Advisors in Central and Eastern Europe.* Budapest, Hungary; 2002.

67. Sabatier PA, Weible CM. The Advocacy Coalition Framework: innovations and clarifications. In: Sabatier PA, ed. *Theories of the Policy Process*. 2nd ed. Cambridge, MA: Westview Press; 2007.

68. Breton E, Richard L, Gagnon F, Jacques M, Bergeron P. Coalition advocacy action and research for policy development. In: Clavier C, De Leeuw E, eds. *Health Promotion and the Policy Process*. Oxford, UK: Oxford University Press; 2013.

69. De Leeuw E, Keizer M, Hoeijmakers M. Health policy networks: Connecting the disconnected. In: Clavier C, De Leeuw E, eds. *Health Promotion and the Policy Process*. Oxford, UK: Oxford University Press; 2013.

70. Adam S, Kriesi H. The network approach. In: Sabatier P, ed. *Theories of the Policy Process*. Boulder, CO: Westview Press; 2007.

71. Howlett M. Do networks matter? Linking policy network structure to policy outcomes: Evidence from four Canadian policy sectors, 1990–2000. *Can J Polit Sci*. 2002;35(2):235–267.

72. Rogers EM. *Diffusion of Innovations*. 5th ed. New York, NY: Free Press; 2003.

73. Shipan CR, Volden C. Bottom-up federalism: the diffusion of antismoking policies from U.S. cities to states. *Am J Pol Sci*. 2006;50(4):825–843. doi:10.1111/j.1540-5907.2006.00218.x.

74. Rogers EM. Diffusion of preventive innovations. *Addict Behav*. 2002;27:989–993.

75. Berry FS, Berry WD. Innovation and diffusion models in policy research. In: Sabatier P, ed. *Theories of the Policy Process*. 2nd ed. Cambridge, MA: Westview Press; 2007.

76. Green LW, Ottoson JM, García C, Hiatt R a. Diffusion theory and knowledge dissemination, utilization, and integration in public health. *Annu Rev Public Health*. 2009;30:151–174. doi:10.1146/annurev.publhealth.031308.100049.

77. National Complete Streets Coalition. Complete Streets. 2015. http://www.smartgrowthamerica.org/complete-streets. Accessed February 1, 2015.

4

Public Health Policy Analysis
and Evaluation

Jamie F. Chriqui and Sabrina K. Young

LEARNING OBJECTIVES

1. Describe public health policy analysis.
2. Describe the steps in conducting a public health policy analysis.
3. Identify tools for use in public health policy analysis.

WHAT IS PUBLIC HEALTH POLICY ANALYSIS?

Policy analysis is both an art and a science.[1] Much like other scientific disciplines, policy analysis is a tradecraft; it is a skill that policy analysts throughout legislatures, governmental agencies, and advocacy organizations utilize on a daily basis. At the most fundamental level, policy analysis fits into several stages of the policymaking process (see Chapter 2 on the policy process). First, when a problem has been identified and deemed worthy of governmental attention, policy analysis is critical in identifying and comparing the range of possible policy solutions that might be proposed for consideration by the authoritative body (e.g., Congress). Second, once a course of action is decided upon by the authoritative body, policy analysis may come into play as part of the policy "feedback loop," during which the chosen course of action is evaluated and decisions are made about whether to recommend (a) no change, (b) a policy revision or amendment, or (c) termination. Finally, policy analysis is critical to the empirical evaluation of the impact of policies. Table 4.1 highlights examples of organizations that conduct policy analysis as a matter of course. In addition, legislative and governmental agency staffers also routinely engage in policy analysis activities.

The Practice of Policy Analysis

In this book, emphasis is placed on the policy analysis that legislative bodies, governmental agencies, think tanks, quasigovernmental bodies, and advocacy groups engage in on a routine basis. Typically, policy analysts in these organizations prepare issue papers and side-by-side analyses comparing alternative policy solutions for addressing the problem at hand. A helpful definition of policy analysis is that it "[. . .] involves

Table 4.1 Examples of Organizations Engaged in Policy Analysis

---

Federal and Congressional Agencies and Offices

U.S. Government Accountability Office (GAO): www.gao.gov
Congressional Budget Office (CBO): www.cbo.gov
Congressional Research Service (CRS): www.loc.gov/crsinfo/about
Policy offices in federal agencies and congressional offices

Think Tanks

American Enterprise Institute for Public Policy Research (AEI): www.aei.org
Brookings Institution: www.brookings.edu
Cato Institute: www.cato.org
Urban Institute: www.urban.org

Other Organizations Conducting Public Health Policy Analyses

The Henry J. Kaiser Family Foundation (KFF): www.kff.org
The Commonwealth Fund: www.commonwealthfund.org/
Professional association legislative/policy offices (e.g., American Public Health
  Association, American Heart Association, American Medical Association,
  American Health Care Association, and America's Health Insurance Plans)

---

looking ahead to anticipate the consequences of decisions and thinking seriously and critically about them."[2]

A useful *policy analysis provides informed advice that is based on facts, data, and evidence; speculation and subjectivity are to be minimized as much as possible.* Because the audience for the policy analysis (i.e., the client discussed below) is usually not an expert on the topic, it is important to write in clear, concise, nontechnical language, using terminology familiar to a lay person. Ideally, the analysis should be as objective and impartial as possible; however, because the process of policy analysis is inherently political and is conducted within a political environment, impartiality may prove challenging. (Political feasibility is discussed further below.)

The consumer of a policy analysis is the "client." The client may be an immediate supervisor, an authoritative decision-maker (e.g., legislator, agency official), or an advocacy organization that is looking to promote various policy options to an authoritative decision-maker. However, the ultimate audience for a policy analysis may include not only the client but supporters and opponents of a policy option;[3] therefore, it is important to prepare a thorough analysis that is able to withstand opposing views.

Understanding the Needs of the Client and/or Targeted Actor(s)

At the outset of embarking on a policy analysis project, it is critical to be very clear about who has requested or paid for the policy analysis and their role in the policymaking process. The client for a given analysis may vary considerably depending on the problem at hand. In many cases, the client is an authoritative decision-maker (e.g., a legislator, legislative committee, regulatory agency official) who possesses the legal authority to make a public policy decision (e.g., to propose or act on a given legislative measure, propose or promulgate new regulations, or appropriate funds). In many cases, however, the client for a policy analysis is an "actor outside of government,"[4] such as an advocacy organization or an interest group. In such cases, the client has requested the policy analysis to present to a targeted actor (i.e., an authoritative decision-maker such as a legislator, legislative committee, or regulatory agency) to present possible courses of action for the decision-maker to consider relative to the given problem. Clarifying the client and/or targeted actor(s) at the outset will help to simplify the remaining steps of the policy analysis process. Being clear on the client's legal authority (whether he or she is an authoritative decision-maker) or on the authority of the targeted actor(s) (e.g., legislators can only make regulations; regulators can only promulgate regulations; advocates can propose or provide input into the legislative and/or regulatory processes) will also be important in various stages of the policy analysis, as described in the sections that follow.

STEPS IN THE POLICY ANALYSIS PROCESS

The seven-step process presented herein is outlined in Figure 4.1. Most public policy and policy analysis textbooks[1,2,5–7] use some combination of these same steps for describing the policy analysis process.

The next section briefly describes each step; the checklist contained in the Appendix at the end of the chapter provides a sample outline for organizing a policy analysis white paper and summarizes key considerations. Readers interested in learning about the policy analysis process in greater depth, particularly the "how," should consult

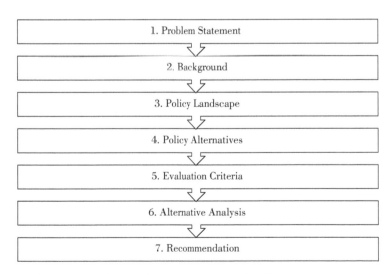

Figure 4.1 Key sections and steps in developing a policy analysis document.

texts specifically focused on conducting policy analysis. Weimer and Vining's classic text approaches the process from an economic analysis perspective.[1] Other scholars[3,5,6] approach it from a more applied perspective including work in public policy settings such as legislatures, governmental agencies, and advocacy organizations.[3,5,6]

Step 1. Problem Statement

Defining the problem is the most critical step in the policy analysis process. Unless the client and/or targeted actor(s) can be convinced that a problem exists and is worthy of governmental attention, it is not likely to move forward on the decisional agenda. Analysts should be sure to communicate with the client up front to understand their perspective on what they consider to be the "problem" or "issue" that they are hoping to address. This will serve as the frame of reference throughout the process.

An effective problem statement should clearly state the magnitude and duration of the problem, provide a comparison to an unaffected or less affected group, and be specific.[7] For example, a sample problem statement might read: *The average annual employer contribution to health insurance premiums for family coverage in the United States significantly increased (p < .05) from $3,791 in 1999 to $15,073 in 2011. This represents a nearly four-fold increase in average employer contributions over the 12-year period.*[8]

Data to support the problem statement should be drawn from epidemiologic, trend, and prevalence data that illustrate the magnitude, extent, and variability in the problem over time and across subpopulations. Importantly, analysts should present data that is relevant for the jurisdiction of interest (based on the client, targeted actor(s), and how the problem is being defined). When addressing national or nationwide health problems, rely on federal or national data sets readily available from federal government agencies (see Table 4.2). Likewise, problems at the state or local levels should be defined based on state (or local) data sources, as applicable and available.

Practical Tips and Considerations When Constructing the Problem Statement

1. Do NOT include the solution (i.e., the recommended course of action identified in Step 7 below) as part of the problem statement.[3,9]
2. The problem statement must be clear as to the affected or target jurisdiction of interest (e.g., federal–United States; state–a specific state; local–county or municipality; school district–a specific school district). This will affect the range of alternatives that may be considered in Step 4 below.
3. When describing the magnitude of the problem, rely on ranges and point estimates; odds and odds ratios are NOT useful for decision-makers.[3] Refer to primary epidemiologic, trend, prevalence, and other key data sources for identifying the problem rather than a scientific article providing odds ratios and results of regression analyses.
4. Recognize that the problem statement is iterative. It likely will evolve through each step in the process, particularly in the alternative specification step (Step 4).

Table 4.2 Examples of Federal Agencies with Health-related Data

Agency Name	Key Data Sources
Department of Health and Human Services Agencies	
Centers for Disease Control and Prevention (CDC) www.cdc.gov	Morbidity and Mortality Weekly Reports (MMWRs) National Vital Statistics System—Mortality (NVSS-M) National Vital Statistics System—Natality (NVSS-N) Behavioral Risk Factor Surveillance System (BRFSS) Youth Risk Behavior Surveillance System (YRBS) School Health Policies and Practices Study (SHPPS) National Health and Nutrition Examination Survey (NHANES) State and Local Area Integrated Telephone Survey (SLAITS) National Health Interview Survey (NHIS) National Immunization Survey (NIS) National Hospital Discharge Survey (NHDS)
Centers for Medicare and Medicaid Services (CMS) www.cms.gov	Medicaid Statistical Information System (MSIS) Medicare Administrative Data Medicare Current Beneficiary Survey (MCBS) Hospital Consumer Assessment of Healthcare Providers and Systems (HCAHPS)
Substance Abuse and Mental Health Services Administration (SAMHSA) www.samhsa.gov	National Survey on Drug Use and Health (NSDUH) Drug Abuse Warning Network (DAWN) National Survey on Substance Abuse Treatment Services (NSSATS) Treatment Episode Data Set (TEDS) National Mental Health Services Survey (N-MHSS)
National Institutes of Health (NIH) www.nih.gov	Panel Study of Income Dynamics (PSID) National Epidemiologic Survey on Alcohol and Related Conditions (NESARC) Surveillance, Epidemiology, and End Results (SEER) cancer database Study data repositories (e.g. National Heart, Lung, and Blood Institute (NHLBI) Biologic Specimen and Data Repository)
Agency for Healthcare Research and Quality (AHRQ) www.ahrq.gov	Medical Expenditure Panel (MEPS) Healthcare Cost and Utilization (HCUP) databases
Selected Other Federal Agencies with Health-related Data	
Bureau of Labor Statistics (BLS) www.bls.gov	Survey of Occupational Injuries and Illnesses (SOII) Employment, Hours, and Earnings databases Employee Benefits Survey (1985 – 2006)/National Compensation Survey—Benefits (from 2010)

(continued)

Table 4.2 Continued

Agency Name	Key Data Sources
Selected Other Federal Agencies with Health-related Data	
Census Bureau www.census.gov	National census data including information on disability, fertility, HIV/AIDS, health insurance, health, expenses and investments, education, employment, families, housing, and income, among other categories.
Department of Agriculture (USDA) www.usda.gov	Economic Research Service (ERS) National Agricultural Statistics Service (NASS) Rural Business-Cooperative Service Rural Development (RD) data School Nutrition Dietary Assessment Study (SNDA)
Department of Housing and Urban Development (HUD) www.hud.gov	Public Housing Physical Inspection Scores Multifamily Housing Physical Inspection Scores Low-Income Housing Tax Credit (LIHTC) Qualified Census Tract (QCT) Community Planning and Development (CPD) Appropriation Fair Market Rents For The Section 8 Housing Assistance Payments Program HUD Insured Multifamily Properties HUD Insured Hospitals
Occupational Safety and Health Administration (OSHA) www.osha.gov	Employee Benefits Security Administration Mine Safety and Health Administration Office of Federal Contract Compliance Programs OSHA Enforcement Data Wage and Hour Compliance Action Data

Step 2. Background Section

Once the problem has been defined, it is important to provide evidence (i.e., qualitative and quantitative data)[10–12] to support the breadth and depth of the problem. This section of the policy analysis helps to make the case for why the problem is worthy of governmental attention, how it came to be a problem, the magnitude of the problem, etc. Key questions to consider are:

- *Why* is this a problem worthy of governmental attention? Here, it is important to consider which market and governmental failures provide the rationale for a public policy solution. Clarify which failure(s) you are seeking to address. (See Chapter 2 on market and government failures.)
- *What is the size* of the problem? Use data to specify the nature and extent or magnitude of the problem.

- *For whom* is this a problem? Provide evidence and data that document the affected population(s). This is also the place to document disparities by race/ethnicity, gender, age, urbanicity, region, etc.
- *How long* has this problem existed? This should build off of the problem statement and should reflect epidemiologic and trend data showing how the problem has grown or changed over time.

Practical Tips for the Background Section

- The background section should be based on research and data. A combination of quantitative and qualitative data can help to "make the case" for the scope and magnitude of the problem and why it is worthy of governmental attention. Inclusion of disparities data (e.g., socioeconomic, gender, racial/ethnic, geography, or urbanicity) relevant to the problem also should be included in this section.
- Be sure to source all facts and data included in this section. This is a research-based product, and sources should be properly cited as is required in a scientific, public health, or social science paper.
- Sources for the background section may come from document research (e.g., peer-reviewed scientific literature reviews; epidemiologic data; or research/issue briefs from think tanks, advocacy organizations, consulting firms, and government agencies) or field research, including case studies, interviews, and the like. (See Table 4.2 in Step 1 for key federal data sources.)
- Rely on primary sources of information to the extent possible. In other words, when describing the magnitude of the problem, utilize the original source of the data rather than a restatement of data from a secondary source such as a journal article, newspaper article, or online article.

Step 3. Policy Landscape Section

In the policy landscape section, attention turns to the key stakeholders and the policy history associated with the problem. This section helps to put a political and policy "frame" around the problem and the alternatives that will be specified later on in Step 4 by clarifying which stakeholders have a vested interest in the problem. A description of the policy landscape examines stakeholder political leanings and resources as well as what policy actions have (or have not) been taken to address the problem to date.

Key Stakeholders. The key stakeholders include not only the client and "targeted actors" (i.e., the authoritative decision-makers; see earlier discussion) but also other decision-makers and/or groups who have a stake and/or standing on the problem at hand. The stakeholders will vary depending on the problem and the jurisdictional focus of the problem statement (i.e., is this a federal, state, or local problem?). Table 4.3 lists key stakeholder groups to consider inside and outside of government.[4,13]

Conducting a stakeholder analysis involves identifying the key stakeholders, including the client and/or targeted actor(s) as well as other key stakeholders both

Table 4.3 Key Stakeholder Groups to Consider

Stakeholder	Authority/Relevance	Examples
	Stakeholders Inside of Government	
Legislative branch	Possess legal authority to engage in policy formation through legislative process; enacted legislation becomes codified law	Individual legislators, Committee chairs, Majority/Minority leaders, Caucus chairs, county/city council members, etc. At the local level may also include elected officials from relevant boards and commissions (e.g., Park Board, Planning and Zoning Commission)
Executives	Can issue executive orders and other policies as delegated by the legislature; oversees executive branch agencies (and the regulatory process)	President, Governor, County/ City Administrator or Executive
Administrative Agencies within Executive Branch	Executes/implements legislation and executive orders; depending on the agency, may possess rulemaking/ regulatory authority to develop regulations; provide technical expertise to legislators and their staff; promulgated regulations become administrative law	Agencies of the 17 cabinet departments at the federal level, such as agencies of the U.S. Department of Health and Human Services (e.g., CDC, HRSA, SAMHSA, NIH) At the state (and local) levels, includes state (and local) agencies
Courts	Determine constitutionality/legality of actions of the legislative and executive branches of government; court decisions are codified as case law; key consideration is whether a given course of action would be deemed legal from a court perspective	U.S. Supreme Court, Appellate Courts, District Courts, etc.
	Stakeholders Outside of Government	
Advocacy organizations	Advocate for specific issues/causes; provide information and expertise in support of a particular position; help to draft legislation	Center for Science in the Public Interest (CSPI); Center for Consumer Freedom

Table 4.3 Continued

Stakeholder	Authority/Relevance	Examples
Interest groups	Lobby on behalf of specific interests; particularly important when political stakeholders rely on relevant parties (e.g., retired persons) for votes; often make large-scale monetary contributions to candidates and fund opposition to or support for specific initiatives (e.g., ballot initiatives)	American Association of Retired Persons (AARP); American Medical Association (AMA); Food Policy Action (FPA); American Beverage Association; National Restaurant Association
Professional membership organizations	Advocate on behalf of individuals or organizations related to a specific profession; prepare policy positions for the organization; assist in drafting new legislation	American Public Health Association (APHA); American Dental Association (ADA); American Congress of Physicians (ACP); National Council for Behavioral Health
Nonprofit organizations	Often advocate for particular policy positions; involved in a range of policy analysis and development	Kaiser Family Foundation (KFF); Bill & Melinda Gates Foundation
Think tanks	Conduct policy impact studies and policy analyses to aid in decision-making	Urban Institute; Brookings Institution; American Enterprise Institute for Public Policy Research (AEI)
For-profit businesses	Relevant as payers (employers) or providers; often provide political donations and, therefore, can be particularly influential in final policy outcomes	Monsanto, Walmart, UnitedHealth Group, Hewlett-Packard

inside and outside of government. This includes identifying their values and motivations, their position on the issue/problem, and the resources that they offer. Resources may include items such as votes or appropriations for legislators, monetary contributions for lobbyists, or information expertise for advocacy groups. This stakeholder analysis also will be useful when considering the political feasibility of each alternative (discussed under Step 6 below).

Policy History. Given that most public policy problems are not "new," but, rather, have existed for some time, chances are that a wide range of policies and/or policy solutions have been considered in the months and/or years leading up to today. Thus, the policy history section focuses on outlining how the problem has or has not been addressed from a public policy perspective (i.e., through enacted/failed bills, enacted laws, proposed/failed regulations, etc.). Timelines are useful tools in this section; they can help to set the stage for describing the current state of affairs in Step 4 (alternative specification). This is the place to outline the chronology of policy action (or inaction). Key considerations include any legislative, executive, and/or judicial decisions or actions that helped to shape the issue and when they occurred.

The policy history should be based on policy actions that are relevant to the jurisdiction for the analysis. For example, if the problem is a national problem, focus on federal policy history or, if relevant, the history of state policymaking that has led to this now becoming a national problem. The policy history can be identified through searches of policy tracking databases (see Chapter 15), including federal, state, and/or local (depending on the jurisdiction of interest) policy tracking databases. At the federal level, the key databases are Thomas, the Federal Digital System, and Regulations. gov. Thomas (http://thomas.loc.gov/home/thomas.php) is maintained by the Library of Congress and includes information on Congressional legislation and bills, appropriations bills, and public laws. The Federal Digital System (FDsys) (http://www.gpo. gov/fdsys/search/home.action) is maintained by the U.S. Government Printing Office. FDsys provides free, online access to official documents from all three branches of government including Congressional legislation, public laws, committee hearing information, and the *Federal Register*, which is where proposed and adopted regulations are published. Regulations.gov (http://www.regulations.gov/#!home) is a repository of all proposed and adopted federal regulations and related documents, including comments submitted in response to proposed regulations. Similar databases often exist at the state level (through the state legislature and the governor's office) and, depending on the local jurisdiction, through local agencies.

Step 4. Policy Alternatives Section

Once the problem has been clearly defined and the policy background and stakeholders clarified, the next key step is to identify a range of policy alternatives or options for addressing the problem. It is important to note here the use of the term "addressing," as opposed to "solving," the problem. Many policy actions are incremental in nature[14] and often will not fully "solve" a problem, but, we can hope, will move things along in the "right" direction.

As with the prior steps we have described, it is important to ensure that the alternatives identified are relevant for the jurisdiction of interest and within the realm of the client's (or targeted actor's) authority. Importantly, the likely impact, outcomes, costs, feasibility, etc. of the alternatives presented should not be included in this section; but instead become a part of the comparison of alternatives in Step 6. Instead, this section focuses on *describing* each alternative; Step 6 focuses on comparing and contrasting the alternatives.

The first alternative that should always be presented is the *status quo* or, in other words, any existing public policies or publicly funded programs that are already in place. The status quo does not include *proposed* policies or programs or *terminated* programs; rather, it includes what is already "on-the-books" and in force. (Whether it is being enforced or implemented is a separate matter, which can be addressed under Step 6 below). If no public policy or publicly funded program exists, then that is the status quo.

The remaining alternatives presented should be based on the policy instruments (e.g., legislation, regulation, appropriation of funding, or program creation) and approaches that are appropriate given the jurisdiction of interest for the problem (i.e., federal, state, or local) and the client's (or targeted actor's) authority. Although it is valuable to think broadly about the "ideal" approach (i.e., a comprehensive solution), such an approach is often not politically, economically, or administratively feasible. In reality, most public policy decisions are incremental[14]—in other words, most policy decisions simply "tinker at the margins" or make small-scale changes to existing policies or programs. When considering alternatives, it is important to consider both comprehensive and incremental approaches. Table 4.4 includes a list of generic policy actions that might be considered, but analysts should also "think outside of the box."

Where to Locate Alternatives

Time is an important factor in all policy analysis projects. Thus, it is typically necessary to draw upon existing alternatives that have been tried elsewhere or for other comparable topics. Furthermore, by considering alternatives that already have been implemented elsewhere, it will be easier to conduct the assessment of the alternatives in Step 6, because information will be available to inform the pros and cons of the given approach. Following is a list of potential starting points for identifying ideas for alternative specification:

- Advocacy and nonprofit organizations (e.g., Center for Science in the Public Interest, Kaiser Family Foundation)
- Current/prior policy proposals (that were not enacted)
- Expert testimony before legislative bodies
- Government agency reports (e.g., Government Accountability Office, Congressional Research Service, Congressional Budget Office)
- Interest groups and lobbyists (e.g., American Association of Retired Persons [AARP], American Medical Association [AMA], or Chamber of Commerce)
- Media and popular press
- Other jurisdictions (e.g., individual states, if addressing a federal issue; other states or local governments, if addressing a state or local issue)
- Scientific literature and reports, particularly policy recommendation sections
- Think tanks (e.g., Brookings Institution, Cato Institute, Urban Institute)

Practical Tips and Considerations for Alternative Specification

- Try to focus on three to five potentially viable options for addressing the problem. If only one or two alternatives come to mind, then the problem statement is too specific; and, if more than five alternatives can be identified, then the problem statement is likely too broad. If necessary, this is a time to revisit the problem statement.
- The first alternative listed should always be the status quo option. This is a legitimate alternative and, in Step 6 (alternative analysis), it may be determined that the current policy is still the best course of action given the criteria specified in Step 6.

Table 4.4 Generic Policy Actions and the Type of Actors Typically Authorized to Pursue the Action

Policy Action	Governmental Branch with Authority for Action	Description and Examples
Education	Executive branch (with funding allocation and/or authorization from legislative branch)	**Description:** To educate and inform the public about a program or public health concern; to provide training and education to service providers or health workers. **Examples:** Social media campaigns (e.g., flu vaccination awareness campaigns, physical activity campaigns, breast cancer screening awareness); requiring the Food and Drug Administration to promulgate regulations that require chain restaurants to post calorie information on menus and menu boards; technical assistance and training to service providers; and training and certification of medical professionals.
Legalization or decriminalization	Legislative branch (to allow) and executive branch (to implement)	**Description:** To remove criminal sanctions associated with use, possession, or purchase of a product. **Example:** Decriminalizing and/or legalizing the purchase and possession of small amounts of marijuana.
Legislation	Legislative branch	**Description:** Includes new measures, amendments to existing measures, or repeal of measures that are no longer working/making sense. Includes appropriations/funding authorization for new programs, creation of new programs, or authorizing an executive branch agency to promulgate regulations on a given topic. **Example:** With the passage of the *Healthy, Hunger-Free Kids Act of 2010*, Congress for the first time authorized the U.S. Department of Agriculture to promulgate regulations governing the sale of snack foods in schools throughout the school day. **Other examples:** Federal/state/local appropriations for individual executive branch agencies or departments; specific set-aside funding for special programs or services, etc.

Policy instrument	Responsible branch	Description and examples
Providing Services or programs	Executive branch (with authorization from legislative branch)	**Description:** May include creating new services/programs, revising existing services/programs, or terminating others. Could expand a program to include new beneficiaries (e.g., expanding eligibility for an assistance program to include a higher income threshold). **Examples:** At the local level, creating shared use agreements for opening school physical activity facilities to the public for use during non-school hours.
Regulation	Executive-branch agencies	**Description:** As with legislation, the regulatory approach may include new regulations, amendments/updates to existing regulations, repeal of existing regulations. **Examples:** In public health, regulations typically will include social regulation (e.g., regulating the safety of tobacco products or regulating the sale of junk foods in schools). Other types of regulation may focus on providers of services (e.g., regulating drug testing laboratories or outpatient treatment service providers), may specify enforcement procedures and authorities (e.g., entities responsible for regulating minors' access to tobacco), may impose/change sanctions for failure to comply with an existing regulation, etc.
Research and evaluation	Executive branch	**Description:** To support or conduct research and development and/or to evaluate federal programs. **Examples:** Funding for NIH grants to support biomedical and behavioral health research; demonstration grants from CMS to study Medicaid waiver implementation; funding to evaluate implementation of the Affordable Care Act (ACA).
Subsidies	Legislative branch (but implemented through executive branch)	**Description:** May include tax incentives/credits, matching funds, vouchers, research and service grants. **Example:** Providing vouchers for low-income households to purchase fruits and vegetables; block grants to states for providing maternal and child healthcare services; tax incentives for business development in "food deserts."
Taxes	Legislative branch	**Description:** Can be applied as a sales tax or as an excise tax, privilege or license fee, etc. In public health, an important consideration with any public health-related taxation is to dedicate at least a portion of the revenue generated from the tax to fund the targeted public health programming (e.g., sugary drink tax revenue dedicated toward childhood obesity prevention programming). **Example:** Raising the excise tax on cigarettes; imposing an excise tax on the sale of sugary drinks.

- Do not set up alternatives that are completely impractical or unfeasible and unlikely to be chosen. Provide realistic choices.
- Identifying alternatives that are mutually exclusive from one another will make it easier to distinguish among the alternatives when comparing them in Step 6.
- Describe each alternative in a succinct, one-sentence write-up using terminology familiar to a lay person. Avoid technical jargon or too many acronyms.
- Consider a range of alternatives including both comprehensive and incremental approaches.

Step 5. Evaluation Criteria Section

Step 4 focused on identifying alternatives, or possible courses of action for ameliorating the problem. Step 5 focuses on specifying standards or metrics by which to evaluate the potential outcomes of each proposed alternative. In this step, a range of possible criteria for evaluating the alternatives should be considered. In the next section, Step 6, we discuss how to utilize the criteria for comparing and contrasting each alternative.

When selecting the criteria for the analysis, be strategic and focus on the ultimate goal or desired outcomes should an identified alternative be selected. When considering criteria, the analyst should consider the political, economic, and social factors that will impact the likely outcomes for each alternative under consideration. In addition, emphasis should be placed on the responsiveness and likely impact that each alternative may have on achieving the overarching goal and/or ameliorating the problem.

Box 4.1 below provides selected criteria that analysts often consider for use in their policy analysis. To make the analysis as manageable as possible, analysts are encouraged to minimize the number of criteria employed. The criteria used should be the most appropriate ones for the analysis at hand, in addition to ones that are particularly important to policymakers, namely, political feasibility and cost.

Practical Tips and Considerations for Identifying the Criteria for Evaluation

- Identify criteria that will be most useful to the client, the targeted actor(s), and/or key stakeholders, who will ultimately have to make a decision as to which course of action to pursue.
- Be clear about client, targeted actor(s), and/or key stakeholders' values.
- Always include criteria related to political feasibility and monetary cost to implement the course of action.
- If the client, targeted actor(s), and/or key stakeholders are particularly interested in addressing disparities, include criteria that will address the extent to which each alternative will help to reduce and/or eliminate disparities.
- Choose a manageable number of criteria; three is probably too few and 10 is probably too many, unless an in-depth policy analysis is being conducted. For an academic exercise, five to seven criteria is often appropriate, particularly given that political feasibility and cost should always be selected as two of the criteria.

Box 4.1 Selected Criteria for Assessing Public Health Policy Alternatives

Administrative or Technical Feasibility: How feasible or challenging will it be for governmental agencies to implement the alternative? Do they have the resources (financial, staff, infrastructure, etc.) necessary to facilitate implementation?

Cost: This refers to the monetary cost associated with implementing the alternative (i.e., how much will this alternative cost taxpayers?).

Cost-benefit*: Ratio of costs to benefits—ideally seeking to maximize benefits to the affected population at the least possible cost.

Cost-effectiveness*: Assesses the costs of the policy alternative and measures the alternative's effect in a unit other than dollars (e.g., years of life lost, reduced cancer risk, reduced smoking rates).

Effectiveness: Will the alternative help to ameliorate the problem in the jurisdiction of interest and for the key target populations? This is also referred to as **targeted impact** and relates to the **evidence-based** criterion.

Evidence-based*: Is there a scientific basis for this alternative? Has it been tested and proven to be impactful? This relates to the **effectiveness** criterion.

Equity (or Fairness): Are the groups affected by the alternative treated equally, fairly, and justly? Another approach to equity includes targeted universalism (i.e., designing universal programs with targeted impacts for specific populations[15]).

Legality: Is there a legal basis for the alternative? For example, if an alternative proposes new regulations, has the legislature granted the regulatory agency the legal authority to regulate on the given topic?

Political Feasibility*: Will the given alternative be supported or adopted by the client and/or targeted actor(s) (i.e., policymakers) and key stakeholders? Consider their positions when considering political feasibility.

Timeliness: How quickly can the alternative be implemented? And how long will it take for it to have an effect on the problem and target population?

*See section below, "Tools for Policy Analysis," for a more in-depth discussion of these topics.

Step 6. Alternative Analysis Section

Now that the criteria are identified, the next step is to critically assess each alternative identified in Step 4 by the criteria selected under Step 5. This is where the hard work really takes place. This is the stage in the policy analysis process where the analyst will compare and contrast the various policy alternatives against the status quo and ask the key question: "Will this alternative help to ameliorate the problem, make it worse, or make little difference as compared to the status quo (i.e., the base case)?" The answer to this question will be based on a detailed analysis of each alternative by the criteria *using research and evidence.*

The goal of this step is to identify the pros and cons of each policy option (including the status quo) based on the criteria identified in Step 5. This step (Step 6) usually is presented both in text (paragraph) and tabular format, with a summary side-by-side table typically presented at the end of the analysis. *It is important to note that wherever possible, the analyst should rely on documentary and other evidence, facts, and data to back up each point.* This stage of the process is based on research (often through literature and Internet searches, but it also may include qualitative research) that the analyst must conduct in order to accurately assess the pros and cons and the likely impact of each alternative. This is NOT a subjective exercise. Rather, this is the heart of the analysis and is intended to be mainly an OBJECTIVE analysis. One critical tool used by policy analysts throughout governmental agencies, advocacy organizations, interest groups, and think tanks to evaluate the policy alternatives is a *side-by-side table,* which is described and illustrated below.

Tools for Policy Analysis

This section briefly describes some helpful tools for analyzing policy alternatives. These tools have varying uses, including considering the financial (cost-effectiveness analysis and cost-benefit analysis) and health (health impact assessment) ramifications of a policy decision, as well as the scientific basis or evidence-base for a given policy action. These tools may be utilized to get a better picture of what the existing evidence indicates. For example, a city's planning department may wish to use a health impact assessment to consider whether action should be taken to prevent asthma in children by developing new affordable housing regulations. First, we turn to the side-by-side table, a framework that will help in comparing policy alternatives. We will then share some analytic tools that will provide information to populate the side-by-side tables.

Side-by-Side Tables

Side-by-side tables are an essential tool in any policy analyst's arsenal to compare and contrast policy options. Although some side-by-side tables are *descriptive* (i.e., simply describe each policy option), we recommend creating and using an *analytic* side-by-side table that presents a detailed assessment of each alternative by the specified criteria. Although the side-by-side table is intended to supplement the textual analysis, it actually is the primary source of information for the textual analysis. We recommend that analysts prepare two versions of their side-by-side tables: (1) a detailed, in-depth table that cites appropriate sources and populates each cell of the table with detailed evidence/data; and (2) a simplified summary version for presentation. The more detailed table can also be included as an appendix to the final paper.

Regardless of whether the analyst is preparing an analytic or summary side-by-side table, it is helpful to include a summary term or indicators to describe how each alternative "ranks" for the given criterion. Summary terms may be based on Likert-type scales such as high–medium–low or strong–medium–weak, or analysts may employ indicators such as "+" and "–" symbols or arrows such as "↑" "↓" "↔" (neutral). Notwithstanding the summary approach taken, the intention is to tell the story as simply as possible while minimizing the text in the table. Even with the large, detailed tables developed to inform the analysis, it is useful to include the summary terms or indicators, because this will make the development of the summary table much easier.

Table 4.5 provides a sample of a summary side-by-side table using the example of legislative options for reducing sugary drink consumption among children and youth in one state. In each cell, include a summary statement (symbol or phrase) with citations from the documentary research to support the analysis (where available). For the detailed analytic side-by-side table, include detailed explanations to support the summary statement in addition to the citations. Use meaningful headers for the alternative titles.

Determining the Evidence-base for a Policy

An important criterion listed in Step 5 is the evidence-base for the policy alternative. It is imperative that proposed policy actions are supported by the best available evidence on the impact of the policy for similar populations. Readers are encouraged to consult the extensive literature on the topic of evidence-based policymaking.[10,11,42,43] However, for the current volume, we briefly touch on some of the key considerations when determining the evidence-base for a given policy alternative.

At the outset, while evidence-based medicine maintains a strict standard order of importance based on study type,[10,44] evaluating evidence for policy is less straightforward. In particular, studies that provide strong scientific evidence may not easily be generalized to the broader population. There are three main types of studies for generating evidence—experimental, quasiexperimental, and observational[45]—each with its own strengths and weaknesses.

Although *experimental studies*, including randomized controlled trials (RCTs), are considered the "gold standard" for generating causal evidence and providing high degrees of internal validity (i.e., a high level of confidence that the observed outcome is caused by the intervention), they are often not practical for determining effectiveness in real-world settings, such as studying the impact of a public policy (i.e., a natural experiment).[10,45,46]

Quasiexperimental studies are often better suited to describing how an intervention fares in the real world. Quasiexperimental studies are typically not randomized but still allow for some researcher control in the study design.[10] The *natural experiment*—a type of study in which the researcher has no control over the distribution of an intervention across subpopulations—is particularly relevant to the current discussion.[47] Natural experiments are routinely conducted in public health to assess changes in health behaviors (i.e., cigarette purchases or soda consumption) before and after a policy (e.g., cigarette excise tax rate increase) is enacted. Natural experiments are particularly strong in describing real-world effectiveness and external validity (i.e., generalizability) because they indicate how an intervention may affect other, similar populations. Additionally, natural experiments may provide real-world information about the feasibility of implementing the policy intervention. Thus, policy analysts may turn to scientific studies based on natural experiments to assess the potential impact that a given alternative may have on the outcomes of interest.

Table 4.5 Sample of Summary Side-by-Side Table Comparing State Legislative Options for Reducing Sugary Drink Consumption among Children and Adolescents

Criteria	Status Quo (already on the books): Ban sugary drinks in schools	Alternative 1: Impose a 1-cent per ounce excise tax on sugary drinks	Alternative 2: Social marketing campaign to raise awareness about the consequences of overconsumption	Alternative 3: Require nutrition education for all grades that educates students about healthy eating habits, including the consequences of overconsumption of sugary drinks
Impact on overall consumption	Minimal (only in school)[16,17]	High[18-20]	Minimal–Moderate[21-23]	Minimal–Moderate[24-27]
Cost to implement	Neutral (already implemented)	Moderate initially but then minimal once systems in place[18-20]	Minimal (materials already developed by other states and CDC)[28-30]	Moderate (depends on scope of intervention, i.e., number of schools, for how long, etc.)[31-33]
Revenue generation to support childhood obesity programs	None	High[18-20]	None	None
Political feasibility	High (already in place)	Low[34-41]	High	Moderate
Administrative ease to implement	High (already in place)	Moderate (once system in place)[18-20]	High	High[31-33]

Finally, *observational studies* (i.e., qualitative research) can be combined with the above to provide a more comprehensive framing of the issue as it relates to the targeted community. Observational studies are particularly useful for health impact assessments and for providing "stories" for use by authoritative decision-makers. In observational studies, variables are observed rather than manipulated. Thus, the researcher has little control over the study.

Several tools exist for evaluating evidence. One commonly used tool is the *systematic review*. Systematic reviews provide an overview of the literature on a particular problem or intervention. In such a review, systematic methods are used to evaluate the body of evidence (usually includes peer-reviewed and gray literature) to answer the carefully formulated research question. Methods include the identification, selection, and critical appraisal of relevant research on a specific question, as well as the collection and analysis of data from the studies that are included in the review.[48] Statistical methods (*meta-analysis*) may or may not be used to analyze and summarize the results of the included studies.[49]

Systematic reviews are increasingly being compiled on a wide range of public health policy interventions. A number of organizations provide access to published systematic reviews including, but not limited to, the Cochrane Collaboration,[50,51] the Campbell Collaboration,[52] the Community Guide,[53] and the U.S. Preventive Services Task Force.[54]

Assessing Political Feasibility of Alternatives

Political feasibility is one of the most important criteria for policy analysis. If the recommended alternative is not going to garner support from the authoritative decision-makers (e.g., legislators), then the alternative will not move forward. The matrix provided below is a simplified template for assessing political feasibility using the example of legislative options for reducing sugary drink consumption presented in Table 4.6. For illustrative purposes, only three stakeholders are listed below; however, for a full policy analysis, a wide range of stakeholders would typically be included and grouped according to their most appropriate classification, such as key decision-makers (e.g., key legislators, committee chairpersons), advocacy groups, and interest groups. Within each cell, include the given stakeholder's stated or likely position (for/against) on each alternative, along with resources the stakeholder brings to the table. Be sure to cite to documentation (where available) to back up the stakeholders' positions.

Cost-Effectiveness Analysis

Cost-effectiveness analysis (CEA) is a tool in which the costs and benefits are quantified for a number of policies or programs with the same goal. Costs of alternatives are measured in terms of their requisite estimated dollar expenditures. Effectiveness is the degree to which an intervention achieves its goal. For example, the goal of a tax increase on alcoholic beverages may be to decrease incidence of liver disease. The effectiveness, or benefits, of a program are set at a numerical unit, such as the Quality Adjusted Life-Year (QALY) or a biomarker for improvement or remission of a particular disease

Table 4.6 Hypothetical Matrix for Assessing Stakeholder Positions Relative to State-level Policy Options for Reducing Sugary Drinks Consumption among Children and Adolescents

Stakeholder		Alternatives			
Name	*Resource(s)*	*Status Quo: Ban Sugary Drinks in Schools*	*1: Excise Tax on Sugary Drinks*	*2: Social Marketing Campaign*	*3: Nutrition Education in Schools*
American Beverage Association	Financial resources and lobbying	Supportive – federal regulations already in place which create one nationwide standard in schools	Opposed because it would raise the price of beverages they sell	Somewhat supportive as long as it is not critical of industry	Supportive – would be the best option
Center for Science in the Public Interest	Information expertise, policy maker relationships, ability to mobilize advocacy community	Supportive – federal regulations already in place	Supportive – would be best way to reduce consumption	Supportive but only as a starting point to raise awareness	Supportive but would need to be a sequential, grade-specific program with specific number of hours dedicated to didactic learning
Democratic Legislator (would be named in the analysis)	Legislative voting and ability to rally fellow legislators for/ against a given alternative committee and chamber discussions	Supportive – federal regulations already in place	Supportive but wants money dedicated to child obesity prevention programs	Supportive	Supportive but would likely need to be done at the state level to ensure consistency across districts
Republican Legislator (would be named in the analysis)	Legislative voting and ability to rally fellow legislators for/against a given alternative committee and chamber discussions	Opposed – does not believe the federal government should regulate in this area; it should be left to state, districts, and parents to decide	Opposed – would be regressive and unfair to marginalized populations	Supportive as long as not critical to industry	Supports nutrition education as long as it does not take away from core subjects. No additional time should be allocated.

(e.g., an intervention for diabetes prevention may use decrease in blood glucose levels). The interventions are then compared in order of effectiveness, and those interventions that are both higher in cost and lower or equal in effectiveness to another intervention (i.e., those that are less cost-effective) are eliminated. The final set of interventions can then be used to determine the most effective method for achieving a program or policy goal, based on a set budget or willingness-to-pay.[55] Previously completed cost-effectiveness analyses can be found online in the CEA Registry.[56]

Cost-Benefit Analysis

The cost-benefit analysis (CBA), like the CEA, is useful for quantifying both causes and effects to determine cost-effectiveness. Unlike a CEA, the CBA approach assigns a monetary value to both costs and benefits, and thereby attributes monetary value to person-time and life-years-lost. The costs are then subtracted from the benefits, and the end result is the net present value (NPV), or net health benefit (NHB), of an intervention. If several interventions are being considered, the process is to calculate the NPV for each intervention and, finally, to compare these numbers.

Health Impact Assessment

The Health Impact Assessment (HIA) is a newly developed tool that is growing in use. Its goal is to evaluate the impact or potential impact of a policy or program on the health of a population. HIAs typically are used to assess the impact of a policy decision that is not necessarily within the purview of a health department or organization. For example, decisions made in environmental and public planning departments may affect human health, and these decisions may first be reviewed with an HIA to determine what this impact might be. One of the main concerns of the HIA is to assess whether the policy or program disproportionately affects minority members of the population.[57,58]

There is currently no standardized process for developing a health impact assessment, but the procedure typically has six parts. First, a screening, such as checklists or community surveys, should be done to determine whether an HIA is required. Second, scoping sets up the HIA by determining goals, measurement methods, and a plan of action for the assessment. After scoping takes place, the appraisal is completed. Information from the appraisal is then used to provide recommendations. Finally, the HIA is evaluated (often informally) to gauge its success and suggestions for future HIAs. Guides to conducting health impact assessments, as well as HIA registries, can be found through several organizations, including the International Health Impact Assessment Consortium at the University of Liverpool,[59] the Health Impact Project,[60] and the Health Impact Assessment Clearinghouse at the University of California, Los Angeles.[61]

Step 7. Make a Recommendation

Once the difficult task of comparing and contrasting the alternatives is complete, it is time to make a recommendation. At this stage, it is not only important to assess how each alternative (including the status quo) "stacked up" in the comparison stage (Step 6) but, also, to weigh the body of evidence, particularly in relation to "key" criteria identified in Step 4 (in particular, political feasibility). For example, suppose that one particular alternative (let us call it, "Alternative X") meets all of the criteria related to impact, timeliness, and reducing disparities, but it is not politically feasible or is exorbitantly expensive to implement. Chances are great that Alternative X may not be the best course of action. Instead, the analyst may opt for a different course of action but note that "in the ideal" world she or he would recommend Alternative X should the political and/or economic conditions change.

The recommendation section should be fairly short and straightforward. There should be no surprises, because it should be based entirely on the objective assessment conducted in Step 6. The analyst should explain how he or she arrived at the given recommendation (e.g., which criteria were deemed critical), particularly in cases where two alternatives seemed to be comparable on several criteria.

CONCLUSION

This chapter discussed policy analysis as a profession, as well as the methods and tools with which it is conducted. Information in this chapter should be particularly useful for public health students seeking to pursue careers in public health advocacy and public health policy. Although this chapter attempts to provide a broad but detailed overview of the critical steps necessary for conducting public health policy analysis, readers are encouraged to refer to the myriad resources and volumes cited in this chapter for more in-depth exploration of public health policy analysis as a profession.

REFERENCES

1. Weimer DL, Vining AR. *Policy Analysis: Concepts and Practice*. 5th ed. Boston, MA: Longman; 2011.
2. Kraft ME, Furlong SR. *Public Policy: Politics, Analysis, and Alternatives*. 5th ed. Thousand Oaks, CA: CQ Press; 2014.
3. Bardach E. *A Practical Guide to Policy Analysis: The Eightfold Path to More Effective Problem Solving*. Thousand Oaks, CA: CQ Press; 2012.
4. Kingdon JW. *Agendas, Alternatives, and Public Policies*. 2nd ed. New York, NY: Addison-Wesley Educational Publishers, Inc.; 2003.
5. Seavey JS, McGrath RJ, Aytur S. *Health Policy Analysis: Framework and Tools for Success*. New York, NY: Springer Publishing Company; 2014.
6. McLaughlin CP, McLaughlin PEKF, McLaughlin CD. *Health Policy Analysis*. 2nd ed. Burlington, MA: Jones & Bartlett Learning; 2014.
7. Bhattacharya D. *Public Health Policy: Issues, Theories, and Advocacy*. San Francisco, CA: Wiley 2013.
8. Kaiser Family Foundation, Health Research and Educational Trust. *Employer Health Benefits: 2011 Annual Survey*. https://kaiserfamilyfoundation.files.wordpress.com/2013/04/8225.pdf. Updated 2011. Accessed March 5, 2015.

9. Teitelbaum JB, Wilensky SE. *Essentials of Health Policy and Law*. 2nd ed. Burlington, MA: Jones & Bartlett Learning; 2013.

10. Institute of Medicine. Committee on an Evidence Framework for Obesity Prevention Decision Making. *Bridging the Evidence Gap in Obesity Prevention: A Framework to Inform Decision Making*. Washington, DC: National Academy of Sciences; 2010.

11. Brownson RC, Chriqui JF, Stamatakis KA. Understanding evidence-based public health policy. *Am J Public Health*. 2009;99:1576–1583.

12. Brownson RC, Chriqui JF, Burgeson CR, et al. Translating epidemiology into policy to prevent childhood obesity: the case for promoting physical activity in school settings. *Ann Epidemiol*. 2010;20:436–444.

13. Anderson JE. *Public Policymaking*. 6th ed. Boston, MA: Houghton Mifflin Company; 2006.

14. Lindblom CE. The science of muddling through. *Public Administration Review*. 1950;19: 79–88.

15. Powell JA. Post-racialism or targeted universalism. *Denver University Law Review*. 2008;86: 785–806.

16. Taber DR, Chriqui JF, Powell LM, et al. Banning all sugar-sweetened beverages in middle schools: reduction of in-school access and purchasing but not overall consumption. *Arch Pediatr Adolesc Med*. 2012;166:256–262.

17. Blum JE, Davee AM, Beaudoin CM, et al. Reduced availability of sugar-sweetened beverages and diet soda has a limited impact on beverage consumption patterns in Maine high school youth. *J Nutr Educ Behav*. 2008;40:341–347.

18. Chaloupka FJ, Wang YC, Powell LM, Andreyeva T, Chriqui JF, Rimkus LM. *Estimating the Potential Impact of Sugar-Sweetened and Other Beverage Excise Taxes in Illinois*. http://www. preventobesityil.org/f/Study___Tax_on_sugar_loaded_drinks_reduces_obesity_and_ healthcare_costs.pdf. Updated 2011. Accessed December 31, 2011.

19. Chaloupka FJ, Powell LM, Chriqui JF. Sugar-sweetened beverages and obesity prevention: policy recommendations. *J Policy Anal Manage*. 2011;30:662–664.

20. Chriqui JF, Chaloupka FJ, Powell LM, et al. A typology of beverage taxation: multiple approaches for obesity prevention and obesity prevention-related revenue generation. *J Public Health Policy*. 2013;34:403–423.

21. Gase LN, Robles B, Barragan NC, et al. Relationship between nutritional knowledge and the amount of sugar-sweetened beverages consumed in Los Angeles County. *Health Educ Behav*. 2014;41:431–439.

22. Robles B, Blitstein JL, Lieberman AJ, et al. The relationship between amount of soda consumed and intention to reduce soda consumption among adults exposed to the Choose Health LA 'Sugar Pack' health marketing campaign. *Public Health Nutr*. 2015;7:1–10.

23. Boles M, Adams A, Gredler A, et al. Ability of a mass media campaign to influence knowledge, attitudes, and behaviors about sugary drinks and obesity. *Prev Med*. 2014;67(Suppl 1):S40–S45.

24. Connell DB, Turner RR. School Health Education Evaluation. The impact of instructional experience and the effects of cumulative instruction. *J Sch Health*. 1985;55:324–331.

25. DeVault N, Kennedy T, Hermann J, et al. It's all about kids: preventing overweight in elementary school children in Tulsa, OK. *J Am Diet Assoc*. 2009;109:680–687.

26. Simons LA, Simons J. Health lifestyle education in high schools. A three-year follow-up study. *Med J Aust*. 1984;141:158–162.

27. Johnson CC, Li D, Galati T, et al. Maintenance of the classroom health education curricula: results from the CATCH-ON study. *Health Educ Behav.* 2003;30:476–488.

28. California Department of Public Health. *Rethink Your Drink Campaign Resources.* http://www.cdph.ca.gov/programs/cpns/Pages/RethinkYourDrink-Resources.aspx. Updated 2015. Accessed April 28, 2015.

29. New York City Department of Health and Mental Hygiene. *Pouring On the Pounds Ad Campaign.* http://www.nyc.gov/html/doh/html/living/sugarydrink-media.shtml. Updated 2015. Accessed April 28, 2015.

30. Centers for Disease Control and Prevention. *Rethink Your Drink.* http://www.cdc.gov/healthyweight/healthy_eating/drinks.html. Updated 2011. Accessed April 28, 2015.

31. Hoelscher DM, Feldman HA, Johnson CC, et al. School-based health education programs can be maintained over time: results from the CATCH Institutionalization study. *Prev Med.* 2004;38:594–606.

32. Hoelscher DM, Kelder SH, Murray N, et al. Dissemination and adoption of the Child and Adolescent Trial for Cardiovascular Health (CATCH): a case study in Texas. *J Public Health Manag Pract.* 2001;7:90–100.

33. Johnson CC, Li D, Galati T, et al. Maintenance of the classroom health education curricula: results from the CATCH-ON study. *Health Educ Behav.* 2003;30:476–488.

34. Dinkelspiel F. *Why Berkeley passed a soda tax while other cities failed.* http://www.berkeleyside.com/2014/11/05/why-berkeley-passed-a-soda-tax-where-others-failed/. Updated 2014. Accessed March 23, 2015.

35. Dinkelspiel F. *Around $3.4m spent on Berkeley soda tax campaign.* http://www.berkeleyside.com/2015/02/05/around-3-4m-spent-on-berkeley-soda-tax-campaign/. Updated 2015. Accessed March 23, 2015.

36. Knight H. *Why Berkeley passed a soda tax and S.F. didn't.* http://www.sfgate.com/bayarea/article/Why-Berkeley-passed-a-soda-tax-and-S-F-didn-t-5879757.php.%20Updated%20November%207. Updated 2014. Accessed March 23, 2015.

37. Mejia P, Nixon L, Cheyne A, Dorfman L, Quintero F. *Issue 21: Two communities, two debates: News coverage of soda tax proposals in Richmond and El Monte.* http://www.bmsg.org/resources/publications/news-coverage-soda-tax-proposals-Richmond-El-Monte-California. Updated 2014. Accessed March 23, 2015.

38. Nixon R. Nutrition group lobbies against healthier school meals it sought, citing cost. *New York Times.* July 2, 2014;A18.

39. Oatman M. *The soda tax lost. Now what?* http://www.motherjones.com/blue-marble/2012/11/soda-taxes-fail-california-richmond-ritterman. Updated 2012. Accessed March 23, 2015.

40. Zigas E. *Why did Berkeley pass a soda tax and not San Francisco?* http://www.spur.org/blog/2014-11-25/why-did-berkeley-pass-soda-tax-and-not-san-francisco. Updated 2014. Accessed March 23, 2015.

41. Zingale D. *Gulp! The high cost of Big Soda's victory.* http://articles.latimes.com/2012/dec/09/opinion/la-oe-zingale-soda-tax-campaign-funding-20121209. Updated 2012. Accessed March 31, 2015.

42. Anderson LM, Brownson RC, Fullilove MT, et al. Evidence-based public health policy and practice: promises and limits. *Am J Prev Med.* 2005;28:226–230.

43. Brownson RC, Jones E. Bridging the gap: translating research into policy and practice. *Prev Med.* 2009;49:313–315.

44. Biller-Andorno N, Lie RK, ter Meulen R. Evidence-based medicine as an instrument for rational health policy. *Health Care Anal.* 2002;10:261–275.

45. Mercer SL, DeVinney BJ, Fine LJ, et al. Study designs for effectiveness and translation research:identifying trade-offs. *Am J Prev Med.* 2007;33:139–154.

46. Brownson RC, Hartge P, Samet JM, et al. From epidemiology to policy: toward more effective practice. *Ann Epidemiol.* 2010;20:409–411.

47. Petticrew M, Cummins S, Ferrell C, et al. Natural experiments: an underused tool for public health? *Public Health.* 2005;119:751–757.

48. Bambra C. Real world reviews: a beginner's guide to undertaking systematic reviews of public health policy interventions. *J Epidemiol Community Health.* 2011;65:14–19.

49. Jacobs JA, Jones E, Gabella BA, et al. Tools for implementing an evidence-based approach in public health practice. *Prev Chronic Dis.* 2012;9:E116.

50. Cochrane Public Health Group. http://ph.cochrane.org/. Updated 2015. Accessed March 5, 2015.

51. The Cochrane Collaboration. http://www.cochrane.org/. Updated 2015. Accessed March 5, 2015.

52. The Campbell Collaboration. http://www.campbellcollaboration.org/lib/. Updated 2015. Accessed March 5, 2015.

53. The Community Preventive Services Task Force. *The Guide to Community Preventive Services.* http://www.thecommunityguide.org/. Updated 2015. Accessed March 5, 2015.

54. U.S. Preventive Services Task Force. http://www.uspreventiveservicestaskforce.org/. Accessed March 5, 2015.

55. Drummond F. *Methods for the Economic Evaluation of Health Care Programmes.* New York: Oxford University Press; 2005.

56. Tufts Medical Center. Cost-Effectiveness Analysis Registry. https://research.tufts-nemc. org/cear4/Home.aspx. Updated 2015. Accessed March 5, 2015.

57. Brownson RC, Royer C, Ewing R, et al. Researchers and policymakers: travelers in parallel universes. *Am J Prev Med.* 2006;30:164–172.

58. Kemm J. Health impact assessment: a tool for healthy public policy. *Health Promot Int.* 2001;16:79–85.

59. University of Liverpool. International Health Impact Assessment Consortium. http:// www.liv.ac.uk/psychology-health-and-society/research/impact/about/. Updated 2015. Accessed April 28, 2015.

60. The Pew Charitable Trusts. Health Impact Project. http://www.pewtrusts.org/en/projects/health-impact-project/research-and-analysis/hia-reports. Updated 2015.

61. UCLA Health Impact Assessment Project. UCLA Health Impact Assessment Clearinghouse Learning and Information Center. http://www.hiaguide.org. Updated 2015.

APPENDIX: POLICY ANALYSIS WHITE PAPER CHECKLIST

☐ Problem Statement: Define the problem.
  ☐ Clearly state the magnitude of the problem using point estimates and ranges.
  ☐ Clearly state the duration of the problem (i.e., how long it has been a problem).
  ☐ Include a target (affected) population and a comparison to an unaffected or less-affected population.
  ☐ Be specific.
  ☐ Utilize data that is relevant to the jurisdiction of interest.
  ☐ Do not include solution.
  ☐ Ask a question with a reasonable number (three to five) of viable options.
  ☐ Revise continually throughout the process.
☐ Background Section: Provide evidence to support the problem statement.
  ☐ Why is this a problem worthy of governmental attention?
  ☐ What is the size of the problem?
  ☐ For whom is this a problem?
  ☐ How long has this problem existed?
  ☐ Use data, tables, and figures to support the problem statement and be sure to cite to sources of the data/tables/figures (ideally primary sources).
☐ Policy Landscape: Capture key stakeholders and policy history.
  ☐ Determine key stakeholders and their standing or proposed solutions to this problem.
    ☐ Be mindful of the client and targeted actor(s) positions, values, and political philosophy.
  ☐ Describe the history of the problem and any prior policy activity on the topic.
    ☐ Ensure policy history is relevant to jurisdiction.
    ☐ Utilize primary legal sources.
☐ Comparing Policy Alternatives
  ☐ Identify policy alternatives: Be objective; fully source and cite to the sources for your alternatives
    ☐ Include the status quo.
    ☐ Consider both sides of the policymaking spectrum.
    ☐ Ensure alternatives are relevant to jurisdiction.
    ☐ Ensure alternatives are within realm of authority for the target actor.
  ☐ Select criteria for comparing alternatives.
    ☐ Specify criteria for analysis.
    ☐ Include potential political, economic, and social influences.
    ☐ Consider likely impact on outcomes.
  ☐ Compare each alternative by the specified criteria.
    ☐ Provide evidence base for each alternative; cite to research and evidence documenting expected outcomes of each alternative
    ☐ Include a side-by-side table.
    ☐ Be objective.
    ☐ Utilize other tools for analyzing the criteria (i.e., CEA, CBA, HIA).
☐ Recommend a course of action.
☐ Include References list with full citations using standard citation format (e.g., American Medical Association, American Psychological Association)

5

Policy Implications of Social Determinants of Health

Jason Q. Purnell, Sarah Simon, Emily B. Zimmerman,
Gabriela J. Camberos, and Robert Fields

LEARNING OBJECTIVES

1. Describe the policy implications of social and economic determinants of health.
2. Explain the how Education Health Initiative and *For the Sake of All* projects relate to improving social and economic determinants of health in the target population.
3. Describe the stakeholder groups that need to be involved with policies related to social and economic determinants of health.

INTRODUCTION

In many ways, policies affecting social and economic determinants of health are the ultimate prevention policies. Widely recognized as "fundamental causes" of health,[1] factors like education, poverty, housing, and employment help to shape the contexts in which individuals live their lives, with significant consequences for health. Despite a recent increase in attention to what are called upstream social determinants of health (i.e., nonmedical, social, and economic factors, as well as environmental conditions) among academic researchers, government agencies, and major private foundations,[2] policymakers and individual consumers continue to invest most of their attention and resources in payment for, and delivery of, health care. Indeed, the United States spends more money on health care than any country in the world but lags behind many of its wealthy peer nations on such indicators as life expectancy, chronic and communicable disease, disability, low birth weight, infant mortality, injuries, and homicides.[3] An Institute of Medicine panel investigating the health of the United States relative to other wealthy nations recently concluded that the gap in life expectancy between the United States and other nations has been widening for years. Although there are likely several explanations for the relative health disadvantage of the United States, the panel noted that

"The public health literature certainly documents the health benefits of strengthening systems for health and social services, education, and employment; promoting healthy life-styles; and designing healthier environments. These functions are not solely the province of government: effective policies in both the public and private sector can create incentives to encourage individuals and industries to adopt practices that protect and promote health and safety. In countries with the most favorable health outcomes, resource investments and infrastructure often reflect a strong societal commitment to the health and welfare of the entire population." (p. 6)[3]

Effective policies that consider not only the delivery of health care services, but also social services, education, employment, and the built environment hold the most promise for preventing illness, injury, and premature death.

This view is consistent with a framework offered by Centers for Disease Control and Prevention director, Thomas Frieden. The Health Impact Pyramid (see Figure 3.2 in Chapter 3) is a framework intended to broaden the focus of public health intervention beyond clinical care and to direct public health activities toward high-impact interventions that improve population health.[4] At the top of the pyramid are interventions focused mainly on individual behavior change and maintenance. These activities have the smallest impact on population health, according to Frieden, largely because they are so dependent on individual behavior, which is incredibly difficult to alter even under the best of circumstances. In fact, Frieden notes that the activities with the least impact on population health also require the greatest effort on the part of individuals. The next tiers of the pyramid, by contrast, require relatively little in terms of individual time or effort. Instead they provide long-lasting benefits from a single intervention (e.g., vaccination or colonoscopy) at the middle tier, alter contexts in which multiple individual choices are made (e.g., fluoridation of drinking water and smoke-free laws) at the next level, and influence the distribution of social and economic resources at the bottom level of the pyramid. The key insight of the model is that the largest impact on population health comes from changing the contexts in which behavior occurs and providing equal access to fundamental resources for living a healthy life, including income and wealth, education, and quality neighborhoods. Frieden also notes that intervening at the bottom of the pyramid is the most politically charged and challenging work within public health, precisely because the distribution of social and economic resources is highly controversial. This is particularly so in the United States, where an ethic of individualism emphasizes personal responsibility. Indeed, this strong cultural current likely explains both the less-generous support for social and economic well-being (e.g., education, health care, family leave policies) and the porous social safety net that distinguish the United States from other wealthy countries with better health outcomes.

This chapter will briefly describe the rationale, in terms of prevention, for policies directed at the social and economic determinants of health by reviewing the evidence that such policies do, in fact, result in better health outcomes. Recognizing that this evidence alone is unlikely to move the actors most directly responsible for enacting social and economic development policy, the chapter also presents two different approaches (one national and one local) designed to mobilize public and policymaker support for policies and interventions that address social and economic determinants. The chapter will conclude with recommendations for future research and action in this important area.

SOCIAL AND ECONOMIC POLICY
AND PREVENTIVE HEALTH

Research has shown that emerging and established social and economic policy interventions may have implications for health and may improve the well-being of children, youth, and families. Examples of social and economic policies in the areas of early childhood, education, asset building, and community and economic development are discussed in this section. Rather than an exhaustive review, what follow are necessarily brief, general overviews of several broad and complex fields of research, policy, and practice.

Early Childhood

Socioeconomic disadvantages often begin early in life. One study on the relationship between poverty and school readiness found that only 48% of children living in poverty were ready for school at age five years compared with 75% of children from moderate- or high-income households.[5] Children who are born into poverty not only have worse outcomes in childhood, but often these disadvantages follow them into adulthood. Compared with children from households with incomes of at least twice the poverty line, children who live in poverty complete fewer years of schooling, work fewer hours, receive food stamps at higher rates, are more likely to report poor health, and are almost 50% more likely to be overweight in adulthood.[6]

High-quality early childhood programming can have lasting health benefits. The Abecedarian project, a randomized, controlled study in which the intervention consisted of full-time, early educational programming with individualized activities; a focus on social, emotional, and cognitive development; and an emphasis on language, is one of the most widely cited studies on the benefits of high-quality early childhood programming. There is evidence that children who were assigned to the Abecedarian project intervention group had lower prevalence of risk factors for chronic diseases such as heart disease, stroke, and diabetes by their mid-thirties.[7]

Policies have been developed and implemented to make early childhood care and education more accessible for low-income families. Two examples of federally funded programs include Head Start and the Child Care Development Fund. Head Start is administered by the Office of Head Start, Administration for Children and Families within the Department of Health and Human Services, and federal spending is authorized by Congress each year. The Child Care Development Fund provides funding to assist low-income families in obtaining child care. The high cost of high-quality child care can make it difficult for low-income families to access child care. Although child care subsidy programs provide support for working families, eligibility requirements (e.g., household income) for these subsidies vary widely across states and many families struggle to afford quality child care. Policies that increase child care subsidies and relax income eligibility requirements have the potential to improve health and well-being among low-and-middle income families.

Education

Policies that help prevent school dropout and support higher educational attainment can also function as preventive health interventions. Americans with more years of education live longer and healthier lives compared with those who complete fewer years of education,[8] and the gap in life expectancy has been widening between those with high levels of education and low levels of education.[9] Implications of educational attainment for health outcomes are described in more detail later in this chapter (see Education and Health Initiative). Researchers from the Education and Health Initiative led by the Virginia Commonwealth University Center on Society and Health have studied the connections between education and health and suggest the need for policies that set children up for success in education. The Education and Health Initiative also provides evidence of how these policies can save not only lives but also save money. For example, a 1% increase in the percentage of Americans with some college education could save $1.3 billion per year in avoidable medical care for diabetes alone.[10]

The relationship between education and health is bidirectional. More years of education translates into better health, but students' health also influences their ability to learn and to complete their education. Examining school dropout as a public health issue, Freudenberg and Ruglis[11] recommend a number of health interventions that may lead to improvements in school dropout rates. Health-related interventions suggested as part of school-based programs to prevent dropout include:

- School-based health clinics
- Mental health programs
- Substance abuse prevention programs
- Sex, HIV infection, and pregnancy prevention programs
- Services for pregnant and parenting teens
- Violence prevention programs
- Policies to improve the school climate (e.g., reduce stigmatization).[11]

Policies to develop, fund, and implement these programs at the school district, community, state, or federal level play an important role in improving students' health and school completion rates.

School-based healthcare programs have been shown to improve both health and academic outcomes. For example, school-based health clinics/centers (SBHCs) have been shown to improve access to services students might otherwise find challenging to obtain (e.g., counseling and family planning services).[12] Compared with students who were not served by a SBHC, users of SBHCs had higher completion rates for immunization series,[13] reported greater satisfaction with their health, and engaged in a greater number of health-promoting behaviors.[14] Additionally, access to SBHCs was associated with a decrease in the rate of hospitalization and a gain of three days of school for children with asthma.[15] SBHC programs have been implemented to varying degrees from state to state. In the school year 2010–2011, the range of SBHCs by state was quite large, ranging from one SBHC each in Nebraska, New Hampshire, South Carolina, and Wisconsin to 224 total in Florida.[16]

Asset Building

Household-income poverty is consistently associated with a range of negative outcomes for children and youth, including poorer educational, behavioral, and health outcomes.[17–19] There is growing recognition that asset poverty, or a lack of household wealth, is also implicated in negative child development, with recent interest in wealth inequality fueling this line of research.[20] Policies that support asset-building among low-to-moderate income families have the potential to act as prevention strategies to address social and economic disparities and improve health and well-being. Recent evidence has demonstrated the benefits of policies that encourage asset-building. For example, children with college savings accounts in their names are up to three times more likely to attend college and four times more likely to graduate from college compared with students who lack savings.[21] Research also has begun to link specific asset-building policy interventions such as Child Development Accounts (CDAs) to health outcomes. CDAs are savings or investment accounts opened as early as birth and intended to ensure that children have the resources to reach key developmental milestones such as postsecondary education, homeownership, or starting a business.[22] In a longitudinal, randomized experiment in the state of Oklahoma, researchers have found that having a CDA leads to better social and emotional development for the most socially disadvantaged young children who received a $1,000 CDA at birth.[23] Mothers of children with CDAs in the Oklahoma experiment also report significantly lower levels of depressive symptoms.[24]

Currently, there are three states in the United States that automatically deposit funds into their state 529 plans for young children. Maine's Harold Alfond College Challenge was the first statewide universal CDA program in the nation. All newborns in Maine are automatically enrolled in the savings plan and receive a $500 grant. Nevada's College Kick Start program automatically deposits $50 into a 529 account for every public school kindergartner, and the state of Rhode Island provides an opt-in option for parents to enroll their newborns in the CollegeBound*baby* program and receive $100 in the state's 529 savings plan. Similar savings policies have been enacted in Hong Kong, Singapore, South Korea, Taiwan, and the United Kingdom. As this policy innovation continues to gain acceptance in states and cities throughout the United States, there will be opportunities to examine more long-term health impacts of asset building as a social and economic development strategy.

Neighborhood, Community, and Economic Development

Policies that impact the social and economic fabric of communities and neighborhoods also can impact the health outcomes of these communities. Mortality is one of the standard metrics used to gauge the health of a community. A large body of evidence has shown that living in a neighborhood with a low socioeconomic status (SES) is associated with increased risk of mortality compared with living in a neighborhood with a high SES.[25] Community development policies that promote better housing options, such as tenant-based rental assistance, have been shown to enhance safety and reduce the likelihood of being exposed to crime.[26]

Under the Affordable Care Act (ACA), the recently established National Prevention Council has issued the National Prevention Strategy, which highlights housing quality and cross-sector collaboration in community development planning as crucial for population health.[27] This is part of a larger move toward a "health in all policies" approach mandated by the ACA and inspired by growing acceptance of the role that social determinants play in population health.[28] Despite the promise of such cross-sector collaborative efforts, the mixed health effects of past interventions by the U.S. Department of Housing and Urban Development (HUD; e.g., "Moving to Opportunity" and HOPE VI neighborhood revitalization) and the willingness to cut funding for the Prevention and Public Health Fund also established by the ACA, point to both practical and political challenges. That HUD has adopted a health in all policies approach even in the face of such challenges, and is actively collaborating on programmatic and data projects with the U.S. Department of Health and Human Services, may help to establish a more robust evidence base for neighborhood and community development strategies to prevent disease and improve population health.[28]

Evidence of effective intervention strategies alone is unlikely to lead to important policy and programmatic change without some concerted effort to translate that evidence for key decision-makers. In the following two sections, both a national and a local model of this type of translation are described. The major components of the "connecting the dots" framework that guides the national Education and Health Initiative are shared in many respects with the *For the Sake of All* project in St. Louis, Missouri.

A NATIONAL EXAMPLE: THE EDUCATION AND HEALTH INITIATIVE

The Education and Health Initiative (EHI), led by the Virginia Commonwealth University Center on Society and Health (CSH), aimed to raise awareness about the implications of educational attainment for health outcomes and to bridge the disconnect that typically exists between researchers and policymakers.[29,30] The message for leaders in health policy was that better education could reduce disease rates and help control the rising costs of health care. The message for education leaders was that the potential health benefits of improved education could bolster their arguments for policies and funding. The initiative, funded by the Robert Wood Johnson Foundation, was part of a larger CSH effort to raise awareness about social determinants of health by connecting the dots between health and upstream factors such as income, poverty, and place.

Employed in this initiative, CSH's Connecting the Dots Model (see Figure 5.1) is a collaborative process that focuses on four key strategies. For EHI, the research component aimed to identify and communicate scientific findings about the impact of education on health. To work toward raising awareness among decision-makers about the links between education and health, the strategic communication component sought to move beyond traditional academic dissemination activities by creatively optimizing communication opportunities through various forms of media tailored to specific audiences. CSH developed a variety of outreach materials for EHI, such as videos, issue briefs, web content, and papers. The stakeholder engagement and policy outreach components involved working with residents of a low-income urban community to create conceptual models of the impact of education on health, and working with decision-makers in order to get feedback on communication strategies and policy priorities. During this latter process, CSH faculty and staff elicited feedback from potential end users on the types of communication that would effectively reach them and how to improve outreach materials.

Research

The EHI team compiled scientific findings about the relationship between education and health in four sets of materials. Each set contained multiple products aimed at specific audiences (e.g., issue briefs, videos, web content). The first set, "Education: It Matters More to Health than Ever Before," explained trends in the relationship between education and health. These trends show that the life expectancy gap between the more educated and the less educated has continued to widen since the 1960s, and since the 1990s life expectancy has actually decreased for some people without a high school education.[31] At the same time, individuals with low levels of educational attainment are now more likely to have major diseases than their better educated peers, are more likely to engage in risky behaviors such as smoking,[32] and experience greater disability.[8] The second set of materials, "Why Education Matters to Health: Exploring the Causes," summarizes potential causal pathways by which education

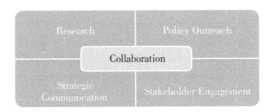

Figure 5.1 The "Connecting the Dots" Model.

may impact health outcomes. Major pathways include opportunities for accruing income and resources, social and psychological benefits, health behaviors, healthier neighborhoods, and the policy context. [33-35] This issue brief brought in viewpoints from local community members who participated in a concept modeling exercise (see next section). The third set of materials, "Health Care: Necessary But Not Sufficient," shows that, even among patients with access to the same health resources, those with lower levels of education tend to have poorer self-rated health, higher rates of diabetes mortality, and higher rates of illness.[36] The fourth set explores the return on investment for education spending in relation to health and explains how budget cuts in education intended to save money may ultimately drive up healthcare costs.

Stakeholder Engagement

The research community increasingly seeks to involve stakeholders in health research to enhance accountability and to improve the quality of research. Community engagement can be a centerpiece of strategies that seek to reduce health disparities through community-based efforts that foster "interplay of civic engagement, political participation, and evidence."[29] EHI utilized a two-pronged approach to stakeholder engagement. Outreach efforts to decision-makers in the fields of education and health policy are described in the next section. In the present section, we describe engagement with residents of a low-income urban community who form part of the "Engaging Richmond" community–university partnership. Participatory research methods have become an important framework for including stakeholders in understanding and addressing health disparities.[37-41] Community researchers on the Engaging Richmond team worked together in a facilitated concept mapping exercise designed to tap into stakeholders' experiences of how education is related to health outcomes. Through this exercise, the team developed a conceptual model of the social, behavioral, environmental, and other factors that link education and health and placed their lived experience into an analytic framework. The group's tasks were to list potential factors influencing the relationship between health and education, and to sketch a diagrammatic model of how determinants are interrelated. The goals of the exercise were to explore whether community stakeholders would develop a causal model that adds to the pathways and mechanisms already hypothesized in the academic literature and to uncover new descriptions and nuances about pathways that are already recognized but are not fully understood.

The community researchers focused on numerous mediators in the link between education and health, many of which mirror the predominant frameworks in the existing literature. For example, Adler and Stewart[42] already have articulated important components of the causal pathway. Some of the community researchers' insights added new perspectives or emphasized different aspects of those causal factors, while highlighting certain specific aspects of the experiences of low-income and minority groups. Potential causal pathways the community researchers focused on included educational opportunities that help to develop non-cognitive skills and attitudes; multiple pathways through which employment experiences may impact health, including exposure to work-related stress, effects on motivation and outlook, and ability to build social networks; the greater risk of exposure to toxins and environmental risks in disadvantaged neighborhoods that are populated by people with limited education; and the intersections between public policy and access to health care.[34]

This stakeholder engagement effort was intended to demonstrate the contributions that community researchers can make to understanding how social determinants of health operate to impact health outcomes in the daily lives of families and communities. The community researchers were involved in the larger EHI effort to raise awareness about the relationship between education and health by collaborating in creating communication materials and participating in dissemination efforts. Their voices and perspectives appear in many EHI materials including videos, issue briefs, and other written materials.

Policy Outreach

Quite often, policy areas such as education, health care, and economic development function in distinct silos, with little space for interaction, despite the fact that research has found these areas of social policy to be inextricable from one another and quite influential on health outcomes. EHI sought to bridge these policy silos, particularly between the areas of education policy and health policy, making decision-makers in both areas more aware of their connection to each other, and encouraging an environment in which each recognizes the other's contributions to shaping health.

The EHI's policy outreach effort was organized to make connections with key influencers in the areas of education policy and health policy, with two main objectives in mind. The first was to introduce the initiative and its aims, soliciting feedback on which topics of discussion and communications tactics would be most compelling and useful in their work. Second, this effort aimed to establish relationships that would help with dissemination of materials and introduce CSH as a resource for information on the connections between social factors and health.

This particular outreach effort involved the development of two matrices—one for education leaders and the other for leaders in healthcare delivery, public health, and health policy—which allowed CSH researchers to target their efforts more deliberately. Each matrix (Table 5.1) featured nine cells for governmental, nongovernmental, and community audiences at the national, state, and local levels. For this initiative, outreach efforts to individuals and organizations representing each of these categories were of equal importance, and audience-specific strategies were developed for communicating and establishing relationships with a wide variety of stakeholders. Organizing

Table 5.1 Policy Outreach Matrix

	National	State	Local
Governmental	√	√	√
Private sector	√	√	√
Community			√

stakeholders into these cells allowed for a more focused effort, which, with additional support from two communications firms,* enabled CSH researchers to meet with influential organizations and policymakers.† These meetings, among other benefits, helped shape a robust strategic communication effort for the Education and Health Initiative.

Strategic Communication

Informed by feedback from policymaker and stakeholder meetings, and with the goal of increasing awareness and understanding of the connections between education and health, CSH researchers employed a multifaceted communications strategy that included the development of a variety of products tailored to different audiences. Communications materials followed a tiered approach, consisting of multimedia products like short videos and graphics to raise awareness of the education–health connection, issue briefs to provide additional insight into the complexities of the relationship, and web-based content allowing users to dig deeper into the data with the goal of inspiring action. In addition to these materials intended for the general public, CSH engaged in more traditional outreach to academic audiences—including presentations at academic conferences and the development of longer written pieces with additional depth on the relationship between education and health.[30,33,34]

To encourage more widespread dissemination of materials, CSH, with the support of the Initiative's funder and two communications firms, engaged in a release strategy for each of the four phases of the project. At each stage, the release of materials involved outreach to relevant media contacts, engagement of more general audiences on social media, and collaboration with key policymakers and organizations.

The strategies and tactics employed in dissemination of materials contributed to significant uptake of the work. For example, the video developed for the first phase of the project currently stands at over 16,800 views and remains one of the Robert Wood Johnson Foundation's ten most viewed videos on YouTube. Media coverage for the briefs included articles in the Huffington Post, Politico, and the local NBC and National Public Radio (NPR) affiliates, and coverage in the newsletters or mailing lists of organizations such as the Committee for Education Funding, The National Conference of State Legislatures, the National Governors Association, the U.S. Senate Committee on Health, Education, Labor, and Pensions, and the American Public Health Association.

---

* The two firms include Burness Communications, which works regularly with the project's funder, the Robert Wood Johnson Foundation, on issues related to public health and social determinants of health, and Vox Communications, which brings expertise in education policy.

† The organizations included, among others, the Alliance for a Healthier Generation, the American Public Health Association, the Committee for Education Funding, the College Board, the Council of Chief State School Officers, Generations United, the National Association of State Boards of Education, the National Conference of State Legislatures, the National Governors Association and the US Senate Committee on Health, Education, Labor, and Pensions. Senators Barbara Mikulski, Bernard Sanders, Elizabeth Warner, and the staff of Senator Tim Kaine and Congressman Eric Cantor were briefed either in one-on-one meetings or in appearances at US Senate hearings.

Likewise, materials from the initiative resulted in a flurry of activity on social media. On Twitter, content was shared by a number of influential voices in the spheres of public health and education, and the Twitter chat that was organized for the release of Phase Three resulted in over 3.3 million impressions.

The Education and Health Initiative served as an important test of principle for CSH's Connecting the Dots Model. The success of the initiative has encouraged the Center to undertake similar work raising awareness of the importance of other social determinants of health, such as income, housing, and environmental conditions. At the time of this writing, efforts to this effect are ongoing at CSH.

A LOCAL EXAMPLE: FOR THE SAKE OF ALL

With funding from the Missouri Foundation for Health, *For the Sake of All* began in March 2013 as a multidisciplinary collaboration between researchers at Washington University in St. Louis and Saint Louis University in partnership with regional leaders representing public health, health care, education, business, community and economic development, and media who constituted the Community Partner Group (CPG). The focus of the project is the health and well-being of African Americans in St. Louis, Missouri, specifically the City of St. Louis and St. Louis County. (Due to a political decision in the late 19th century, the City of St. Louis is a distinct political entity equivalent to a county in the state of Missouri, rather than a city within the larger county. There also are 91 separate municipalities within St. Louis County.)

Goals and Partnerships

In its first phase the goals of the project were to:

1. Inform the public about the social determinants of health as they impact African Americans, as one of the populations most impacted by health disparities.
2. Present the regional economic and health consequences of intervening (or failing to intervene) on social determinants of health.
3. Provide evidence of the impact of persistent disparities on all residents of the region.
4. Influence the policy agenda on health disparities by broadening the conversation beyond personal responsibility and the delivery of medical care.

These goals were developed by the academic researchers and the CPG after careful consideration of the strengths and weaknesses of past efforts to highlight health disparities in the St. Louis region and an assessment of what could be accomplished with the available time and resources. The CPG also advised the research team to intensify already-planned community engagement and outreach efforts, to include consultation with key stakeholders in the issue areas under investigation, and to include opportunities for broader community input on project materials and recommendations.

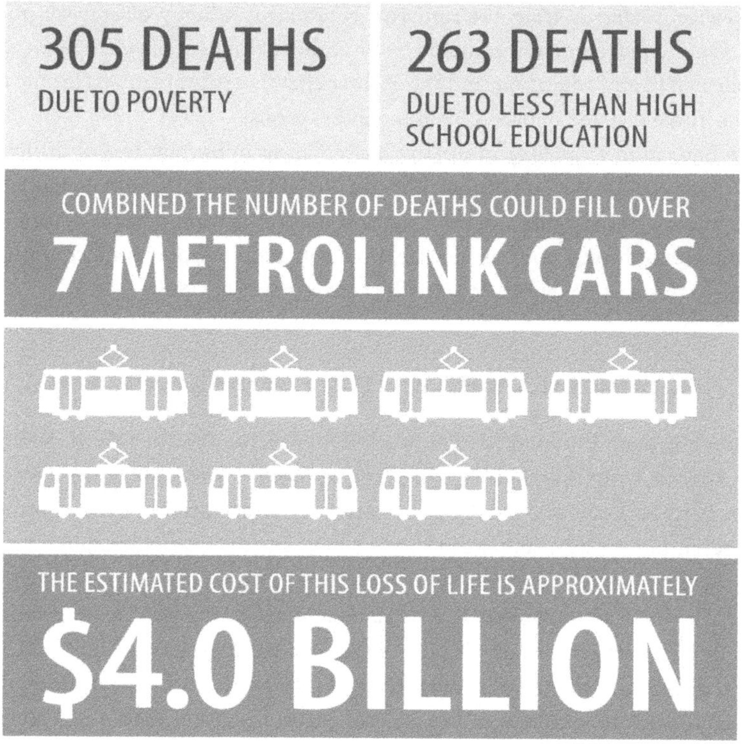

305 DEATHS
DUE TO POVERTY

263 DEATHS
DUE TO LESS THAN HIGH SCHOOL EDUCATION

COMBINED THE NUMBER OF DEATHS COULD FILL OVER
7 METROLINK CARS

THE ESTIMATED COST OF THIS LOSS OF LIFE IS APPROXIMATELY
$4.0 BILLION

Figure 5.2 Estimates of deaths attributable to poverty and low levels of education among African American adults in St. Louis, Missouri.

This turned out to be invaluable advice that greatly enhanced the acceptability and breadth of the final products. In addition to regional leaders, there were also important institutional partners, including the nationally recognized African American weekly newspaper, the *St. Louis American*; an independent, nonprofit online news journal, the *St. Louis Beacon*; the Policy Forum, a program of the George Warren Brown School of Social Work at Washington University that fosters public discourse on social and health policy; and the Institute for Public Health at Washington University, which brings together scholars from across the university whose work involves public health. Both the individual and institutional partners helped leverage their networks of influence to disseminate information about the project through internal communication and by featuring it in local print, radio, and television media.

Dissemination and Engagement

The main first-phase products of *For the Sake of All* were five policy briefs released between August and December of 2013 and a final report released at a community conference in May of 2014. The first brief was released on August 28, 2013 exactly 50 years after the historic March on Washington for Jobs and Freedom and the iconic keynote now known as the "I Have a Dream" speech by Dr. Martin Luther King, Jr.

This symbolism, like the title of the project itself (based on an unfinished 1915 composition by St. Louis resident and ragtime impresario, Scott Joplin), helped to elevate the visibility and broad applicability of the brief for the general public. Titled, "How can we save lives—and save money—in St. Louis? Invest in economic and educational opportunity," the first brief included estimates of the number of deaths in 2011 attributable to poverty and low levels of education among African American adults ages 25 years and older in St. Louis (see Figure 5.2). These estimates were based upon population-attributable fractions for these factors reported by Galea and colleagues[43] in a study on mortality attributable to social factors in the United States. This first brief also provided an estimate of the economic impact of this loss of life using the value of a statistical life method employed by federal agencies like the Environmental Protection Agency to determine economic impact of policy. Community stakeholders who reviewed early drafts of the brief provided information on ongoing activities to support economic and educational opportunity in low-to-moderate income households in the St. Louis region. They also informed the recommendations to "invest in quality early childhood development for all children" and "help low-to-moderate income families create economic opportunities."[44] The project team also contracted with a health literacy consultancy to ensure that language was accessible to a broad audience and worked with a professional design firm to develop a visually compelling and consistent "look and feel" for the presentation of data, text, and graphics. The project coordinated media dissemination of the brief with Washington University's Office of Public Affairs and media partners at the *St. Louis American* and the *St. Louis Beacon*, which resulted in extensive print, radio, and television coverage of its release on the project's website, "forthesakeofall.org." As of February 2015, the brief had been downloaded over one thousand times.

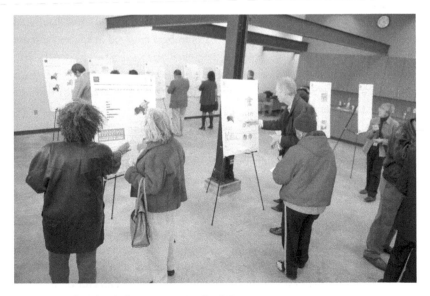

Figure 5.3 *For the Sake of All* Community Feedback Forum.

This same general pattern of preparation and presentation was followed for each of the four subsequent briefs. The second brief examined mental and physical health factors influencing eventual high school dropout in St. Louis.[45] An exploration of the social and economic factors associated with mental health was the topic of the third brief.[46] The fourth brief described how residential segregation in St. Louis by both race and income impacts neighborhood resources that are needed to promote health.[47] Progress toward Healthy People 2010 goals on cardiovascular disease, diabetes, and cancer mortality for St. Louis and the state of Missouri was presented in the fifth brief.[48] In total, these briefs had been downloaded more than 2,900 times as of February 2015, and they received significant coverage in radio, television, and print media.

In March of 2014, community members were invited to attend a Community Feedback Forum (see Figure 5.3). Nearly 100 people, representing a broad cross-section of the St. Louis region provided their reactions to poster-board-sized draft elements of the final report, including data and graphics presented in the briefs as well as new data on historical trends, neighborhood violence, and other topics. All of the evidence-based and community stakeholder-informed recommendations made in each of the briefs also were collected on a poster board. Individual responses were reviewed for common themes, and where appropriate and feasible, modifications were made to data presentation, topic coverage, and the final recommendations. For example, extended coverage of HIV/AIDS was added to the report, and recommendations were added to enhance neighborhood resources for youth development and address violence as a public health issue.

Even before release of the final report, project team members and partners began engagement with key policymakers at the state and local level. In March, a briefing was held for the Mayor of the City of St. Louis and his Cabinet. The presentation included an overview of each of the five briefs as well as a table showing the alignment between *For the Sake of All* recommendations and the City of St. Louis Sustainability Plan. A similar briefing was held the same month with the Missouri Legislative Black Caucus in the state capitol of Jefferson City. Caucus members engaged in spirited discussion with the project team and partners about the policies necessary to advance the recommendations. Members of the team also met with the governor's staff to brief them on the work at that stage. Subsequent meetings with the President of the City of St. Louis Board of Aldermen and its Health and Human Services Committee and the Treasurer of the City of St. Louis also served to acquaint key local leaders with the project, its findings, and its recommendations. Efforts to engage St. Louis County leadership at this stage in the project were made more difficult by a contentious election for county executive. However, leaders and staff of the St. Louis County Department of Health and Department of Planning were active participants in partnership and community engagement activities.

The final report was released at a community conference in May of 2014. Nearly 300 community members gathered for the conference, hearing from representatives from both City and County government, project leaders, and a keynote address by the Senior Vice President for Policy and Washington Bureau Director of the National Urban League. Panels of project partners and community stakeholders discussed

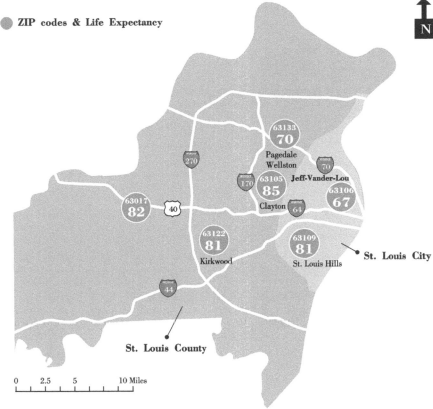

Figure 5.4 Life expectancy map by St. Louis, Missouri zip codes.

education and health, social and economic factors related to mental and physical health, and healthy neighborhoods. They reacted to the report findings and offered examples of their own work in the St. Louis region to address health disparities.

The 77-page final report[49] provided a comprehensive overview of the economic, educational, and health status of African Americans in the St. Louis region, with an introduction providing the rationale for considering these major factors alongside one another; a section devoted to historical and current demographics; an examination of the impact of place on health outcomes, including a life expectancy map by representative zip codes in the St. Louis region (see Figure 5.4); an infographic story of the life trajectory of a character named "Jasmine" told from two different starting points (see Figure 5.5); an in-depth look at educational outcomes for African Americans and their implications for health; a health profile of African Americans in St. Louis with key disparities noted; and finally, recommendations in the following six major areas:

1. Invest in quality early childhood development for all children.
2. Help low-to-moderate income families create economic opportunities.

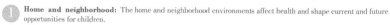

① **Home and neighborhood:** The home and neighborhood environments affect health and shape current and future opportunities for children.

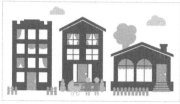

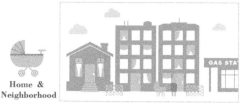

Home & Neighborhood

Jasmine is born to college-educated parents, who have stable jobs and income. When she is born, they start a college savings account to prepare for her future. Jasmine grows up in a neighborhood that provides healthy food options and safe places to play.

Jasmine is born to a single mother. Her mother works two jobs but struggles to make ends meet. She wishes she could spend more time reading to and interacting with Jasmine, but her work schedule makes it difficult. Jasmine's neighborhood doesn't have many places to buy fresh and healthy foods. **We could help Jasmine by making college savings accounts available for all children and investing in quality neighborhoods for all families.**

② **Early childhood:** High-quality early childhood programs allow children to grow and develop in a nurturing environment. This prepares them for future academic and job success and healthy adulthoods.

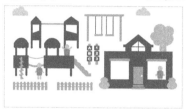

Early Childhood

Jasmine's parents pay for her to attend a high-quality early childhood education center. She grows up in a nurturing environment, exposed to many fun learning activities and opportunities to explore her world.

Jasmine stays with her grandmother during the day, and spends many hours inside because her family worries that it is not safe to play outside. Although her grandmother loves Jasmine very much, she also watches other grandchildren and doesn't have resources to do learning activities with Jasmine. She is also limited in what she can do by her own health problems. **We could help Jasmine by investing in quality early childhood education and development for all children.**

Figure 5.5 Excerpt from the "Two Lives of Jasmine" infographic.

3. Invest in coordinated school health programs for all students.
4. Invest in mental health awareness, screening, treatment, and surveillance.
5. Invest in quality neighborhoods for all in St. Louis.
6. Coordinate and expand chronic and infectious disease prevention and management.

Response

The final report was hailed by a variety of local media as a "landmark study" immediately after it was released in May 2014. Media partners at the *St. Louis American* and the *St. Louis Beacon* (now merged with the local NPR affiliate, St. Louis Public Radio) featured prominent coverage, but the work also drew coverage from the large daily newspaper, the *St. Louis Post-Dispatch,* and inspired a series of blog posts and Letters to the Editor. In total, over 65 news stories have referenced *For the Sake of All.* While averaging approximately 1,000 views and 380 visitors per month from August 2013 through April 2014, views of the forthesakeofall.org website increased to 1,963 in May

2014 and 2,772 in June, with 816 and 1,191 visitors respectively. As of February 2015, the website had been viewed over 35,000 times by nearly 13,000 visitors in the United States and over 90 other countries. The report alone had been downloaded more than 2,500 times. Materials related to the project have been used by local nonprofits in their grant writing, by secondary and postsecondary instructors in classrooms, and by local advocacy organizations in their messaging. The Gateway Center for Giving, a group of major philanthropies in the region, is currently using *For the Sake of All* to analyze its coordinated funding priorities in the six areas of recommendation. Dissemination to academic audiences has included presentations at annual meetings of the American Public Health Association and the Society of Behavioral Medicine, and publication (in collaboration with colleagues at the Virginia Commonwealth University Center on Society and Health) in the *Annual Review of Public Health*.[30]

It must be noted that *For the Sake of All* has taken on even greater resonance in the St. Louis region following the fatal shooting of unarmed teenager, Michael Brown, in the St. Louis County suburb of Ferguson on August 9, 2014. The report was almost immediately referenced by national and international media seeking explanations for the protests and unrest that ensued over several weeks. Outlets covering the project in the wake of events in Ferguson were as varied as the *Washington Post, Bloomberg Business News*, NPR, *Vox.com*, and *Colorlines* in the United States and *Maclean's* magazine in Canada and the *Korea Times* in Seoul, South Korea. Website views spiked again to over 2,700 (1,200 visitors) in August and reached an all-time high of 4,200 (1,300 visitors) in October. There were 2,750 average views per month from August 2014 to February 2015, with an average of just under 1,000 visitors per month. The project and recommendations have also been referenced by civic, political, and philanthropic leaders as a potential blueprint for transformation and have been formally included in the deliberations of the Ferguson Commission appointed by the governor to address the underlying social and economic factors that led to the summer's protests and demands for change.

Second Phase

Having begun its second phase in June 2014 with an additional round of funding from the Missouri Foundation for Health, the project is now focused on implementation of recommendations through broad community mobilization and engagement of key stakeholder groups, policymakers, and other leaders at the state and local levels. This includes a partnership with a local civic leadership development organization called FOCUS St. Louis to produce discussion guides and action toolkits associated with each of the six areas of recommendation. These guides distill the information shared in the briefs and report and provide concrete steps that community members can take along a continuum of intensity from information sharing to voluntarism and philanthropy to organization and advocacy. Versions of these materials are being produced for both general audiences and youth.

Broad dissemination also continues in the second phase to groups including churches, schools, businesses, and social and civic organizations. To date, over one hundred presentations and meetings have been held with interested community organizations and leaders. With the release of each set of discussion guides and action toolkits, the project team is hosting "Community Action Forums" that bring community members together with stakeholders and experts in the six recommendation areas to discuss effective strategies. Efforts also are planned for specific mobilization of faith-based and youth-serving organizations using "train the trainer" models to equip community members to lead discussions and action. In addition to community engagement, policymakers also have been engaged in dissemination efforts. The project team provided copies of the final report to all members of the City of St. Louis Board of Aldermen, the Mayor of St. Louis, members of the St. Louis County Council, the newly elected St. Louis County Executive, all state representatives and senators serving the St. Louis area, and the federal Congressional delegation serving the City of St. Louis and St. Louis County. The team is also following up with those policymakers to identify areas of recommendation that are aligned with legislative and executive agendas. Outreach is also being targeted at local corporate and civic leaders and organizations that are influential in setting the agenda in St. Louis.

In the first year of the second phase, the emphasis has been on recommendations to (1) create economic opportunity for low-to-moderate income households, (2) invest in quality early childhood development, and (3) invest in coordinated school health. Specific policy and programmatic proposals include universal CDAs for children born in the City of St. Louis and St. Louis County (intended as both an economic opportunity and early childhood intervention), as well as school-based clinics in the most vulnerable schools and districts in the region. Partners in the Center for Social Development at Washington University have had extensive national and international experience with implementation of CDA policies and have been instrumental in helping to make the case for such a policy in St. Louis. A key supporter of *For the Sake of All*, the Treasurer of the City of St. Louis, also has taken up child savings, and with the beginning of the 2015–2016 school year, will introduce college savings accounts for kindergarteners in St. Louis Public Schools and charter schools in the City of St. Louis. An evaluation currently underway of a school-based clinic operated by a major health care system in a public high school in the City of St. Louis will also inform the recommendation regarding coordinated school health and school-based health care.

CONCLUSION

Though there is growing recognition that upstream social determinants exert considerable influence on population health, the policy agenda in this area remains underdeveloped. Far more focus has been placed on health care and health insurance, both essential but insufficient to address persistent disparities and overall population health. In part, this is because the complex causal chain from early childhood experiences and K–12 education to the prevention of chronic disease and premature death may be difficult to explain to lay audiences and policymakers. The imperative to translate research evidence on the social determinants of health is beginning to be taken up by researchers, major philanthropies, and government agencies. As the Education and Health Initiative and *For the Sake of All* illustrate, these are by no means simple or short-term undertakings. They require not only an understanding of the social determinants literature, but also an ability to communicate effectively, to engage communities and key stakeholders, and to interact with policymakers and their staffs in ways that are responsive to their professional domains.

Ultimately, it will be necessary to evaluate these initiatives carefully in order to establish the efficacy of the "key ingredients" for community mobilization and policy change. The primary outcome will be changes in funding priorities to match attention to upstream determinants as a preventive strategy. There are also shorter-term and intermediate outcomes, such as increased awareness among the media, the public, and policymakers; increased community and other stakeholder coordination and action; and an increase in the number of new pieces of legislation filed that are aligned with recommendations. Following the enactment of new policies, there also will be a need to rigorously evaluate the impact of investments in specific areas on health and health-related outcomes and to communicate these findings on a regular basis to the community and key stakeholders.

ADDITIONAL RESOURCES

- Center on Society and Health at Virginia Commonwealth University. Education and Health Initiative. http://societyhealth.vcu.edu/work/the-projects/education-health.html
- Robert Wood Johnson Foundation Commission to Build a Healthier America (2014). Time to Act: Investing in the Health of Our Children and Communities. http://www.rwjf.org/content/dam/farm/reports/reports/2014/rwjf409002
- Washington University in St. Louis. *For the Sake of All.* http://forthesakeofall.org.

REFERENCES

1. Phelan JC, Link BG, Tehranifar P. Social conditions as fundamental causes of health inequalities. *J Health Soc Behav.* 2010;51(1 Suppl):S28–S40.
2. Braveman P, Egerter S, Williams DR. The social determinants of health: coming of age. *Annu Rev Public Health.* 2011;32:381–398.
3. National Research Council, Institute of Medicine. *Shorter Lives, Poorer Health.* Washington, DC: The National Academies Press; 2013.
4. Frieden TR. A framework for public health action: the health impact pyramid. *Am J Public Health.* Apr 2010;100(4):590–595.
5. Issacs J. *Starting School at a Disadvantage: The School Readiness of Poor Children.* Washington, DC: Center on Children and Families at Brookings; 2012.
6. Duncan GJ, Ziol-Guest KM, Kalil A. Early-childhood poverty and adult attainment, behavior, and health. *Child Dev.* Jan–Feb 2010;81(1):306–325.
7. Campbell F, Conti G, Heckman JJ, et al. Early childhood investments substantially boost adult health. *Science.* 2014;343:1478–1485.

8. Crimmins EM, Saito Y. Trends in healthy life expectancy in the United States, 1970-1990: gender, racial, and educational differences. *Soc Sci Med*. Jun 2001;52(11):1629-1641.

9. Meara ER, Richards S, Cutler DM. The gap gets bigger: changes in mortality and life expectancy, by education, 1981-2000. *Health Aff (Millwood)*. Mar-Apr 2008;27(2):350-360.

10. Center on Human Need. County Health Calculator. Virginia Commonwealth University; 2015. http://countyhealthcalculator.org/. Accessed March 3, 2015.

11. Freudenberg N, Ruglis J. Reframing school dropout as a public health issue. *Prev Chronic Dis*. Oct 2007;4(4):A107.

12. Soleimanpour S, Geierstanger SP, Kaller S, McCarter V, Brindis CD. The role of school health centers in health care access and client outcomes. *Am J Public Health*. Sep 2010;100(9):1597-1603.

13. Federico SG, Abrams L, Everhart RM, Melinkovich P, Hambidge SJ. Addressing adolescent immunization disparities: a retrospective analysis of school-based health center immunization delivery. *Am J Public Health*. Sep 2010;100(9):1630-1634.

14. McNall MA, Lichty LF, Mavis B. The impact of school-based health centers on the health outcomes of middle school and high school students. *Am J Public Health*. Sep 2010;100(9):1604-1610.

15. Webber MP, Carpiniello KE, Oruwariye T, Lo Y, Burton WB, Appel DK. Burden of asthma in inner-city elementary schoolchildren: Do school-based health centers make a difference? *Arch Pediatr Adolesc Med*. Feb 2003;157(2):125-129.

16. Lofnik H, Kuebler J, Juszczak L, et al. *2010-2011 School-Based Health Alliance Census Report*. Washington, DC: School-Based Health Alliance; 2013.

17. Brooks-Gunn J, Duncan GJ. The effects of poverty on children. *The Future of Children*. 1997;7(2):55-17.

18. Duncan GJ, Brooks-Gunn J, Klebanov PK. Economic deprivation and early childhood development. *Child Development*. 2008;65(2):296-318.

19. Evans GW. The environment of childhood poverty. *American Psychologist*. 2004;59(2):77-92.

20. Williams Shanks TR. The impacts of household wealth on child development. *Journal of Poverty*. 2007;11(2):93-116.

21. Elliott W, Beverly SG. The role of savings and wealth in reducing 'wilt' between expectations and college attendance. *Journal of Children & Poverty*. 2011;17(2):165-185.

22. Sherraden M. *Assets and the Poor: A New American Welfare Policy*. Armonk, NY: M.E. Sharpe, Inc.; 1991.

23. Huang J, Sherraden M, Kim Y, Clancy M. Effects of child development accounts on early social-emotional development: an experimental test. *JAMA Pediatr*. Mar 2014;168(3):265-271.

24. Huang J, Sherraden M, Purnell JQ. Impacts of Child Development Accounts on maternal depressive symptoms: Evidence from a randomized statewide policy experiment. *Soc Sci Med*. Jul 2014;112:30-38.

25. Meijer M, Rohl J, Bloomfield K, Grittner U. Do neighborhoods affect individual mortality? A systematic review and meta-analysis of multilevel studies. *Soc Sci Med*. Apr 2012;74(8):1204-1212.

26. Anderson LM, Charles JS, Fullilove MT, Scrimshaw SC, Fielding JE, Normand J. Providing affordable family housing and reducing residential segregation by income. A systematic review. *Am J Prev Med*. Apr 2003;24(3 Suppl):47-67.

27. National Prevention Council. *National Prevention Strategy: America's Plan for Better Health and Wellness*. Washington, DC: U.S. Department of Health and Human Services; 2011.

28. Bostic RW, Thornton RL, Rudd EC, Sternthal MJ. Health in all policies: the role of the U.S. Department of Housing and Urban Development and present and future challenges. *Health Aff (Millwood)*. Sep 2012;31(9):2130–2137.

29. Cacari-Stone L, Wallerstein N, Garcia AP, Minkler M. The promise of community-based participatory research for health equity: a conceptual model for bridging evidence with policy. *Am J Public Health*. Sep 2014;104(9):1615–1623.

30. Woolf SH, Purnell JQ, Simon SM, et al. Translating evidence into population health improvement: strategies and barriers. *Annual Review of Public Health*. January 12, 2015.

31. Olshansky SJ, Antonucci T, Berkman L, et al. Differences in life expectancy due to race and educational differences are widening, and many may not catch up. *Health Aff (Millwood)*. Aug 2012;31(8):1803–1813.

32. Schiller JS, Lucas JW, Ward BW, Peregoy JA. Summary health statistics for U.S. adults: National Health Interview Survey, 2010. *Vital Health Stat 10*. Jan 2012(252):1–207.

33. Zimmerman EB, Woolf SH. *Understanding the Relationships Between Education and Health*. Washington, DC: Institute of Medicine; 2014.

34. Zimmerman EB, Woolf SH, Haley A. Understanding the relationship between education and health: a review of the evidence and an examination of community perspectives. *Review of Behavioral and Social Sciences Research Opportunities: Innovations in Population Health Metrics*. Bethesda, MD: National Institutes of Health. Office of Behavioral and Social Sciences Research; 2015.

35. Cutler D, Lleras-Muney A. Education and health. In: Culyer A, ed. *Encyclopedia of Health Economics*. Vol 1. San Diego, CA: Elsevier; 2014:232–245.

36. Marmot Report Team. *Fair Society, Healthy Lives*. London: UCL Institute of Health Equity; 2010.

37. Israel B, Eng E, Schulz A, Parker E, eds. *Methods in Community-based Participatory Research for Health*. San Francisco, CA: Jossey-Bass; 2005.

38. Israel BA, Schulz AJ, Parker EA, Becker AB. Community-based participatory research: policy recommendations for promoting a partnership approach in health research. *Educ Health (Abingdon)*. 2001;14(2):182–197.

39. Simonds VW, Wallerstein N, Duran B, Villegas M. Community-based participatory research: its role in future cancer research and public health practice. *Prev Chronic Dis*. 2013;10:E78.

40. Tandon SD, Phillips K, Bordeaux BC, et al. A vision for progress in community health partnerships. *Prog Community Health Partnersh*. Spring 2007;1(1):11–30.

41. Wallerstein NB, Duran B. Using community-based participatory research to address health disparities. *Health Promot Pract*. Jul 2006;7(3):312–323.

42. Adler NE, Stewart J. Health disparities across the lifespan: meaning, methods, and mechanisms. *Ann N Y Acad Sci*. Feb 2010;1186:5–23.

43. Galea S, Tracy M, Hoggatt KJ, Dimaggio C, Karpati A. Estimated deaths attributable to social factors in the United States. *Am J Public Health*. Aug 2011;101(8):1456–1465.

44. Purnell JQ. *How Can We Save Lives—and Save Money—in St. Louis? Invest in Economic and Educational Opportunity*. St. Louis, MO: Washington University in St. Louis and Saint Louis University; 2013.

45. Tate W. *How Does Health Influence School Dropout?* St. Louis, MO: Washington University in St. Louis and Saint Louis University; 2013.

46. Hudson D. *How Can We Improve Mental Health in St. Louis? Invest in Our Community and Raise Awareness.* St. Louis, MO: Washington University in St. Louis and Saint Louis University; 2013.

47. Goodman M, Gilbert K. *Segregation: Divided Cities Lead to Differences In Health.* St. Louis, MO: Washington University in St. Louis and Saint Louis University; 2013.

48. Drake B, Elder K. *Chronic Disease in St. Louis: Progress for Better Health.* St. Louis, MO: Washington University in St. Louis and Saint Louis University; 2013.

49. Purnell JQ, Camberos GJ, Fields RP, eds. *For the Sake of All: A Report on the Health and Well-being of African Americans in St. Louis—and Why It Matters for Everyone.* St. Louis, MO: Washington University in St. Louis and Saint Louis University; 2014.

Part 2
Policy Illustrations for Specific Public Health Issues

6

Public Policy and Tobacco

Sarah Moreland-Russell and Shelley D. Golden

LEARNING OBJECTIVES

1. Describe patterns of tobacco use and their implications.
2. Examine how policies have been used in tobacco control efforts.
3. Identify key stakeholders in public policy related to tobacco use.
4. Describe barriers to using policy in tobacco control efforts.

IDENTIFYING THE PROBLEM: TOBACCO USE AND CONSEQUENCES

Tobacco has been deeply ingrained in American culture for over a century. From the development of the cigarette in the early 1900s to today's modern version, the e-cigarette, the tobacco industry has utilized production, advertising, design, and social behavior to permeate social norms and create a culture around tobacco use. Over the past century, the tobacco industry has both celebrated success as a business monopoly and been disparaged as patterns of death and disease associated with tobacco use have emerged.

Over the past 50 years, public health prevention strategies used by tobacco control proponents have been integral to the changing social norms that spur the decline of tobacco use. The 1964 Surgeon General's Report, *Smoking and Health*, was the first comprehensive review of research linking lung cancer and other diseases to tobacco use.[1] This report transformed the public debate about smoking from an issue of consumer choice to a serious health issue.[2] It also spurred national advocacy and education efforts to transform social norms around smoking. In the wake of this initial report, scientists engaged in further research on the ramifications of using tobacco; smoking, other tobacco use, and exposure to secondhand smoke are now believed to cause more than 20 types of cancer, as well as other heart and lung diseases.[3] As evidence of health consequences emerged, policy strategies, beginning with smoke-free policy, were implemented to reduce secondhand smoke exposure and encourage smoking cessation.[4] Tobacco control policy expanded to include excise taxes, funding for media campaigns, development of state-supporting telephone quitlines, and product regulation, and is now considered the most effective intervention for combatting tobacco use and initiation and promoting cessation.[5,6]

Efforts to promote policy change continue to play a critical role in tobacco control[2] and are the primary prevention strategy in countering the tobacco industry, reducing tobacco use and secondhand smoke exposure, and enhancing existing tobacco control policies.[2] Despite the addictive nature of tobacco and the economic forces promoting its use, these policy efforts have been very successful, with few parallels in public health history.[3]

This chapter provides a perspective on the tobacco epidemic, describes some of the factors driving continued tobacco use, and outlines the importance of tobacco control policy in preventing initiation, decreasing consumption, and ultimately eliminating tobacco use as a social norm in this country.

Descriptive Epidemiology

Tobacco use has long been a leading cause of morbidity and mortality worldwide and currently accounts for an estimated 9% of deaths across the globe. In the United States, smoking is the leading preventable cause of premature death and disease. Smoking has been causally linked with a host of diseases, including many types of cancer, coronary heart disease, chronic obstructive pulmonary disease, diabetes, asthma, and stroke. Nonsmokers who are exposed to secondhand smoke suffer from tobacco-related illnesses as well; since the United States Surgeon General began reporting on smoking more than 50 years ago, almost 2.5 million nonsmokers have died from smoking-related diseases.[3]

In 1965, 42% of Americans smoked cigarettes. As the health risks of smoking have become better understood since the release of the first Surgeon General's Report, tobacco prevention and cessation efforts have been established and various tobacco control policies implemented. By 2013, smoking prevalence rates dropped to 18% of adults and under 13% of youth.[7] Tobacco control practitioners, however, are concerned that the rate of decline has slowed recently, remaining well above Healthy People 2020 goals. The emerging growth of non-cigarette tobacco product use also poses health risks. When accounting for people who use non-cigarette tobacco products either alone or in addition to cigarettes, more than one in five adults and high school students report using tobacco. The most commonly used non-cigarette tobacco products are smokeless products (e.g., snuff), little or regular cigars, pipes, hookah (water pipes), and electronic cigarettes.[8]

Disparities

Despite overall reductions in tobacco use, differences in tobacco use exist across multiple dimensions, including gender, race and ethnicity, educational and poverty status, and sexual orientation (Figure 6.1).[7] Other groups that use tobacco at disproportionately high rates include military workers (e.g., active service members and civilian employees), construction workers, people with a history of mental health problems, people

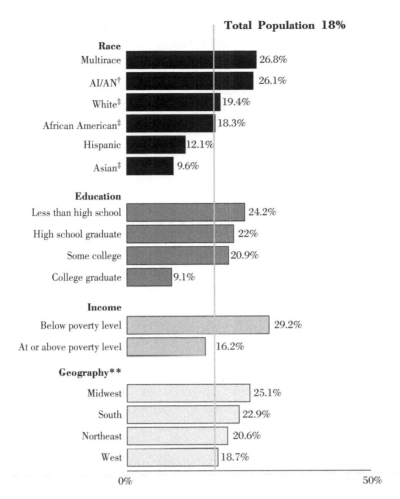

Figure 6.1 Current smoking prevalence among adults 18 years and older.*

Graphic reprint from the Centers for Disease Control and Prevention. Best Practices User Guide: Health Equity in Tobacco Prevention and Control.

Data Source: Current Cigarette Smoking Among Adults—United States, 2011.[7]

Current smoking is defined as smoking in the 30 days before the survey and having used 100 cigarettes or more in lifetime. [†]American Indian/Alaska Native, non-Hispanic, [‡]Non-Hispanic.

who are homeless, and incarcerated individuals. These groups are more likely to use tobacco, less likely to successfully quit, and experience poorer health outcomes.[3,9,10]

There is also significant geographic variation in tobacco use. International comparisons of adult smoking rates indicate that the United States ranks slightly better than average. In a 2010 comparison, United States smoking rates were lower than those in many countries like Norway, Egypt, China, and Chile, but remained higher than those in other places like Mexico, Australia, Kenya, and India.[11] Within the United States there are differences as well. Fewer than one in ten Utah residents smoke cigarettes, whereas more than one in four people in Kentucky, Arkansas, and West Virginia do. (See Figure 6.1 for regional variation.)[12]

Several factors result in health disparities related to tobacco control, including excessive exposure to tobacco product promotion, tobacco industry targeting, and lack of comprehensive policies.[13] Health equity in tobacco control can be achieved, however, by eliminating differences in tobacco use and in exposure to tobacco smoke among certain groups. Well-enforced, comprehensive tobacco control policies can help reduce these differences. Unlike traditional direct-service interventions that target individual behaviors, tobacco control policies focus on large-scale, population-level changes. They have the potential to influence and change social norms related to tobacco initiation, use, and exposure.[14]

PUBLIC POLICY STRATEGIES IN TOBACCO CONTROL

A variety of tobacco control policies or protocols have been implemented at the international, federal, state, and local levels. In 2003, the World Health Organization adopted the Framework Convention on Tobacco Control, which establishes international tobacco control guidelines for countries to implement. Targeted policy areas in the Convention include raising prices and taxes on tobacco products, along with other measures to reduce the demand for tobacco; ensuring protection from exposure to tobacco smoke; regulating tobacco product contents, packaging, labeling, advertising, and promotion; and providing education, training, and public awareness. Although U.S. officials signed the Framework Convention in 2003, the United States has not joined the more than 150 countries that have ratified the Convention. Yet tobacco policy goals described in many national documents in the United States mirror and extend Convention goals. The Institute of Medicine's report *Ending the Tobacco Problem: A Blueprint for the Nation*, recent Surgeon General's Reports on tobacco, and information from the Centers for Disease Control and Prevention(CDC)[15] all emphasize the need to (1) raise product prices, (2) create smoke-free places, (3) restrict marketing, packaging, and youth access, and (4) support cessation attempts. In fact, the CDC's 2014 *Best Practices for Comprehensive Tobacco Control* outlines these four core strategies as the suggested foundation of state and community tobacco control program efforts.

Creating Smoke-free Environments

Smoke-free laws protect employees and the public from the dangers of secondhand smoke, including cancer, heart disease, and respiratory diseases.[3] These laws also encourage people to quit,[16] help prevent smoking initiation, and change social norms around tobacco use and exposure.[17,18] The inception of policy as a tobacco control strategy was with smoke-free policy efforts. Many tobacco control policy advocates today use lessons learned from smoke-free policy efforts and utilize some of the same grassroots groups established as a result of the smoke-free movement.

Smoke-free policies can be designed to impact public areas, private areas, or both. Figure 6.2 illustrates the state and local comprehensive smoke-free laws enacted as

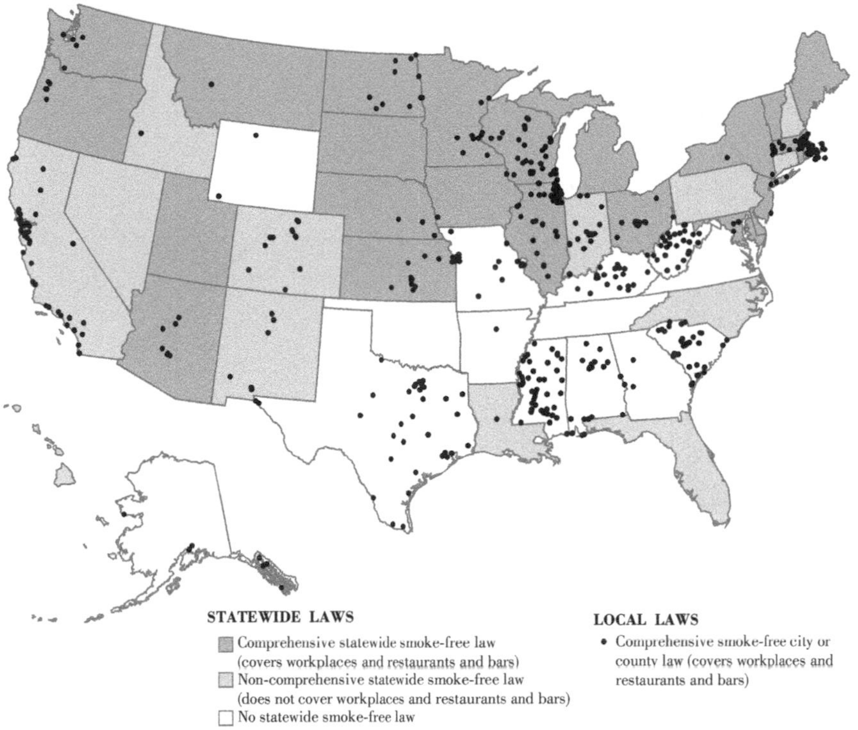
STATEWIDE LAWS
Comprehensive statewide smoke-free law (covers workplaces and restaurants and bars)
Non-comprehensive statewide smoke-free law (does not cover workplaces and restaurants and bars)
No statewide smoke-free law
LOCAL LAWS
Comprehensive smoke-free city or county law (covers workplaces and restaurants and bars)

Figure 6.2 United States Map of Comprehensive Smoke-free laws.
Graphic reprint from Policy Strategies: A Tobacco Control Guide, Center for Public Health Systems Science and the Tobacco Control Legal Consortium.
Data source: Americans for Nonsmokers' Rights 2013.

of 2013. In the past, smoke-free laws have focused specifically on publically accessed indoor workplace settings. Today, smoke-free laws are being expanded to include publically accessed outdoor areas (e.g., restaurant patios, parks, playgrounds, and beaches) and private settings such as multiunit housing and cars. Smoke-free laws can be adopted voluntarily within organizations, or more formally through legal processes at the state or local level. Although voluntary adoption is considered a step in the right direction, a legislated policy is preferred because it serves to mandate the rules for consistency, fairness, and maximum protection, and closes the gaps in secondhand smoke protection that result from voluntary adoption.[4] In addition, voluntary policies may have fewer resources and limited accountability for implementation and enforcement.

Raising the Price of Tobacco Products through Tax Increases

Policies designed to raise the price of tobacco products make tobacco less affordable, reducing tobacco use (Figure 6.3) and changing social norms.[18,19] Studies find that higher tobacco prices prevent youth initiation,[20] decrease tobacco-related healthcare

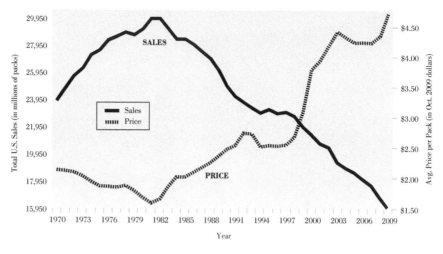

Figure 6.3 Impact of Cigarette Prices Increases on Cigarette Sales (1969–2009).
Graphic reprint from Policy Strategies: A Tobacco Control Guide, Center for Public Health Systems Science and the Tobacco Control Legal Consortium. Data source: Cigarette Smoking Prevalence and Policies in the 50 States: An Era of Change–The Robert Wood Johnson Foundation ImpacTeen Tobacco Chart Book, Tax Burden on Tobacco 2010, and Pricing Strategies for Tobacco, Healthy Eating, and Physical Activity.

costs, and can reduce tobacco-related health disparities.[21,22] When implemented as taxes (the most common type of price policy), price policies also can generate revenue for governments.[23,24] Tax-based pricing policies can be implemented at the local, state, and federal levels, through legislative or ballot measures (Box 6.1), and can be applied in a number of ways, including (1) per item or pack, (2) as a percentage-of-price, (3) as a percentage of weight, and (4) as a percentage-of-price with an additional minimum tax based on weight or dose. The largest increase in federal cigarette taxes was passed as part of the reauthorization and expansion of the Children's Health Insurance Program in 2009, bringing the total federal tax to $1.01 per cigarette pack.[25] In 2014, the total per pack excise taxes ranged from $4.35 in New York to only $0.17 in Missouri.[26]

Box 6.1 A Note about Ballot Initiatives

In tobacco control, ballot measures have been used to pass state and local smoke-free laws, excise tax initiatives, and laws authorizing the use of Master Settlement funds in states in which such legal mechanisms are allowed. Though perhaps the best-publicized mechanisms, ballot measures are not the preferred method for enacting state and local tobacco control policies because they are costly and require a significant amount of political and legal expertise. Implementing ballot initiatives also can provide the tobacco industry with a significant advantage, given the industry's surplus of resources. Ballot measures are also not an option in all states due to state regulations.

The expanding tobacco product market has forced policymakers and advocates to re-examine tax-based policy. Today, tobacco tax policies should not just increase cigarette taxes, but should also include language that imposes similar tax rates on all tobacco products; complements state tax increases with local tax increases (where allowed); and dedicates, through an earmark, a portion of revenue to enforcement and tobacco control initiatives.

The Institute of Medicine's Committee on Tobacco Use also recommends that tobacco taxes be indexed to inflation.[2] Adding an inflation adjustment (by linking the tax level to the Consumer Price Index) would help avoid erosion of the impact of the tax over time and help maintain tobacco-related revenues as cigarette consumption decreases.[27] Some researchers and legal scholars also recommend pairing high excise taxes with non-tax price strategies to maintain high prices. Other price-based strategies include minimum price policies that set price mark-ups or floor prices beneath which products cannot be sold, and efforts to limit the use of coupons, multipack offers, or other price reduction marketing tools.[28,29]

Restrictions on Marketing, Packaging, and Youth Access

The tobacco industry spends more than $9 billion dollars each year to promote its products in the United States alone.[30,31] Since tobacco advertising has been banned on television, the radio, billboards, and public transportation, the bulk of the industry's marketing budget is spent in the tobacco retail environment, also known as the point-of-sale. Smoking and other tobacco use is promoted through advertisements, special price offers, tobacco branding on other products, and on the tobacco product packaging itself. Exposure to tobacco-related marketing at the point-of-sale has been associated with higher odds of initiation and regular daily smoking among youth and young adults,[32–34] as well as the unplanned purchase of cigarettes[35] and relapse among former smokers.[36] Internal industry documents reveal that specific marketing efforts have been made to attract youth smokers by introducing products with appealing flavors and integrating images of smoking into activities and places popular among youth and young adults.[37]

Addressing these concerns has been the focus of several pieces of federal legislation (Table 6.1).[38] Together, these bills require cigarette packages and smokeless tobacco products to carry health-related warning labels, ban advertising of some tobacco products on the radio and on television, require states to enforce laws prohibiting the sale and distribution of tobacco products to minors, ban the sale of packages of fewer than 20 cigarettes, ban free cigarette samples, and give the Food and Drug Administration (FDA) the authority to regulate the manufacture, distribution, and marketing of tobacco products.

With the exception of the Synar agreement (Table 6.1), the retail setting was relatively untouched as a setting for state and local public health prevention policy development until recently. Increasing evidence now suggests that point-of-sale strategies should be implemented alongside traditional tobacco control policy interventions (such as smoke-free and tax-based policy), particularly for states that have made

Table 6.1 Federal Marketing and Packaging Legislation[36]

Legislation	Key Provisions
Federal Cigarette Labeling and Advertising Act (FCLAA) of 1965 (amended in 1969, 1984, 2009)	• Requires manufacturers, importers, or distributors to place health-related warning labels on cigarettes • Bans advertising of cigarettes on television and radio • Requires reporting of ingredients added to tobacco in cigarettes
Comprehensive Smokeless Tobacco Health Education Act of 1986	• Requires manufacturers, importers, or distributors to place health-related warning labels on smokeless products • Bans advertising of smokeless products on television and radio
Synar Amendment to the Alcohol, Drug Abuse and Mental Health Administration Reorganization Act of 1992	• Requires states to enact and enforce laws prohibiting the sale and distribution of tobacco products to minors
Family Smoking Prevention and Tobacco Control Act (TCA) of 2009 and subsequent FDA regulations	• Gives the U.S. Food and Drug Administration (FDA) the authority to regulate the manufacture, distribution, and marketing of tobacco products • Gives the FDA the authority to review new products before they go to market • Requires proof of age to purchase tobacco products • Bans the distribution of free cigarette samples and sales of packages fewer than 20 cigarettes
Prevent All Cigarette Trafficking (PACT) Act of 2010	• Prohibits mailing cigarettes and smokeless tobacco through the U.S. Postal Service • Requires Internet and mail-order sales retailers to verify customer ages

progress in these core areas of tobacco control.[39–41] The Tobacco Control Act gave states and communities some legal authority to pursue point-of-sale strategies, opening the door for states and communities to pursue interventions in the retail setting that go beyond implementing and enforcing youth access restrictions, and that allow for legislation restricting the time, place, and manner (but not the content) of cigarette advertising and promotion.[42,43] Primary types of point-of-sale strategies focus on:

1. Reducing (or restricting) the number, location, density, and types of tobacco retail outlets (e.g., prohibiting the sale of tobacco in retail establishments near schools, child care centers, or other places youth visit).
2. Adding prevention and cessation messaging to retail outlets or on tobacco products (e.g., requiring that a quitline sign be posted on tobacco vending machines and in all locations selling tobacco products).

3. Restricting the placement or amount of advertising inside and outside of tobacco retail stores (e.g., amending a jurisdiction's sign code to reduce the window area that can be covered by temporary and permanent signs).
4. Restricting product placement (e.g., requiring retailers to cover product displays with screens).

In addition to the areas above, other restrictions on marketing, products, and access is permissible at state and local levels, if not already explicitly regulated by the FDA or legislated at the federal level (Table 6.1). For example, in absence of FDA regulation of electronic cigarettes, 22 states passed restrictions on youth access to the product by 2013.[44] Similarly, the Tobacco Control Act bans the sale of flavored cigarettes other than menthol, but does not regulate other flavored tobacco products (e.g., flavored little cigars), leaving room for local jurisdictions to do so. Since the Tobacco Control Act went into effect, several local governments including New York City, New York, Providence, Rhode Island, and Santa Clara County, California, have adopted a ban on sales of cigars, hookah, cigarillos, pipe and chewing tobacco, and e-cigarettes flavored with tastes that might appeal to youth (e.g., apple, grape, or mint) in establishments where youth could be present.[39]

There are many point-of-sale policy options to consider with legal feasibility varying greatly. State and local governments can sometimes leverage the power they have to regulate area businesses to place restrictions on tobacco retailers through the use of licensing and zoning laws and conditional use permits (Box 6.2).

Because point-of-sale policy is an emerging area of tobacco control, careful evaluation studies are needed to build the evidence base for these approaches. Time will tell which of these strategies are both effective and able to withstand industry challenge.

Cessation Support

More than two thirds of current smokers report that they want to quit completely.[45] But because tobacco products contain addictive ingredients like nicotine, many smokers find it difficult to quit without help. More than half of smokers try to quit each year, but less than 7% are successful.[45] The United States Department of Health and Human Services recommends individual and group counseling services as well as several cessation medications as the strongest strategies for helping people stop using tobacco.[46] Most of these are provided through the healthcare system, but two primary policy strategies have been used to help ensure people can access these services. First, the federal government and some states can require insurance programs to cover cessation medications and counseling. For example, through the Affordable Care Act and Medicaid regulations, the federal government requires both public and private insurers to cover some services[47] that support attempts to quit. States can make similar requirements for public insurance programs over which they have some control. Many states, for example, include some sort of cessation coverage benefits for some Medicaid enrollees. However, in 2014, only seven states covered all of the FDA-approved tobacco cessation medications

Box 6.2 Regulating Tobacco Retailers

State and local governments have the authority to regulate the locations and practices of businesses through several policy instruments that have been used in tobacco control work.

Licensing laws require retailers or other businesses to obtain a license to operate a certain type of business. Licensing laws can be used to help enforce point-of-sale policies if continued licensing is tied to policy compliance. Most states already license tobacco retailers, but the ability of local governments to adopt tobacco retailer licensing laws, or to place conditions on retailers within existing local licensing laws depends on the amount of authority given to local governments by state law.[28]

Zoning laws govern various activities within a local community by dividing the community into areas called zones. Zoning laws can include restrictions on where facilities for living, shopping, manufacturing, and farming can be established and maintained, as well as rules about how businesses can post signs. St. Paul, Minnesota used zoning to implement a sign code that limits all outdoor and outward-facing indoor ads, regardless of content, to no more than 25% of a retailer's window space.[82] This "content-neutral" sign code improved public safety and additionally resulted in a reduction of tobacco advertising.

Conditional use permits (CUPs) are special use permits that specify the conditions that a business must meet to operate in an area where it may not normally be allowed. CUPs allow for tailored restrictions to reduce negative impacts that certain businesses might have on the surrounding area.[83] These restrictions can be developed to support other tobacco control policies related to youth tobacco-access laws, including the Tobacco Control Act's restrictions on tobacco sales to youth.[84,85]

and counseling for all Medicaid patients, and many states have recently erected barriers to care, including limiting the number of times a smoker can try to quit with treatment each year, adding prior authorization requirements, or adding copays.[48]

Second, as part of their tobacco control programs many states provide funding for telephone quitline services, which allow smokers to access evidence-based behavioral counseling and support by telephone, usually at no personal cost to the caller. Some quitlines provide additional help, like mailed materials, integrated web-based support, follow-up text messaging or phone calls, or assistance accessing medications.[49] A recent review of research about quitlines finds them to be both effective and cost-effective cessation programs.[50] Funding the quitlines, as well as the marketing and outreach programs to ensure smokers are aware of the quitlines and the services they offer, can be part of state budgeting efforts. States also may establish public-private partnerships with health plans and employers who reimburse the state quitline for services provided to their members or employees. The CDC issues recommendations on state funding for quitlines based on the proportions of smokers who access them in a state and estimates of costs per call.[51]

TOBACCO CONTROL SUPPORT AND OPPOSITION

Policy Rationale

Public interests have been the main drivers of national, state, and local implementation of tobacco control policies. Chief among these concerns is the financial burden associated with tobacco use born by government programs, and in turn, by American taxpayers. In 2010, nearly 9% of annual healthcare costs nationwide were attributable to smoking, and 60% of these were paid by public programs like Medicare or Medicaid.[52] Governments also have had to assume costs associated with pollution or public housing contamination from tobacco products[53] and disposal of tobacco-related litter.[54] Offsetting these costs is one justification for the implementation and maintenance of tobacco taxation or other fees.[55]

The protection of high-risk populations like youth is another strong rationale for tobacco control policies. The vast majority of smokers try their first cigarettes before the age of 18 years, and in 2012, 6.7% of middle school students and 23.3% of high school students reported using tobacco products.[8] If these rates continue, 5.6 million of children younger than 18 years are projected to die prematurely from a smoking-related illness.[3] Prevention efforts focused on youth are particularly promising strategies for reducing these future tobacco-related mortalities and cost. As a result, many tobacco control policies, including those found in the Tobacco Control Act, focus on preventing marketing to youth and limiting product availability in places youth frequent.

Governments also can take action to ensure the public receives clear and accurate information about tobacco products.[56] The harmful health and addictive effects of tobacco are now well documented, but research finds that tobacco manufacturers have taken (and continue to take) many measures to convince their consumers otherwise. Following lawsuits against the tobacco industry at the end of the last century, the industry was forced to release internal documents that exposed its efforts to hide information and misguide policymakers about the health risks associated with smoking, the addictive qualities of nicotine, the dangers of secondhand smoke, and marketing targeted to youth.[37,57,58] The industry's efforts to misrepresent scientific findings continue today, especially in low- and middle-income countries.[59] To combat this deceptive marketing, funding collected from the tobacco industry as a result of lawsuits and through product taxation sometimes is used to fund tobacco control programs designed to provide more accurate information about tobacco use and its risks.

Finally, several tobacco control policies, especially those designed to create smoke-free places, are based on concern about the consequences of tobacco use for nonsmokers,[56] especially through secondhand smoke.

As new tobacco products enter the market, the rationales used to support cigarette-specific legislation are often applied. Box 6.3 highlights how such arguments have been used in new legislation to regulate electronic cigarettes.

Political Support

The active participation of multiple sectors of the community, state and national level advocacy groups, and legal organizations has been a fundamental vehicle for

Box 6.3 Tobacco Control Rationale Extends to E-cigarettes

After electronic cigarettes were first made available for purchase in the United States in 2007, many states considered and implemented regulations on product advertising, sale, and use. Proponents of these laws raised many of the same arguments applied to earlier tobacco control policies:

Advertising to Youth—Dr. Scott Barton of the Utah Tobacco Free Alliance, during a 2015 debate about regulating and taxing e-cigarettes in that state, proclaimed:[86]

Our message to big tobacco is this: Don't mess with us. Not in our state. Not with our kids.

Regulating sale—Connecticut state Representative Jeff Berger, speaking in support of a 2015 proposal to implement e-cigarette licensing and fees, argues:[87]

We would know who is selling them and what's in the product because there would be a labeling process there.

Smoke-free air—The Hawaii state health department released the following statement in response to 2015 legislation extending smoke-free air laws to e-cigarettes:[88]

The use of e-cigarettes in existing smoke-free locations has had the potential to expose non-smokers and vulnerable populations, such as children and pregnant women, to aerosolized nicotine and other toxic substances, which could be dangerous to one's health.

Product regulation—New Jersey state senator Bob Gordon, following a 2010 ban on sales of e-devices to minors, stated:[89]

The liquid used in e-cigarettes often contains flavoring, such as chocolate or cherry. Clearly, the people who make these devices are trying to make them attractive to younger people, all the more reason for us to apply the underage ban to these devices.

There is much work left to be done in the realm of e-cigarette research and policy development. There is limited scientific evidence regarding the human health effects of e-cigarettes. While concerns and issues regarding non-user exposure remain, the impact of e-cigarettes, for users and the public, cannot yet be determined, making policy development in the realm challenging.[90]

comprehensive changes in the tobacco control environment. Often, local and state tobacco control programs do not have the flexibility or authority to influence tobacco control policies that lead to the transformation of tobacco-free norms. Therefore, the active and sustained involvement of national-level voluntary organizations (e.g., American Heart Association, American Cancer Society, American Lung Association), advocacy organizations (Americans for Nonsmokers' Rights, Campaign for Tobacco Free Kids, Counter Tobacco), legal partners (Tobacco Control Legal Consortium), and state and local level coalitions has been integral in advancing state and local tobacco control policy efforts.[60] The 2000 Surgeon General Report, *Reducing Tobacco Use*, cites the emergence of statewide and local coalitions as the most important advancement for comprehensive tobacco control policy, in part for their success in organizing and encouraging policy action through legislation and voter initiatives.[18]

On an individual basis, most opposition to tobacco policy has been by smokers or constituents who oppose government intervention in personal liberties. However, as evidence regarding the harm of tobacco use and the invasive presence of the industry has mounted, public perception has changed and tobacco control policies (specifically smoke-free laws and tax-based policies) have become popular with most Americans, even smokers.

Public support for smoke-free laws is at an all-time high and growing.[61] National and international studies have shown strong public support for smoke-free laws, with levels of support among both nonsmokers and smokers increasing after policy implementation.[62,63] Data from the 2009–2010 National Adult Tobacco Survey indicated that a majority of U.S. adults think workplaces and restaurants should be smoke-free and over half believe bars, casinos, and clubs should be smoke-free.[64]

Tax laws also have gained considerable support. The results of numerous polls conducted throughout the United States have consistently shown broad voter support for tobacco tax increases.[65,66] For example, a 2010 nationwide poll found that 67% of voters favor a $1 increase in their state tobacco tax rates.[65] In addition, statewide polls in more than 40 different states also show strong majority support for tobacco tax increases. In most states, voters favor the proposed tobacco tax increase by more than a two-to-one margin.[65,66]

Political Opposition

The main political influence opposing tobacco control policy efforts is the tobacco industry. The tobacco industry has used a variety of tactics to oppose tobacco control policies at every stage in the policy process and at every level of government.[67] On an ongoing basis, the tobacco industry uses its financial resources and prominent lobbyists to undermine tobacco control efforts in federal and state legislatures.[68] The tobacco industry also recruits decision-makers by providing campaign funding contributions in exchange for their vote against tobacco control policies.[69]

At the local level, where tobacco lobbying has been less effective, the industry uses third parties or creates front groups to lead the fight against the passage of tobacco control policies. These groups may take the form of convenience store associations, hospitality industry groups, or groups that oppose government regulation.[70] The tobacco industry has organized "astroturf" groups—grassroots organizations that are funded, organized, and sometimes run by the tobacco industry.[68] These opposition groups often try to divert the policy debate by bringing up issues of civil liberties, government over-regulation, and unfairness of tobacco control policies.[71] They use these tactics to distract from the real issue: public health. In addition to using front groups to oppose tobacco control policies at the local level, tobacco industry lobbyists often support weak tobacco control laws at the state level that preempt any local efforts.[72]

Legal Debate

As tobacco control policy efforts have moved beyond focusing on smoke-free laws and into the retail setting, the tobacco industry, as well as tobacco retailers, have implemented lawsuits and challenged the constitutionality of policies in court. Tobacco control policies have been challenged on any or all of the following four legal principles: (1) Preemption; (2) First Amendment compelled speech; (3) First Amendment restricted speech; and (4) Takings (Box 6.4).[37] For example, in 2013, New York City enacted an ordinance that regulated the tobacco industry's use of promotional pricing strategies. Among other

---

Box 6.4 Legal Principles Used in Tobacco Control[37]

Preemption

Preemption occurs when a law at the federal or state level prohibits the enactment of more stringent regulations at a lower jurisdiction (e.g., a city or county).[91] In 2010, preemption existed in 27 states, limiting the passage of local ordinances that restrict smoking in certain places, tobacco advertising, or youth access.[92]

First Amendment Compelled Speech

Under the First Amendment compelled speech doctrine, the government is restricted in its ability to require companies to make statements that result in advertising against themselves. The tobacco industry relied on this principle when they argued that the federal government could not require tobacco companies to display graphic health warnings directly on cigarette packages or advertisements.

First Amendment Commercial Speech

Under First Amendment commercial speech protections, the government cannot restrict advertising, branding, and logos, unless the message is misleading or refers to unlawful activity; or unless the government has a substantial interest in restricting it. For instance, even though the Tobacco Control Act mandated larger and stronger warning labels for cigarettes, in order to communicate the health risks of tobacco use more effectively, tobacco companies filed a lawsuit claiming that the regulation violated their First Amendment commercial speech rights. The court found that the specific graphic warnings required were unconstitutional, and the ruling was upheld.

Takings Clause

The Fifth Amendment Takings Clause states that "private property [shall not] be taken for public use, without just compensation."[56] Traditionally, this concept only referred to the government's physical taking of private property. However, the courts have extended the clause to include protection against reduced economic benefits or value derived from a property, known as a "regulatory taking."[57] To determine whether a regulatory taking has occurred, courts weigh the economic impact on the property owner against the purpose of the governmental action (e.g., Does it deprive a business owner of all economic use of the property? Is it in response to an important public health issue?). Some states have adopted additional provisions and regulations addressing the use and/or regulation of private property. These are often more protective of property rights than the federal Takings Clause.[39]

---

rules, the law restricted the sale of tobacco products for less than the advertised price, set a minimum price for cigarettes and little cigars, and prohibited multipack discounts. A year later, retail store associations and tobacco product manufacturers collaborated to file suit against New York City, arguing that the ordinance violated the First Amendment right to commercial speech. They also cited that the city level ordinance was unconstitutional on the grounds of federal and state preemption laws. The court decided in favor of New York City and upheld the regulations, stating that they did not violate the First Amendment, nor state or federal preemption laws.[73]

If the tobacco industry is unable to fight the policy in court, they often still respond by implementing retail measures that undermine the potential public health benefit of policy adoption. For example, after the implementation of a tobacco excise tax increase, the industry often implements retail value-added strategies and merchant incentives to offset the increased price, including advertising discount brands that provide a quality product for a better value; adding coupons and discounts on multipacks; and creating toll-free numbers smokers can call to receive coupons.[74] These strategies comprise more than 90% of tobacco company promotional expenditures.[75]

CASE STUDY

The first United States tobacco-free pharmacy policy reduces local level tobacco-related disparities and sets the stage for state and national tobacco-free pharmacy efforts.

Centers for Disease Control and Prevention.
Best Practices User Guide: Health Equity. Atlanta, GA:
U.S. Department of Health and Human Services, Centers for Disease
Control and Prevention, National Center for Chronic Disease
Prevention and Health Promotion, Office on Smoking and Health; 2015.

In 2003, the California Department of Public Health/Tobacco Control Section funded a statewide coalition, the California Lesbian Gay Bisexual and Transgender (LGBT) Tobacco Education Partnership to work on initiatives to reduce tobacco-related disparities in California. Research has shown that tobacco use in LGBT communities is high[76,77] and that LGBT individuals are more often targeted by tobacco industry marketing.[3] The Partnership is particularly focused on educating LGBT communities and partners about policies limiting tobacco industry donations and reducing the availability of tobacco products. Led by project director Bob Gordon, the group began exploring the sale of tobacco in pharmacies in San Francisco in 2007.

The idea for the pharmacy ban came from observations made by the Partnership about two Walgreens pharmacies in the Castro district of San Francisco, one of the nation's largest and most active gay communities. A traditional Walgreens store located at the busy corner of 18th and Castro sold medications and other products, including tobacco. At one time, this store was known to have the highest revenue of the Walgreens chain. Gordon worried that this high sales revenue translated to a high volume of cigarette sales to community members. A second Walgreens located just half a block away, was a "specialty pharmacy," that sold only medications; no greeting cards, food items, or office supplies—and no cigarettes. The difference in sales practices between the two stores prompted the Partnership to consider whether community members could have a say about what items were sold in their neighborhoods, and particularly in their pharmacies. Because the state of California already had encouraged grantees to work on increasing the number of tobacco-free pharmacies, the Partnership decided to begin formally working on this policy.

The Partnership began work by developing a 3-year plan that outlined the activities needed to attain policy change. The Partnership's original goal was to have the San Francisco Board of Supervisors pass a nonbinding resolution (i.e., a written motion that cannot progress into a law) that would help create awareness around and frame the pharmacy tobacco-sales issue. However, the Partnership quickly discovered that other stakeholders (faculty and students at University of San Francisco School of Pharmacy, the San Francisco Department of Public Health, community advocates, and the mayor and city attorney's offices) were also interested in the issue. To assess community support, the Partnership surveyed over 400 community members and found 86% supported tobacco-free pharmacies in their neighborhoods. This initial ground work led to a window of opportunity when the mayor agreed to sponsor a tobacco-free pharmacy ordinance.

The Partnership used several media strategies to move the process along. They launched the *Cigarettes & Pharmacies Don't Mix* awareness campaign (see Figure 6.4), posting ads on buses and inside historic trolley cars. Their goal was not to push for a specific ordinance, but rather to spread awareness of the tobacco-free pharmacy issue. They also distributed flyers to pharmacies and other local businesses, trained advocates to educate the Board of Supervisors, wrote editorial pieces, and encouraged a position statement from a local university. Partners also asked independent pharmacists throughout San Francisco who were already working in tobacco-free pharmacies to write letters of support. These stories were compelling to policymakers as they considered passing the ordinance.

Because of the strength of the broad tobacco control partnership, the mayor's support, and great timing, the ordinance passed quickly in July 2008. Opposition came primarily from Walgreens representatives, individual-rights advocates, and some retailer associations. The ordinance added an amendment to the San Francisco Health

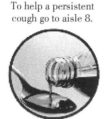
To help a persistent cough go to aisle 8.

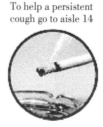
To help a persistent cough go to aisle 14

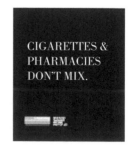
CIGARETTES & PHARMACIES DON'T MIX.

Figure 6.4 Cigarettes & Pharmacies Don't Mix Awareness Campaign.
Source: Centers for Disease Control and Prevention. *Best Practices User Guide: Health Equity.* Atlanta, GA: U.S. Department of Health and Human Services, Centers for Disease Control and Prevention, National Center for Chronic Disease Prevention and Health Promotion, Office on Smoking and Health; 2015.

Code that prevented pharmacies from being issued tobacco retailer licenses after October 1, 2008.

San Francisco's tobacco-free pharmacy ordinance was first challenged by the cigarette and tobacco company Philip Morris USA, which contended that the law violated its freedom of speech by restricting the advertisement of tobacco products in pharmacies.[78] The lawsuit failed; the court held that there was no First Amendment violation. In 2009, San Francisco's pharmacy ban faced its second lawsuit, this time by Walgreens, whose lawyers argued that the law's exemption of supermarkets and big box stores containing pharmacies violated the Equal Protection Clause of the Fourteenth Amendment.[79] San Francisco faced difficulties justifying why the law differentiated between retailer types. As a result, San Francisco amended the law to eliminate the exemptions for supermarkets and big box stores and this revised version passed. The court's decisions in these cases demonstrate that such laws, if written well, do not violate freedom of speech and that laws banning the sale of tobacco in pharmacies should apply equally to all retail establishments that contain pharmacies.

What began as a single local health equity policy initiative in San Francisco has become a national tobacco control movement. As of June 2014, over 100 municipalities (including seven in California and over one hundred in Massachusetts) have implemented tobacco-free pharmacy policies. In addition, major pharmacy chain CVS announced a nationwide policy in 2014 to stop selling all tobacco products, including cigarettes and cigars in its stores. In a statement explaining the change, CVS President Larry J. Merlo said, "We came to the decision that cigarettes and providing health care just don't go together in the same setting." Advocates continue to encourage other large companies to follow suit.

This case study illustrates the many components that have led to effective and comprehensive tobacco control policy in the United States. Similar to the smoke-free movement, the tobacco-free pharmacies movement has developed at the local grassroots level with strong community and diverse stakeholder support. In addition, San Francisco used an existing policy structure, the California licensing law, which allowed for adaptation of an existing policy rather than creation of a new one. As in several of the proceeding tobacco-free pharmacy policy initiatives, the coalition used data on the high LGBT smoking prevalence along with nationwide data to frame the issue and tell a story. As in most tobacco control policy efforts, strong opposition in the form of industry front groups and business associations was also present, and legal battles followed the policy action. However, the coalition successfully educated policymakers and was able to get a comprehensive ordinance passed, paving a path for other localities and states to tackle similar issues and implement strong tobacco control policy.

CONCLUSION

Efforts to implement evidence-based policies in tobacco control over the past 40 years have changed social norms, countered tobacco industry marketing, enhanced tobacco control policies and programs, reduced secondhand smoke exposure, and improved public health.[1,51,80] Many types of tobacco control policies have been implemented successfully at federal, state, and local levels, including those that target product price, marketing, access, and exposure. Bolstered by significant evidence linking tobacco use with morbidity, mortality, and high healthcare costs, public health professionals and their legal partners have leveraged a variety of strategies to encourage policy approaches, even in the face of significant opposition by the tobacco industry. However, tobacco control still has a long way to go. More than one in five adults continues to use tobacco, and declines in prevalence have slowed in recent years. Furthermore, some population groups smoke at particularly high rates, and bear a disproportionate burden of tobacco-related disease. Funding for targeted tobacco control interventions and other efforts to provide cessation support to these groups are important complements to more general policy approaches. Yet funding for tobacco control is continually contested, especially in tight economies. The tobacco industry continues to produce new tobacco products designed to appeal to youth or current smokers, and the regulatory environment cannot always keep up with the market.

Public health partners often serve as the catalysts for policy changes such as increases in tobacco taxes, smoke-free laws, and point-of-sale interventions,[80] but more effort should be focused on educating the public and policymakers about tobacco control policies.[81] Research has shown that unless they are motivated by the potential for increased tax revenue, decision-makers are unlikely to adopt a tobacco control policy without education and encouragement from tobacco control experts.[80] The 2000 Surgeon General's Report notes that "our recent lack of progress in tobacco control is attributable more to the failure to implement proven strategies than it is to a lack of knowledge about what to do."[18]

Although much work is yet to be done, tobacco control policy efforts can certainly celebrate the many successes attained over the past century. Even in the face of limited funding and a formidable opponent, tobacco control continues to evolve. In addition, the expertise gained by the many years of work in the policy arena has been used continually to inform policy development and implementation both within tobacco control policy and in other areas of chronic disease prevention policy. The future goal of tobacco control focuses on the elimination of tobacco use—this goal may be possible, but only with continued and enhanced resources, rigorous research providing evidence for policy strategies, and continuous community mobilization and support of tobacco control policy efforts.

REFERENCES

1. Surgeon General's Advisory Committee on Smoking and Health. *Smoking and Health: Report of the Advisory Committee to the Surgeon General of the Public Health Service.* Washington, DC: U.S. Department of Health, Education, and Welfare, Public Health Service, Office of the Surgeon General; 1964.

2. Institute of Medicine, Bonnie RJ, Stratton K, Wallace RB. *Ending the Tobacco Problem: A Blueprint for the Nation.* Washington, DC: National Academies Press; 2007.

3. U.S. Department of Health and Human Services. *The Health Consequences of Smoking—50 Years of Progress: A Report of the Surgeon General.* 2014:1–978.

4. Hyland A, Barnoya J, Corral JE. Smoke-free air policies: past, present and future. *Tob Control.* 2012;21(2):154–161.

5. Frieden TR. A framework for public health action: the Health Impact Pyramid. *Am J Public Health.* 100(4):590–595. doi:10.2105/ajph.2009.185652.

6. Association of State and Territorial Directors of Health Promotion and Public Health Education and the Centers for Disease Control and Prevention. *Policy and Environmental Change: New Directions for Public Health.* Santa Cruz, CA: Author; 2001.

7. Jamal A, Agaku IT, O'Connor E, King BA, Kenemer, JB, Neff L. Current cigarette smoking among adults—United States, 2011. *MMWR.* 2012;61:889–894. http://www.cdc.gov/mmwr/preview/mmwrhtml/mm6144a2.htm?s_cid=mm6144a2_e.

8. Centers for Disease Control and Prevention. Tobacco product use among middle and high school students—United States, 2011 and 2012. *MMWR.* 2013;62(45):2010–2013. http://www.cdc.gov/mmwr/preview/mmwrhtml/mm6245a2.htm?s_cid= mm6245a2. htm_w.

9. Pierce JP. Tobacco industry marketing, population-based tobacco control, and smoking behavior. *Am J Prev Med.* 2007;33(6):S327–S334. doi:10.1016/j.amepre.2007.09.007.

10. Dwyer-Lindgren L, Mokdad AH, Srebotnjak T, Flaxman AD, Hansen GM & Murray CJL. Cigarette smoking prevalence in U.S. counties: 1996–2012. *Popul Health Metr.* 2014;12(5):1–13.

11. World Health Organization. *WHO Global Report on Trends in Tobacco Smoking 2000–2025;* 2015.

12. Centers for Disease Control and Prevention. Current cigarette smoking prevalence among working adults—United States, 2004–2010. *MMWR.* 2011;60(38):1305–1309.

13. Garrett BE, Dube SR, Babb S, McAfee T. Addressing the social determinants of health to reduce tobacco-related disparities. *Nicotine Tob Res.* 2015;17(8):892–897.

14. Thomas S, Fayter D, Misso K, et al. Population tobacco control interventions and their effects on social inequalities in smoking: systematic review. *Tob Control.* 2008;17(4):230–237. doi: 10.1136/tc.2007.023911.

15. Centers for Disease Control and Prevention. *Targeting the Nation's Leading Killer At A Glance.* Atlanta, GA: Author; 2011. http://www.cdc.gov/chronicdisease/resources/publications/aag/osh.htm.

16. Taurus JA, O'Malley PM, Johnston LD. *Effects of Price and Access Laws on Teenage Smoking Initiation: A National Longitudinal Analysis.* ImpacTeen; 2001. NBER working paper No. 8331.

17. International Agency for Research on Cancer. *Evaluating the Effectiveness of Smoke-Free Policies.* Geneva, Switzerland: World Health Organization; 2009.

18. United States Department of Health and Human Services. *Reducing Tobacco Use: A Report of the Surgeon General.* Atlanta, GA: Centers for Disease Control and Prevention, National Center for Chronic Disease Prevention and Health Promotion, Office on Smoking and Health; 2000.

19. Jha P, Chaloupka FJ, Corrao M, Jacob B. Reducing the burden of smoking world-wide: effectiveness of interventions and their coverage. *Drug Alcohol Rev.* 2006;25(6):597–609.

20. *Toll of Tobacco in the United States of America.* Washington, DC: Campaign for Tobacco-Free Kids; 2009.

21. Thomson CC, Fisher LB, Winickoff JP, et al. State tobacco excise taxes and adolescent smoking behaviors in the United States. *J Public Health Manag Pract.* 2004;10(6):490–496.

22. Chaloupka FJ. Macro-social influences: the effects of prices and tobacco-control policies on the demand for tobacco products. *Nicotine Tob Res*. 1999;1(Suppl 2):S77–S81.

23. Farrelly MC, Nimsch CT, James J. *State Cigarette Excise Taxes: Implications for Revenue and Tax Evasion*. Tobacco Technical Assistance Consortium; 2003.

24. Lindblom E, Boonn A. *Raising State Cigarette Taxes Always Increases State Revenues (and Always Reduces Smoking)*. Washington, DC: Campaign for Tobacco-Free Kids; 2008.

25. Centers for Disease Control and Prevention. Federal and state cigarette excise taxes—United States, 1995–2009. *MMWR*. 2009;58:524–527.

26. Local Government Cigarette Tax Rates & Fees: Most counties and cities do not have their own cigarette tax rates because they are prohibited by state law. Campaign for Tobacco-Free Kids. 2015; (202):2–3.

27. South Carolina Tobacco Collaborative. The value of indexing the cigarette tax to inflation. *Cigarette Tax Briefing Document 2009*. 2009:1–9. http://4info-management.com/pdf/indexingwhitepaper.pdf. Accessed February 9, 2015.

28. Center for Public Health Systems Science. *Point-of-Sale Strategies: A Tobacco Control Guide*. St. Louis, MO: Center for Public Health Systems Science, George Warren Brown School of Social Work at Washington University in St. Louis and the Tobacco Control Legal Consortium; 2014.

29. Counter Tobacco. *Raising Tobacco Through Non-tax Approaches*; 2013. http://counterto-bacco.org/raising-tobacco-prices-through-non-tax-approaches. Accessed April 17, 2013.

30. Federal Trade Commission. *Smokeless Tobacco Report for 2009 and 2010*. Washington, DC: Author; 2012.

31. Federal Trade Commission. *Smokeless Tobacco Report for 2011*. Washington, DC: Author; 2013.

32. Henriksen L, Feighery EC, Wang Y, Fortmann SP. Association of retail tobacco marketing with adolescent smoking. *Am J Public Health*. 2004;94(12):2081–2083. doi:10.2105/AJPH.94.12.2081.

33. Slater SJ, Chaloupka FJ, Wakefield M, Johnston LD, O'Malley PM. The impact of retail cigarette marketing practices on youth smoking uptake. *Arch Pediatr Adolesc Med*. 2007;161(May):440–445. doi:10.1001/archpedi.161.5.440.

34. Soneji S, Ambrose BK, Lee W, Sargent J, Tanski S. Direct-to-consumer tobacco marketing and its association with tobacco use among adolescents and young adults. *J Adolesc Health*. 2014;55(2):209–215. doi:10.1016/j.jadohealth.2014.01.019.

35. Clattenburg EJ, Elf JL, Apelberg BJ. Unplanned cigarette purchases and tobacco point of sale advertising: a potential barrier to smoking cessation. *Tob Control*. 2013;22(6):376–381. doi:10.1136/tobaccocontrol-2012-050427.

36. Kirchner TR, Cantrell J, Anesetti-Rothermel A, Ganz O, Vallone DM, Abrams DB. Geospatial exposure to point-of-sale tobacco: real-time craving and smoking-cessation outcomes. *Am J Prev Med*. 2013;45(4):379–385. doi:10.1016/j.amepre.2013.05.016.

37. Ling PM, Glantz SA. Why and how the tobacco industry sells cigarettes to young adults: evidence from industry documents. *Am J Public Health*. 2002;92(6):908–916.

38. United States Department of Health and Human Services. Federal Laws and Policies. *Be Tobacco Free*. http://betobaccofree.hhs.gov/laws/. Accessed February 14, 2015.

39. Center for Public Health Systems Science. *Point-of-Sale Strategies: A Tobacco Control Guide*. Center for Public Health Systems Science, George Warren Brown School of Social Work at Washington University in St. Louis and the Tobacco Control Legal Consortium;

2014. http://cphss.wustl.edu/Products/Documents/CPHSS_TCLC_2014_PointofSale Strategies1.pdf.

40. World Health Organization. *MPOWER: A Policy Package to Reverse the Tobacco Epidemic.* Geneva, Switzerland: WHO Press; 2008. http://www.who.int/tobacco/mpower/ mpower_english.pdf.

41. National Cancer Institute. *The Role of the Media in Promoting and Reducing Tobacco Use.* Bethesda, MD: Author; 2008.

42. *FDA Authority Over Tobacco Web site.* Campaign for Tobacco-Free Kids; 2011. http:// www.tobaccofreekids.org/what_we_do/federal_issues/fda/. Accessed April 14, 2011.

43. United States Food and Drug Administration. *Overview of the Family Smoking Prevention and Tobacco Control Act.* Washington, DC: Author; 2012. http://www.fda.gov/ TobaccoProducts/GuidanceComplianceRegulatoryInformation/ucm246129.htm. Accessed September 10, 2015.

44. Gourdet CK, Chriqui JF, Chaloupka FJ. A baseline understanding of state laws governing e-cigarettes. *Tob Control.* 2014;23(Suppl 3):iii37–iii40. doi:10.1136/ tobaccocontrol-2013-051459.

45. Centers for Disease Control and Prevention. Quitting smoking among adults—United States, 2001–2010. *MMWR.* 2011;60(44):1518–1528. http://www.ncbi.nlm.nih.gov/ pubmed/22071592.

46. Tobacco Use and Dependence Guideline Panel. *Treating Tobacco Use and Dependence: 2008 Update.* Rockville, MD: United States Department of Health and Human Services; 2008.

47. McAfee T, Babb S, McNabb S, Fiore MC. Helping smokers quit—opportunities created by the Affordable Care Act. *N Engl J Med.* 2014;372(1):5–7. doi:10.1056/NEJMp1411437.

48. American Lung Association. Highlights: State Medicaid Coverage for Tobacco Cessation Treatments and Barriers to Coverage—United States, 2008-2014. 2014. http://www. lung.org/assets/documents/tobacco-control-advocacy/highlights-state-medicaid.pdf. Accessed February 9, 2015.

49. Fiore MC, Jaen CR, Baker TB, Bailey WC, Benowitz NL, Curry SJ. *Treating Tobacco Use and Dependence: Clinical Practice Guideline.* Washington, DC: United States Department of Health and Human Services. Public Health Service; 2008.

50. Guide to Community Preventive Services. *Reducing Tobacco Use and Secondhand Smoke Exposure: Comprehensive Tobacco Control Programs.* www.thecommunityguide.org/ tobacco/comprehensive.html.

51. Centers for Disease Control and Prevention. *Best Practices for Comprehensive Tobacco Control Programs—August 1999.* Atlanta, GA: United States Department of Health and Human Services, Centers for Disease Control and Prevention, National Center for Chronic Disease Prevention and Health Promotion, Office on Smoking and Health; 2014.

52. Xu X, Bishop EE, Kennedy SM, Simpson S a, Pechacek TF. Annual healthcare spending attributable to cigarette smoking. *Am J Prev Med.* 2015 Mar;48(3):326–333.

53. Ong MK, Diamant AL, Zhou Q, Park H-Y, Kaplan RM. Estimates of smoking-related property costs in California multiunit housing. *Am J Public Health.* 2012;102(3):490–493. doi:10.2105/AJPH.2011.300170.

54. Schneider JE, Peterson NA, Kiss N, Ebeid O, Doyle AS. Tobacco litter costs and public policy: a framework and methodology for considering the use of fees to offset abatement costs. *Tob Control.* 2011;20(Suppl 1):i36–i41. doi:10.1136/tc.2010.041707.

55. Lightwood J, Glantz SA. The effect of the California tobacco control program on smoking prevalence, cigarette consumption, and healthcare costs: 1989–2008. *PLoS One.* 2013;8(2):e47145. doi:10.1371/journal.pone.0047145.

56. Jha P, Chaloupka FJ. The economics of global tobacco control. *BMJ: Br Med J.* 2000;321(7257):358–361.

57. Bero L. Implications of the tobacco industry documents for public health and policy. *Annu Rev Public Health.* 2003;24:267–288. doi:10.1146/annurev.publhealth.24.100901.140813.

58. Cummings KM, Morley CP, Hyland A. Failed promises of the cigarette industry and its effect on consumer misperceptions about the health risks of smoking. *Tob Control.* 2002;11(Suppl 1):I110–I117. doi:10.1136/tc.11.suppl_1.i110.

59. Lee S, Ling PM, Glantz SA. The vector of the tobacco epidemic: tobacco industry practices in low and middle-income countries. *Cancer Causes Control.* 2012;23(Suppl 1):117–129. doi:10.1007/s10552-012-9914-0.

60. Centers for Disease Control and Prevention. *Best Practices User Guide: Coalitions—State and Community Interventions.* Atlanta, GA: Centers for Disease Control and Prevention, National Center for Chronic Disease Prevention and Health Promotion, Office on Smoking and Health; 2009.

61. Americans for Nonsmokers' Rights: Going Smoke Free. http://www.no-smoke.org/goingsmokefree.php?id=110.

62. Fong GT, Cummings KM, Shopland DR. Building the evidence base for effective tobacco control policies: the International Tobacco Control Policy Evaluation Project (the ITC Project). *Tob Control.* 2006;15(suppl 3):iii1–iii2. doi:10.1136/tc.2006.017244.

63. Thomson G, Wilson N. One year of smokefree bars and restaurants in New Zealand: Impacts and responses. *BMC Public Health.* 2006;6(1):64. http://www.biomedcentral.com/1471-2458/6/64.

64. Centers for Disease Control and Prevention. Smoke-free policies receive public support. Sept. 10, 2015. http://www.cdc.gov/tobacco/data_statistics/fact_sheets/secondhand_smoke/protection/public_support/index.htm.

65. *Voters in All States Support Significant Increases in State Cigarette Taxes.* Washington, DC: Campaign for Tobacco-free Kids; 2008.

66. Lum KL, Barnes RL, Glantz SA. Enacting tobacco taxes by direct popular vote in the United States: lessons from 20 years of experience. *Tob Control.* 2009;18(5):377–386. doi:10.1136/tc.2009.029843.

67. World Health Organization. *Cancer Control: Knowledge into Action: WHO Guide for Effective Programmes; Module 1.* Geneva, Switzerland; 2006.

68. Monardi F, Glantz SA. Are tobacco industry campaign contributions influencing state legislative behavior? *Am J Public Health.* 1998;88(6):918–923.

69. Bialous SA, Fox BJ, Glantz SA. Tobacco industry allegations of "illegal lobbying" and state tobacco control. *Am J Public Health.* 2001;91(1):62–67.

70. Rights A for N, ed. Front groups and allies. *Am Nonsmok Rights.* December 30, 2009. http://www.no-smoke.org/getthefacts.php?id=62.

71. Levy DT, Chaloupka F, Gitchell J. The effects of tobacco control policies on smoking rates: a tobacco control scorecard. *J Public Health Manag Pract.* 2004; Jul–Aug 10(4)338–353.

72. Americans for Nonsmokers' Rights. Preemption: Tobacco Control's #1 Enemy. 2004. http://www.no-smoke.org/pdf/preemptionenemy.pdf. Accessed October 14, 2011.

73. Tobacco Control Legal Consortium. National Association of Tobacco Outlets, Inc. v. City of New York. 2014.

74. Chaloupka FJ, Cummings KM, Morley CP, Horan JK. Tax, price and cigarette smoking: evidence from the tobacco documents and implications for tobacco company marketing strategies. *Tob Control*. 2002;11(Suppl 1):162–172.

75. Federal Trade Commission. *Federal Trade Commission Cigarette Report for 2009 and 2010*. Washington, DC: Author; 2012.

76. Lee JGL, Griffin GK, Melvin CL. Tobacco use among sexual minorities in the USA, 1987 to May 2007: a systematic review. *Tob Control*. 2009;18(4):275–282.

77. Legacy. *Tobacco Control in LGBT Communities*. Washington, DC: Legacy; 2012. http:// www.legacyforhealth.org/content/download/1469/14683/version/4/file/Tobacco_ Control_LGBT_Communities.pdf.

78. Philip Morris USA v. City and County of San Francisco.

79. Walgreen Co. v. City and County of San Francisco.

80. Institute of Medicine, Bonnie RJ, Stratton K, Wallace RB. *Ending the Tobacco Problem: A Blueprint for the Nation*. Washington, DC: National Academies Press; 2007.

81. Gerlach K, Larkin M. *To Improve Health and Health Care, Vol. VIII: The Robert Woods Johnson Foundation Anthology*. San Francisco, CA: Jossey-Bass; 2005.

82. Brock B. Regulating point-of-sale tobacco advertising: The St. Paul Minnesota experience. Webinar; 2011.

83. Ashe M, Jernigan D, Kline R, Galaz R. Land use planning and the control of alcohol, tobacco, firearms, and fast food restaurants. *Am J Public Health*. 2003;93(9):1404–1408. doi:10.2105/ajph.93.9.1404.

84. Kline R. *Local Land Use Regulation for the Location and Operation of Tobacco Retailers*. Tobacco Control Legal Consortium; 2004.

85. Campaign for Tobacco-free Kids. *FDA Regulation of Tobacco Products: A Common Sense Law to Protect Kids and Save Lives*. 2011. http://www.tobaccofreekids.org/research/factsheets/ pdf/0352.pdf. Accessed June 23, 2011.

86. Leonard W. Utah teens lobby lawmakers for tighter e-cigarette regulations. *Deseret News*. February 12, 2015. http://www.deseretnews.com/article/865621791/Utah-teens-lobb y-lawmakers-for-tighter-e-cigarette-regulations.html?pg=all. February 12, 2015.

87. Davis M. New regulations for E-cigarette sellers coming. *News 8*. 2015. http://wtnh. com/2015/04/27/new-regulations-for-e-cigarette-sellers-coming.

88. Hawaii becomes fourth state with e-cigarette restrictions. *Star Advertiser*. April 24, 2015. http://www.staradvertiser.com/news/breaking/20150424_Hawaii_becomes_fourth_ state_with_ecigarette_restrictions.html?id=301253611].

89. E-cigarette restrictions signed into law. *NJToday.net*. January 14, 2010. http://njtoday. net/2010/01/14/e-cigarette-restrictions-signed-into-law/.

90. Callahan-Lyon P. Electronic cigarettes: human health effects. *Tob Control*. 2014;23 (suppl 2):ii36–ii40. doi:10.1136/tobaccocontrol-2013-051470.

91. Pertschuk M, Pomeranz JL, Aoki JR, Larkin M a, Paloma M. Assessing the impact of federal and state preemption in public health: a framework for decision makers. *J Public Health Manag Pract*. 2012;19(00):213–219. doi:10.1097/PHH.0b013e3182582a57.

92. Griffin M, Babb SD, MacNeil AE. State preemption of local tobacco control policies restricting smoking, advertising, and youth access—United States, 2000–2010. *MMWR*. 2011;60(33):1124–1127.

7

Food, Nutrition, and Obesity Policy

Jamie F. Chriqui and Christina N. Sansone

LEARNING OBJECTIVES

1. Provide an overview of the obesity epidemic in the United States.
2. Describe what is meant by an obesogenic environment and the costs to society of the obesity epidemic.
3. Provide an overview of how the food system has changed over time.
4. Summarize the major federal food and nutrition programs in the United States.
5. Outline the types of public policy strategies used to address the obesity epidemic.

IDENTIFYING THE PROBLEM: OBESITY AND ITS CONSEQUENCES

Obesity may be colloquially referred to as excessive body fat, but there is no clear-cut definition of excessive, nor is there an easy, cost-effective way to measure body fat.[1] As a result, obesity is frequently defined as excess bodyweight, and body mass index (BMI)—a ratio of weight to height, calculated as kilograms divided by meters squared—is often used to categorize an individual as obese.[1] In children, obesity refers to a BMI greater than, or equal to, the 95th percentile of sex-specific Centers for Disease Control and Prevention BMI charts.[2]

Obesity is a major risk factor for type 2 diabetes, cardiovascular disease, and hypertension.[1] Beyond these "big three," obesity confers greater risk for additional comorbid health conditions, including stroke, arthritis, nonalcoholic fatty liver disease, kidney disease, and mental health problems related to social stigma.[1] Obese children are increasingly acquiring multiple comorbid conditions previously associated only with adults, and are increasingly carrying the burden of these conditions into adulthood.[1]

Between 1980 and 2004, obesity prevalence tripled among children aged 2 to 19 years, increasing from 6% to 19%.[1] Overall prevalence has remained fairly stable since 2004, fluctuating only a percentage point or two, with 2011–2012 estimates indicating 17% of children are obese.[1,2] Although overall prevalence has remained stable, significant disparities occur by race/ethnicity, gender, and—to a lesser extent—by age.[1-5] Hispanic children have the highest obesity prevalence, followed by

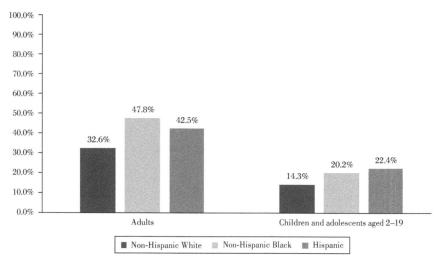

Figure 7.1 Child and adult obesity prevalence, 2011–2012.[3]

Figure created based on data from: Ogden CL, Carroll MD, Kit BK, et al. Prevalence of childhood and adult obesity in the United States, 2011–2012. *JAMA: The Journal of the American Medical Association.* 2014;311:806–814.[3]

non-Hispanic Black and non-Hispanic White children (see Figure 7.1).[2] Black children are more likely to be severely obese than are White children, but linear trends indicate the most pronounced increase of severe obesity in White females and Black males.[6] In addition, 13.9% of all adolescents aged 12–19 years had a BMI greater than or equal to 30,[2] thereby meeting the adult definition of obesity.

Obesity prevalence in adults doubled between 1980 and 2004, increasing from 15% to 33%, and was estimated at 35% in 2011–2012.[1,2] As with children, obesity-related disparities also occur by race/ethnicity, gender, and age, as well as income, urbanicity, and geography.[1–5,7] In adults, obesity is more prevalent in non-Hispanic Blacks and Hispanics than in non-Hispanic Whites (see Figure 7.1) and exists at the highest rate among all adults aged 40 to 59 years, but is increasing fastest among those aged 60 years and older.[2]

Gender- and income-based obesity-related disparities exist among all racial and ethnic groups,[1,2,4,5] but are most pronounced among non-Hispanic Black women across all age categories.[2,4,5,8] Non-Hispanic Black women are more likely to be obese than non-Hispanic Black men,[2] but higher income non-Hispanic Black women are less likely to be obese than those with lower incomes.[4] Interestingly, higher income non-Hispanic Black and Mexican American men have slightly higher obesity prevalence rates than those with lower incomes.[1,2,4,5,8]

Adults in rural areas are significantly more likely to be obese than those in urban areas.[7] Rural residents are more likely to be non-Hispanic White than Hispanic or non-Hispanic Black, but disparities persist even after controlling for race/ethnicity, income, and age.[7] Disparities also exist by state and region of the country (see Figure 7.2), with the South having the highest obesity prevalence and the West having the lowest prevalence.[9]

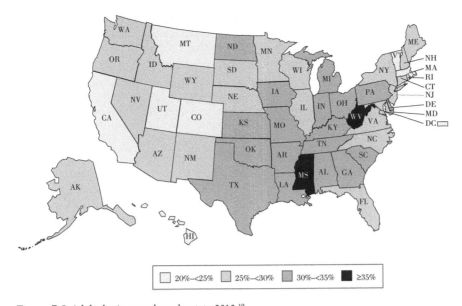

Figure 7.2 Adult obesity prevalence by state, 2013.[10]
Source: Centers for Disease Control and Prevention.[10] Data compiled from self-reported estimates reported by the Behavioral Rise Factor Surveillance System. Data available in the public domain.

The Costs of Obesity

From an economic perspective, obesity comes with a staggeringly high cost. An estimated $315.8 billion[10] was spent on adult obesity-related direct healthcare costs in 2010, with the majority of expenses resulting from the treatment of comorbid health conditions, particularly type 2 diabetes.[10,11]

Research suggests Medicare and Medicaid spending would see decreases of 8.5% and 11.8%, respectively, if obesity-related costs were removed from the analysis.[11] A 2012 study estimated that state-level medical expenditures would be 7% to 11% lower if all obese people were normal weight.[12] Additionally, a substantial portion of state obesity costs are publicly financed through Medicare and Medicaid, ranging from 25% in Virginia to 64% in Rhode Island, with a nationwide mean of 39.44%.[12]

Absenteeism, or absence from work, is a major indirect obesity cost that affects productivity in the workplace.[13] Obese employees miss more work than normal-weight employees (see Table 7.1)[13] and obesity-related absenteeism translates to an estimated cost of $8.65 billion per year in lost productivity.[13] Collectively, both direct and indirect obesity-related costs rise as obesity prevalence increases,[12] as class of obesity increases,[10,13] and when comorbid conditions are present, particularly type 2 diabetes (see Table 7.1).[10,11]

The Obesogenic Environment

Obesity occurs when there is an energy imbalance—i.e., either too much energy consumed (kilocalories) and/or too little energy expended through physical activity.

Table 7.1 Absenteeism and Estimated Obesity-attributed Costs by Weight Classification

Weight Classification	BMI (kg/m²)	Obesity Class	Additional Absent Workdays, Per Year, Compared With Normal Weight Adults (95% CI)	Estimated Annual Obesity-attributable Costs Of Absenteeism
Normal	18.5–24.9	–		
Overweight	25.0–29.9	–	0.22 (0.50, 0.95)	
Obesity	30.0–34.9	I	1.17 (0.01, 2.32)	$216
	35.0–39.9	II	1.71 (0.42, 3.00)	$317
Extreme Obesity	> 40.0	III	1.88 (.042, 3.33)	$348

Source: Adapted from Andreyeva et al.13

Many contend the energy imbalance facing children and adults today is a byproduct of the obesogenic environment found within the areas where they live, work, and play. To this end, the epidemiology of obesity is perhaps best viewed through an ecological framework that emphasizes the interplay between individuals and multiple levels of their environment; when viewed in this context, individuals are impacted by the social interaction and resources—or lack thereof—available in their communities. Put another way, an "obesogenic environment" is one where unhealthy options are frequently more accessible and affordable than healthy options, where physical activity opportunities are limited, and where the marketing of unhealthy options outweighs marketing of healthier options.[14] Figure 7.3 illustrates the complexity of the obesity problem, through the lens of an obesogenic environment, by recognizing the multiple levels and sectors of influence on obesity. As indicated in the figure, obesity is influenced by factors affecting the energy balance. In short, all sectors of society, and all settings where children and adults spend their time, have a role to play in effectuating changes to the food and activity environments to which individuals are exposed.

The built environment is another contributing factor and includes sidewalks, parks and green space, schools, bike lanes or paths, public transportation, and zoning/land use.[14] For example, discontinuous or poorly maintained sidewalks, or lack of parks and green space may contribute to the obesogenic environment, while poor transportation planning could lead to increased dependence on motor vehicle traffic. A poorly structured built environment can impact obesity by providing fewer opportunities for individuals to be physically active while enabling default behaviors that are unhealthy. See Chapter 8 for more information on physical activity.

All of these factors contribute to the obesogenic environment. From a policy perspective, the question remains as to how to address the multitude of factors and issues contributing to obesogenic environments. The Institute of Medicine's (IOM) 2012 report, *Accelerating Progress in Obesity Prevention*, specifically sought to provide a road map for policy and environmental change strategies for obesity prevention efforts nationwide.[14] The IOM Committee envisioned that through engagement, leadership, and synchronous and concerted action across five key environments—physical

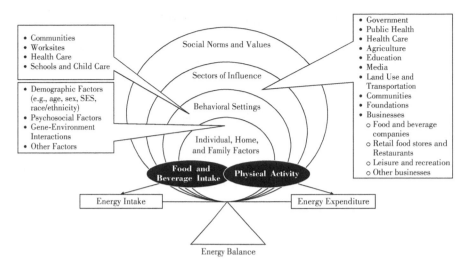

Figure 7.3 Various levels and sectors of influence on obesity in populations.[2]
Source: Institute of Medicine, 2012.[2] Reprinted with permission from the National Academies Press.

activity environments, food and beverage environments, messaging environments, healthcare and work environments, and the school environment—that progress in obesity prevention efforts nationwide would be accelerated.[14] The next section provides examples of a range of policy strategies for addressing the obesity problem.

The U.S. Food System

Over the past 60 years, the American food system has transitioned from one of home-cooked meals to one of prepackaged, processed, convenience foods, and food eaten away from home.[15,16] As food technology advanced (e.g., home refrigeration systems, mechanized industrial processes, microwave technology) food became more processed, faster to prepare, and cheaper while reducing the reliance on scratch-cooked meals.[15] Consequently, Americans consumed more convenience foods at home and also increased the amount of food consumed away from home (FAFH). The amount of household food expenditures on FAFH increased from 25.9% in 1970 to 43.1% in 2012, and FAFH is generally of lower nutritional quality than foods consumed at home.[16]

Some contend the packaged food industry further perpetuates obesity and associated health disparities by selling convenience foods and beverages higher in sugar, salt, and/or fat[17] than unprocessed foods. These additives are required to extend the shelf life of the products and may contribute to their ready availability in low food-access areas,[18,19] thereby increasing obesity prevalence in low-income Black and Hispanic urban neighborhoods, as well as low-income, predominately White rural areas. Additionally, unhealthy processed foods include those available at fast-food outlets, which are also cheaper to purchase than healthy, whole foods. As with packaged foods, fast food retailers are more prevalent in low food-access areas.[18,20]

Federal Food and Nutrition Programs

The U.S. Department of Agriculture (USDA) operates a number of food and nutrition programs related to food distribution, child nutrition, and/or food assistance.[21] Table 7.2 lists the federal programs that are most relevant from a public health policy perspective.

One aspect of federal nutrition-related policymaking that has garnered extensive media, public, and policymaker attention since the mid-2000s (given the heightened focus on obesity among our nation's youth) is the federal Child Nutrition Programs. For example, the *Child Nutrition and Women, Infants, and Children Reauthorization Act of 2004*,[22] provided the USDA with the authority to routinely update the National School Lunch Program (NSLP) and School Breakfast Program (SBP) nutrition standards (which had not been updated since the mid-1990s) to align them with the most current scientific evidence and each issuance of the *Dietary Guidelines for Americans*.[23] Similarly, other than restrictions on foods of minimal nutritional value (i.e., certain candies and carbonated beverages), the sale of foods and beverages in schools, aside from the NSLP and SBP, were not regulated at the federal level until the passage of the *Healthy, Hunger-Free Kids Act of 2010*.[24,25] The Act provided the USDA with the authority it needed to impose nutrition standards for all foods and beverages sold outside of the meal programs. These are commonly referred to as "competitive foods and beverages" because their sale competes with meal programs. In 2013, USDA issued the *Smart Snacks in School* interim final rule, which provides science-based nutrition standards for all foods sold on school campuses during the school day, with implementation commencing at the beginning of the 2014–2015 school year.[26] Importantly, the *Smart Snacks* regulation does not apply to foods offered to children during the school day in classroom parties or celebrations, as a reward for good behavior, or to events occurring on campus during non-school hours or off-campus events.

Table 7.2 Federal Food and Nutrition Programs Operated by the U.S. Department of Agriculture[21]

Food Distribution Programs	Child Nutrition Programs	Food Assistance and Nutrition Programs
• Commodity Supplemental Food Program • Food Distribution Program on Indian Reservations • The Emergency Food Assistance Program	• Child and Adult Care Food Program (CACFP) • Fresh Fruit and Vegetable Program (FFVP) • National School Lunch Program (NSLP) • School Breakfast Program (SBP) • Special Milk Program (SMP) • Summer Food Service Program (SFSP)	• Supplemental Nutrition Assistance Program (SNAP) • Women, Infants, and Children (WIC) • Farmers' Market Nutrition Program for WIC recipients (FMNP) • Senior Farmers' Market Nutrition Program (SFMNP)

Additionally, the *Smart Snacks* standards allow for "infrequent" fundraisers, but do not define "infrequent" and instead allow for determination of special exemptions in each state. As a result, policymaking on these non-federally regulated issues will be left to the states and school districts nationwide. Early evidence on the fundraising exemption indicates wide variation in states' interpretation of "infrequent," ranging from 0 exempt fundraisers in 29 states to 30 exempt fundraisers per semester, per school in Oklahoma.[27]

Another example of federal food and nutrition policy that has attracted heightened attention in recent years because of the obesity epidemic is the federal Supplemental Nutrition Assistance Program (SNAP; formerly referred to as the Food Stamp Program). Although SNAP includes "nutrition" in its title, the Program does not regulate what foods and beverages can be purchased with SNAP dollars. In fact, the only items prohibited from purchase with SNAP dollars are cleaning supplies, tobacco, and alcohol. Given the prevalence of obesity among low-income populations (who may also be SNAP recipients), advocates and policymakers at all levels have called on the USDA to limit SNAP food and beverage purchasing to nutrient-dense foods and non-calorically sweetened beverages. For example, Minnesota applied for an exemption to prohibit the purchase of candy and soft drinks with food stamps, as they were then known, and, more recently, New York City applied to conduct a 2-year demonstration project to remove sugar-sweetened beverages from SNAP coverage.[28,29] To date, all requests from states and localities to restrict SNAP purchases have been denied by the USDA.

PUBLIC POLICY STRATEGIES RELATED TO OBESITY

At the same time, state and local legislatures and regulatory agencies also have taken an active role in pursuing numerous policy strategies to address the energy imbalance; change the overall food and beverage environment; and create programs, insurance mandates, and funding streams to support obesity prevention and treatment efforts. The policy strategies pursued thus far include a full range of policy instruments including legislative approaches (such as ballot initiatives), regulatory approaches, executive orders, and, even case law (see Table 7.3).

The Politics of Obesity

Political support for food and obesity policy is largely tied to policymakers' beliefs about the root causes of obesity, as well as their views on the proper role of government in dealing with the problem. Liberal policymakers tend to frame their approach as an issue of social responsibility, and to present the need to regulate the food industry as an effort that dovetails with decreasing the economic burden of publicly funded healthcare.[30,31] Conservatives and libertarians tend to emphasize personal responsibility, favor fewer regulations, and resent what they perceive as government interference with the market.[30-33] They may argue that obesity/food-based polices are a

Table 7.3 Examples of State and Local Public Policy Strategies Related to Food and Nutrition

Policy Strategy (Listed Alphabetically)	Example	Typical Jurisdiction(s) Where Policy May Be Adopted	Typical Policy Instrument(s) Legislative/Statutory Includes Ordinances and Zoning at Local Levels Employed
Banning inclusion of toy gifts in children's meals	Banning inclusion of toys in children's meals sold through fast food outlets	Local	legislative/statutory, regulatory/ administrative law
Body Mass Index (BMI) screening, assessment, and reporting requirements	Requiring BMI screening for all students entering a certain grade with aggregate school-level reporting and confidential reporting to parents	State, District	legislative/statutory, regulatory/ administrative law
Dedicated tax revenue for obesity prevention efforts	Dedicating a portion of sugar-sweetened beverage (SSB) tax revenue to childhood obesity prevention programming	State, Local	legislative/statutory, regulatory/ administrative law
Farm-to-institution policies	Farm-to-school or -cafeteria (including worksites and hospitals) source locally grown fruits and vegetables	State, Local, District	legislative/statutory, regulatory/ administrative law
Financial incentives for purchasing fruits and vegetables	Women, Infants, and Children (WIC) vouchers; Electronic Benefit Transfer (EBT) acceptance at farmers' markets	State, Local	legislative/statutory
Financial incentives for selling fruits and vegetables	Healthy food financing initiatives; tax incentive financing/tax credits	State, Local	legislative/statutory
Insurance coverage	Medicaid coverage for weight management counseling; mandated insurance coverage for obesity treatment; mandated insurance coverage for gym memberships	State	legislative/statutory, regulatory/ administrative law
Menu/calorie labeling	Nutrition and calorie labelling for retail store shelves, menus, and menu boards	State, Local	legislative/statutory, regulatory/ administrative law

Table 7.3 (Continued)

Policy Strategy (Listed Alphabetically)	Example	Typical Jurisdiction(s) Where Policy May Be Adopted	Typical Policy Instrument(s) Legislative/Statutory Includes Ordinances and Zoning at Local Levels Employed
Minimum age restrictions on purchase of certain beverages	Age restrictions on purchasing energy drinks	State, Local	legislative/statutory
Nutrition education standards	Minimum nutrition education curricular requirements for elementary and secondary school students	State, District	legislative/statutory, regulatory/ administrative law
Nutrition standards for foods sold or served on property at: • Before/after school programs • Child care • Hospitals • Schools • Worksites	Nutrition standards for licensed child care providers in a given state	State, Local, District	legislative/statutory, regulatory/ administrative law
Nutrition training/ certification for food service providers	Nutrition training/ certification requirements for school food service directors; nutrition certification requirements for local government cafeteria managers	State, Local, District	legislative/statutory, regulatory/ administrative law
Portion size restrictions on beverages for retail sale (beyond nutrition standards for specific locations of sale)	Limiting the sale of SSBs to 16 ounces or less	State, Local	legislative/statutory, regulatory/administrative law, case law
Preemption of local ordinances related to food policy	State preemption laws that prohibit local governments from levying a tax on SSBs	State	legislative/statutory, case law
Prohibiting "open campuses"	Prohibiting students from leaving school campuses during their lunch hour	State, District	legislative/statutory, regulatory/ administrative law

(*continued*)

Table 7.3 (Continued)

Policy Strategy (Listed Alphabetically)	Example	Typical Jurisdiction(s) Where Policy May Be Adopted	Typical Policy Instrument(s) Legislative/Statutory Includes Ordinances and Zoning at Local Levels Employed
Prohibiting use of food as a reward or incentive	Prohibiting teachers from providing candy or other food as a "reward" for good behavior or to incentivize students to do something	State, District	legislative/statutory, regulatory/ administrative law
Requiring healthy food and beverage marketing or restricting advertising of unhealthy food and beverages	Banning advertising of SSBs on school campuses; requiring that vending machine fronts on public property only advertise water; prohibiting marketing or advertising of foods/beverages on school buses	State, Local, District	legislative/statutory, regulatory/ administrative law, case law
School wellness policies	School district creation of the Congressionally mandated local school wellness policy	State, District	legislative/statutory, regulatory/ administrative law
Taxation of sugary drinks and certain snack foods	SSB taxes; removing sales tax exemptions on the sale of candy	State, Local	legislative/statutory, regulatory/ administrative law, ballot initiative
Zoning and licensing prohibitions, restrictions on retail outlets selling foods and/or beverages	Fast-food restaurant moratorium; restricting food trucks within a certain distance of school property; density restrictions on the number of fast food outlets within a certain geographic area	State, Local, District	legislative/statutory, regulatory/ administrative law
Zoning permitted uses for certain types of food outlets and or agriculture	Zoning ordinance permitting community gardens in a community; zoning ordinance permitting gardens on building rooftops in urban neighborhoods	State, Local	legislative/statutory

government intrusion that creates a nanny-state whereby lawmakers seek to control personal food choices.

Advocacy groups and professional organizations are also influential actors, bringing expertise, consumer outreach, and grassroots influence to the political landscape, but they do not leverage direct financial influence. One of the most prominent advocacy groups in the obesity arena is the Center for Science in the Public Interest (CSPI), an organization that leads science-backed, evidence-based public health initiatives and is nationally recognized as a top consumer advocate.[34] CSPI represents public interests before legislative and regulatory bodies, and also provides direct consumer education through newsletters and facilitation of local events. Other prominent nationwide organizations are described in Table 7.4.[35]

Professional organizations such as the American Medical Association, American Heart Association, American Diabetes Association, and the Academy of Nutrition and Dietetics also assume an advocacy role on behalf of consumers as well as their members. They frequently issue position statements and treatment guidelines for obesity and related comorbidities.

Although advocacy groups have a national presence, they do not have the loudest voice on the political front. Perhaps the most pronounced voice is that of the food and beverage industry. They have an enormous financial stake in any policy that would regulate their industry, and they favor voluntary approaches over government regulation.[36] A particularly thorny issue is that of financial contributions and lobbying efforts. Food and beverage industry interests are extremely well funded and provide substantial financial support to policymakers from both political parties.[17] In 2014 alone, organized food and beverage interests made 13,833 contributions totaling $28,478,657 to federal, state, and local candidates and committees during the 2014 election cycle.[37] More than one half of these contributions went to Republican Party and/or Democratic Party candidates or committees. Contributions to Republican Party candidates and committees was 80% greater than that provided to Democratic Party candidates and committees—$9,154,225 (Republican) as compared with $5,034,387 (Democratic).[37]

Given the amount of money and influence involved, it is not surprising that policymakers indicate industry lobbying presents a barrier to passing obesity prevention policy[38,39,40,41] It is interesting and important to note the influence of industry extends beyond political candidates. The food and beverage industry often funds professional organizations—including the Academy of Nutrition and Dietetics (AND) and School Nutrition Association (SNA)—through sponsorship agreements. This presents a potential conflict of interest for the organizations and their members. As a result, AND and SNA leadership have been subjected to member pressure to cut ties with food and beverage industry groups as sponsorship is increasingly viewed as counterproductive to the public's health and detrimental to professional credibility.[42-46]

Public Support for Obesity Policy Interventions

The public overwhelmingly agrees obesity is a major health concern. National public opinion polling estimates 75%–91% of Americans indicate overweight and obesity

Table 7.4 Examples of Food and Obesity Advocacy Groups

Organization	Description	URL
Action for Healthy Kids	Focuses on school-level change	http://www.actionforhealthykids.org/
Alliance for a Healthier Generation	Provides evidence-based resources and best practices to facilitate environmental-level change	https://www.healthiergeneration.org/
Berkeley Media Studies Group	Collaborative group that researches how the media portrays health issues and provides media advocacy training	http://www.bmsg.org/
California Center for Public Health Advocacy	Advocacy group focusing on childhood obesity in California with an emphasis on addressing underlying factors contributing to obesity	http://www.publichealthadvocacy.org/
Center for Science in the Public Interest	Consumer advocate group with an emphasis on nutrition and using science for public good	https://www.cspinet.org/index.html
Food Research and Action Center	Focuses on policy and public–private partnerships to eliminate hunger	http://frac.org/
The Public Health Advocacy Institute	Supports public health policy through collaborative work at the intersection of public health and law	http://www.phaionline.org/
Share our Strength	Connects hungry children to nutritious food and teaches families how to cook healthy, affordable food	http://www.nokidhungry.org/
Voices for Healthy Kids	Advocates, promotes, and supports policy and environmental change strategies to help children and youth eat healthier and be physically active.	http://www.heart.org/HEARTORG/Advocate/Voices-for-Healthy-Kids_UCM_453195_SubHomePage.jsp

is an extremely or very serious health concern.[47–49] There is similar near-universal agreement that childhood obesity is a major health issue.[47–52] Nevertheless, there is little public consensus about who bears responsibility for addressing and solving the obesity crisis— individuals, governments, communities, or a combination of entities[47–55]—even as expert groups such as the IOM[14] recommend a multisectoral approach to accelerating progress in obesity prevention.

Public support for government action on obesity is closely tied to political affiliation and personal views about obesity. Conservatives exhibit lower support for government responsibility to address obesity than do liberals,[56,57] although a quick scan of states with higher obesity prevalence[9] indicates that they voted for the Republican candidate in the 2012 presidential election.[58] Importantly, although political affiliation and obesity may be related, the nature of the association is complex and the interplay between the two is more likely correlational rather than causal.

As with the political landscape, the food and beverage industry plays a role in public support, especially in the arena of sugar-sweetened beverage (SSB) taxation. Exceptionally well-funded, industry-led campaigns against SSB taxes played a prominent role in defeating local tax initiatives in El Monte and Richmond, California and Telluride, Colorado in 2012; and in San Francisco, California in 2014. Although there is less public support for restrictive policies, public opinion may be changing in the area of sugar-sweetened beverage (SSB) taxes. Statewide polling data from Kentucky—a historically conservative state—released in March 2015 indicate 51% of adults favor taxing SSBs when the revenue is used for school nutrition and school physical activity programs.[59] The case study at the end of this chapter presents an in-depth review of SSB tax initiatives and industry opposition.

Message Framing Regarding the Obesity Issue

Regardless of political affiliation, numerous public opinion polls found that conservatives, moderates, and liberals rated childhood obesity as a serious health issue, and public support increases when policies are tied to improving outcomes for childhood obesity.[50–52,60] A 2013 study found that message framing had a significant impact on public support for childhood obesity policies; in addition, the study found that the most resonant message among conservatives framed childhood obesity as a threat to military readiness.[60] Such results reinforce the importance of framing obesity in the context of health and non-health consequences to broaden public support for government intervention.[31,60,61]

Other research on message framing found that media coverage mentioning a specific obese child emphasized individual factors (e.g., behavior/lifestyle choices) over environmental factors (e.g., neighborhood characteristics), which led to decreased public support for obesity prevention policies.[62] Framing media campaigns to focus on population-level obesity could have the opposite effect and serve to increase public support.

In addition, message framing can be used to shift the conversation from the "nanny-state" frame to the "savvy-state" frame.[63] For example, emphasizing the burden of publicly funded healthcare costs associated with obesity (savvy-state) can serve as a counter-frame to the argument that individual-level unhealthy behaviors are not a public health problem (nanny-state).[63] Such a complex, multilevel approach to framing obesity policy could facilitate a shift in public perception of obesity, and thus increase support for food and obesity policy intervention.

The Case of Sugar-sweetened Beverage Taxation

In this case study, sugar-sweetened beverages (SSBs) are defined as: all carbonated soft drinks, fruit and vegetable beverages containing less than 100% juice, sports drinks, ready-to-drink sweetened teas and ready-to-drink coffee drinks, flavored waters, and other beverages containing caloric sweeteners.

SSB consumption has been linked to weight gain in children and adults,[64,65] as well as to comorbidities including metabolic syndrome and type 2 diabetes,[64] hypertension,[64,66] increased cardiovascular-disease risk,[64] and increased risk of coronary heart disease even after controlling for BMI and additional unhealthy dietary factors.[67] The link between SSB consumption and weight gain is the most immediate, tangible consequence as obesity is an independent risk factor for many of the poor health outcomes listed above.

As discussed in the overview section, overall obesity prevalence rates doubled among adults and more than tripled among children between 1980 and 2004, and then leveled off between 2004 and 2012, although disparities in prevalence occur.[1,2,4,6,8] During roughly the same time periods, SSB consumption increased, then leveled off with consumption decreasing in some subcategories of beverages, and increasing in others. Daily per capita caloric consumption of all SSBs more than doubled from 1977 to 2002, increasing from 69 calories to 203 calories.[68] During this time calories from soda/cola were the largest contributor, with daily consumption more than tripling from 41 calories in 1977, to 143 calories in 2002.[68] A 2011 study estimated daily SSB consumption between 2005 and 2008 at 178 calories for males and 103 calories for females; this represents 62% (men) and 57% (women) of the average daily limit for empty calories.[69] The same 2011 study found that males consumed significantly more calories than females across all age groups except children aged 2 to 5 years.[70] Additionally, overall soda consumption fell across all races/ethnicities.[71]

Non-Hispanic Black and Hispanic children and adults consumed a greater percentage of calories from SSBs than non-Hispanic Whites, and consumed more fruit drinks than soda, whereas non-Hispanic Whites consumed more soda and sports/energy drinks than Hispanics or non-Hispanic Blacks.[70-72] Lastly, less educated and low-income populations are more likely to consume regular soda than are better educated or high-income groups, but low-income children and adolescents are less likely to consume sports/energy drinks.[71] In other words, populations with higher obesity prevalence disparities consume more calories from SSBs, and from different categories of beverages than populations with lower obesity prevalence rates.

Clearly, SSBs remain a major source of excess calories in the American diet while directly contributing to poor health outcomes.[14] As a result, taxation of SSBs can be an attractive policy mechanism to decrease SSB consumption and generate revenue to fund obesity-prevention initiatives, particularly efforts to decrease childhood obesity prevalence.[73-76] There are two tax schemes available to policymakers: (1) sales taxes levied at the register (i.e., not included in the purchase price) and (2) excise taxes included in the shelf or purchase price.[75] Lessons learned from tobacco taxation suggest excise taxes are the preferable approach because consumers are aware of the increased cost at the point-of-purchase.[77]

Thirty-five states currently impose small sales taxes on the sale of soda at retail; fewer states tax other SSBs like isotonics or sport drinks, less than 100% juice drinks, and ready-to-drink teas.[75] The average sales tax rate on regular sodas across all states and the District of Columbia is 3.55% and the average tax rate in taxing states was 5.17% as of January 1, 2015.[78] Additionally, seven states levy additional excise taxes or equivalent fees on manufacture, distribution, wholesale, and/or retail sale of sodas.[75] However, none of the existing taxes were imposed with the intention of reducing consumption of SSBs. For the most part, the small sales taxes have been levied entirely for revenue generation purposes and some of the non-sales taxes have been adopted to fund other state programs. For example, in 1994, a referendum in Arkansas imposed a privilege tax per gallon of soft drinks (bottles, powder, base products, syrups) on distributors, manufacturers, wholesalers, and retailers, with the revenue generated used to fund the Arkansas Medicaid Trust Fund, but there was no declared intent to decrease SSB purchases or impact obesity prevalence.[78–80]

Momentum in this area has been increasing steadily in recent years, particularly with the tremendous advocacy efforts focused on the issue. Between 2010 and early 2015, SSB-specific excise taxes have been proposed in 19 states, 6 municipalities, and the District of Columbia; in addition, a federal SSB tax was proposed in 2014.[81]

Industry Opposition to Sugar-sweetened Beverage Taxes

Of all recently proposed SSB taxes, only the 2014 City of Berkeley excise tax was approved via voter referendum. The tax was not earmarked for a specific purpose and required a simple majority vote, but passed with 75% approval.[82] In contrast, the 2014 San Francisco referendum received a majority vote of 55%, but did not meet the 2/3 majority required under California law for earmarked taxes.[83] In both cities, the American Beverage Association (ABA) poured money into opposition campaigns at much higher rates than supporters of the tax financed campaign efforts.[84,85] ABA spending in San Francisco and Berkeley was patterned after the approach employed during 2012 elections in El Monte and Richmond, California; measures in both cities failed largely as a consequence of the tremendous amount of money spent by the ABA (see Table 7.5).[86,87]

In particular, opposition groups funded local antitax coalitions composed of a wide range of community members, which were not identified as industry-funded. Beverage-industry interests deftly used these groups to exploit existing community attitudes and political issues in each municipality.[88] In Richmond, a history of racial tension was used to frame the tax as White City Council members imposing a tax on the Black community.[88,89] In El Monte, antigovernment sentiment was used to portray

Table 7.5 Amounts Spent by Opponents and Supporters of Sugar-sweetened Beverage Tax Initiatives

Location in California	Year	American Beverage Industry/Opposition	Public Health/Supporters
Berkeley[84]	2014	$2,445,107	$929,048
San Francisco[85]	2014	$9,100,000	$275,000
El Monte[86,87]	2012	$4,100,000 combined	$114,000 combined
Richmond[86,87]	2012		

the tax as balancing the budget at the expense of residents.[88,89] Subsequent media analyses of these campaigns suggest the bills were poorly framed at the local level,[88] indicating that policymakers could do more to engage constituents and reframe the conversation along the lines of "savvy state" messaging.[63]

Another argument frequently presented by the ABA is framed in the context of economic harm; this was the single most common antitax position reported in news coverage of the 2012 proposals in El Monte and Richmond.[88,89] However, an economic analysis published in April 2014, found that with a 20% tax imposed on SSBs in California, beverage industry jobs would be offset by new employment opportunities in other sectors; thus, there was essentially a net zero change in employment in California.[90]

Public Support for Sugar-sweetened Beverage Taxes

Polling data suggests lower public support for SSB taxes in conservative areas, and limited-to-moderate support in liberal areas.[57,60] As mentioned previously, conservatives tend to believe an SSB tax is an infringement on personal choice and not an appropriate use of government regulation, while liberals slightly favor an SSB tax as a mechanism to generate revenue for obesity interventions.[48,57,60,91,92] However, as with other policy options, support increases substantially across both parties when tax revenue is earmarked for obesity prevention measures aimed at children.[50–52,59,91,93–95] Support also increases when tax revenue would be used to fund new healthcare initiatives or avoid service reductions in existing healthcare.[51,55]

An emerging example of changing opinions is underway in Kentucky, a historically conservative Republican state. The 2014 Kentucky Health Issues Poll asked adults

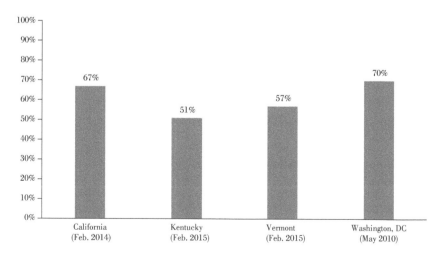

Figure 7.4 Percentage of adults favoring sugar-sweetened beverage taxes in California,[94] Kentucky,[59] Vermont,[95] and Washington, DC.[52]

Created by the authors based on data available from public sources; note year of poll varies by location; refer to the year for each location in the bar chart labels.

whether they favor or oppose an SSB tax to fund school-based nutrition and physical activity programs and found that opinion was divided, with a slight 51% majority favoring SSB taxes.[59] Women and African Americans were more likely than men or White adults to favor the tax, and Louisville and Lexington area residents were more likely than residents in the rest of the state.[59] Kentucky has an adult obesity prevalence of 31%[9] and the polling data could represent a deviation from conservative norms and concurrent desire to curb the obesity epidemic among children. Recent polls in other states show similar trends, as illustrated in Figure 7.4.

It may be that public perception is changing after the Berkeley SSB-tax initiative passed in 2014, generating enough momentum to increase support in other areas of the country. The Berkeley tax may have created a window of opportunity[96] for policymakers in other regions to curb consumption while simultaneously raising revenue for prevention; the framing issues discussed in California can serve as an important start for policymakers to frame their strategies for maximum public support.

CONCLUSION

This chapter aimed to describe the obesity epidemic in the United States and to provide insight into the complexity of the obesity problem through multiple lenses—systems or ecologic, policy, economic, and political. Additionally, we sought to provide examples of a wide range of obesity and food-related policy strategies that have been or are being considered by state and local governments nationwide. Because so much of the policymaking in this domain is left to states and localities, they have a particular role to play in effectuating key policy changes. To this end, we concluded the chapter with a case study that provides a detailed overview of the political and policy issues associated with one hotly debated public policy issue—SSB taxation.

REFERENCES

1. Ogden CL, Yanovski SZ, Carroll MD, et al. The epidemiology of obesity. *Gastroenterology.* 2007;132:2087–2102.
2. Ogden CL, Carroll MD, Kit BK, et al. Prevalence of childhood and adult obesity in the United States, 2011–2012. *JAMA: The Journal of the American Medical Association.* 2014;311:806–814.
3. Flegal KM, Carroll MD, Ogden CL. Trends in obesity and extreme obesity among U.S. adults—reply. *JAMA: The Journal of the American Medical Association.* 2010;303: 1695–1696.
4. Ogden CL. *Obesity and socioeconomic status in adults: United States, 2005–2008.* http:// stacks.cdc.gov/view/cdc/11833/cdc_11833_DS3.pdf. Updated 2010. Accessed March 23, 2015.
5. Fryar CD, Carroll MD, Ogden CL. *Prevalence of overweight, obesity, and extreme obesity among adults: United States, trends 1960–1962 through 2009–2010.* http://198.246.102.49/nchs/ data/hestat/obesity_adult_09_10/obesity_adult_09_10.pdf. Updated 2012. Accessed March 23, 2015.

6. Skinner AC, Skelton JA. Prevalence and trends in obesity and severe obesity among children in the United States, 1999–2012. *JAMA Pediatr.* 2014;168:561–566.

7. Befort CA, Nazir N, Perri MG. Prevalence of obesity among adults from rural and urban areas of the United States: findings from NHANES (2005–2008). *J Rural Health.* 2012;28:392–397.

8. Flegal KM, Carroll MD, Ogden CL, et al. Prevalence and trends in obesity among U.S. adults, 1999–2008. *JAMA: The Journal of the American Medical Association.* 2010;303:235–241.

9. Centers for Disease Control and Prevention. *Obesity Prevalence Maps.* http://www.cdc.gov/obesity/data/prevalence-maps.html. Updated 2014. Accessed March 23, 2015.

10. Cawley J, Meyerhoefer C, Biener A, Hammer M, Wintfeld N. Savings in medical expenditures associated with reductions in body mass index among U.S. adults with obesity, by diabetes status. *Pharmacoeconomics.* In press.

11. Finkelstein EA, Trogdon JG, Cohen JW, et al. Annual medical spending attributable to obesity: payer- and service-specific estimates. *Health Aff.* 2009;28:w822–w831.

12. Trogdon JG, Finkelstein EA, Feagan CW, et al. State- and payer-specific estimates of annual medical expenditures attributable to obesity. *Obesity (Silver Spring).* 2012;20:214–220.

13. Andreyeva T, Luedicke J, Wang YC. State-level estimates of obesity-attributable costs of absenteeism. *J Occup Environ Med.* 2014;56:1120–1127.

14. Institute of Medicine. Committee to Accelerate Progress in Obesity Prevention. *Accelerating Progress in Obesity Prevention: Solving the Weight of the Nation.* Washington, DC: The National Academies Press; 2012.

15. Cutler D, Glaeser E, Shapiro J. *Why have Americans become more obese?* http://www.nber.org/papers/w9446.pdf. Updated 2003. Accessed September 3, 2015.

16. United States Department of Agriculture. *Food Away-from-Home.* http://www.ers.usda.gov/topics/food-choices-health/food-consumption-demand/food-away-from-home.aspx. Updated 2015. Accessed April 25, 2015.

17. Kiener R. Food policy debates: Should the government regulate unhealthy foods? *CQ Researcher.* 2014;24:817–840.

18. Hilmers A, Hilmers DC, Dave J. Neighborhood disparities in access to healthy foods and their effects on environmental justice. *Am J Public Health.* 2012;102:1644–1654.

19. Zenk SN, Powell LM, Rimkus L, et al. Relative and absolute availability of healthier food and beverage alternatives across communities in the United States. *Am J Public Health.* 2014;104:2170–2178.

20. Powell LM, Chaloupka FJ, Bao Y. The availability of fast-food and full-service restaurants in the United States: associations with neighborhood characteristics. *Am J Prev Med.* 2007;33:S240–S245.

21. United States Department of Agriculture. *Programs and Services.* http://www.fns.usda.gov/programs-and-services. Updated 2014. Accessed April 24, 2015.

22. Child Nutrition and WIC Reauthorization Act of 2004. P.L. 108–265. 2004.

23. *Dietary Guidelines for Americans* (6th ed.). 2005. Washington, DC, U.S. Department of Health and Human Services and U.S. Department of Agriculture.

24. Categories of Foods of Minimal Nutritional Value, 7 C.F.R. 210, Appendix B.

25. Healthy, Hunger-Free Kids Act of 2010 § 208, 42 U.S.C. § 1779. http://www.gpo.gov/fdsys/pkg/USCODE-2011-title42/pdf/USCODE-2011-title42-chap13A-sec1779.pdf. Updated 2011. Accessed February 24, 2014.

26. United States Department of Agriculture. National School Lunch Program and School Breakfast Program: nutrition standards for all foods sold in school as required by the Healthy, Hunger-Free Kids Act of 2010: interim final rule. *Federal Register.* 2013;78:39068–39120.

27. School Nutrition Association. *Smart Snacks: State Fundraising Exemptions.* https://school-nutrition.org/uploadedFiles/Legislation_and_Policy/State_and_Local_Legislation_and_Regulations/SmartSnacksFundraisingExemption.pdf. Updated 2015. Accessed April 24, 2015.

28. United States Department of Agriculture. *Supplemental Nutrition Assistance Program (SNAP): Historical Waivers Database.* http://www.fns.usda.gov/snap/waivers-rules. Updated 2015. Accessed April 24, 2015.

29. New York City Department of Health & Mental Hygiene. *Removing SNAP Subsidy for Sugar-Sweetened Beverages.* http://www.nyc.gov/html/doh/downloads/pdf/cdp/cdp-snap-faq.pdf. Updated 2010. Accessed April 24, 2015.

30. Kersh R, Morone JA. Obesity, courts, and the new politics of public health. *J Health Polit Policy Law.* 2005;30:839–868.

31. Kersh R. The politics of obesity: a current assessment and look ahead. *Milbank Q.* 2009;87:295–316.

32. CATO Institute. *The Nanny State.* http://www.cato.org/cato-handbook-policymakers/cato-handbook-policy-6th-edition-2005. Updated 2005. Accessed March 23, 2015.

33. Snowdon C. *The Slippery Slope of Food Regulations.* http://www.cato-unbound.org/2015/01/27/christopher-snowdon/slippery-slope-food-regulations. Updated 2015. Accessed March 23, 2015.

34. *Center for Science in the Public Interest.* http://www.cspinet.org/about/index.html. Updated 2014. Accessed March 23, 2015.

35. *Voices for Healthy Kids.* http://www.heart.org/HEARTORG/Advocate/Voices-for-Healthy-Kids_UCM_453195_SubHomePage.jsp. Updated 2015. Accessed March 23, 2015.

36. Mantel B. Preventing obesity. *CQ Researcher.* 2010;20:797–820.

37. National Institute on Money in State Politics. Selected food and beverage industry contributions to candidates and committees in elections in 2014. www.followthemoney.org. Updated 2015. Accessed March 30, 2015.

38. Nestle M. Dieticians put seal on Kraft Singles (you can't make this stuff up). http://www.foodpolitics.com/2015/03/dietitians-put-seal-on-kraft-singles-you-cant-make-this-stuff-up/. Updated 2015. Accessed March 23, 2015.

39. Nestle M. Dieticians in turmoil over conflicts of interest: it's about time. http://www.foodpolitics.com/2015/03/dietitians-in-turmoil-over-conflicts-of-interest-its-about-time/. Updated 2015. Accessed March 23, 2015.

40. Dodson EA, Fleming C, Boehmer TK, et al. Preventing childhood obesity through state policy: qualitative assessment of enablers and barriers. *J Public Health Policy.* 2009;30(Suppl 1):S161–S176.

41. Robbins R, Niederdeppe J, Lundell H, et al. Views of city, county, and state policy makers about childhood obesity in New York State, 2010–2011. *Prev Chronic Dis.* 2013;10:E195.

42. Strom S. A cheese "product" gains kids' nutrition seal. *New York Times.* March 13, 2015;B3.

43. Evich HB. Behind the school lunch fight. http://www.politico.com/story/2014/06/michelle-obama-public-school-lunch-school-nutrition-association-lets-move-107390.html. Updated 2014. Accessed March 23, 2015.

44. Change.org. *Petitioning The Academy of Nutrition and Dietetics/Kids Eat Right Foundation.* https://www.change.org/p/the-academy-of-nutrition-and-dietetics-kids-eat-right-foundation-repealtheseal?just_created=true. Updated 2015. Accessed March 23, 2015.

45. Dieticians for Professional Integrity. FAQ. http://www.integritydietitians.org/about-us/faq. Updated 2013. Accessed March 23, 2015.

46. Nixon R. Nutrition group lobbies against healthier school meals it sought, citing cost. *New York Times.* July 2, 2014;A18.

47. Field Research Corporation. Nationwide findings from the 2013 Kaiser Permanente Childhood Obesity Prevention Survey. http://xnet.kp.org/newscenter/pressreleases/nat/2013/downloads/2013-KP-Childhood-Obesity-Prevention-Survey-Findings.pdf. Updated 2013. Accessed March 23, 2015.

48. Tompson T, Benz J, Agiesta J, et al. Obesity in the United States: public perceptions. http://www.apnorc.org/PDFs/Obesity/AP-NORC-Obesity-Research-Highlights.pdf. Updated 2014. Accessed March 23, 2015.

49. Mendes E. Americans' concerns about obesity soar, surpass smoking. http://www.gallup.com/poll/155762/americans-concerns-obesity-soar-surpass-smoking.aspx. Updated 2012. Accessed March 23, 2015.

50. DiCamillo M, Field M. Most Californians see a direct linkage between obesity and sugary sodas. http://www.uconnruddcenter.org/files/Pdfs/CA_Field_Poll_2_13.pdf. Updated 2013. Accessed March 23, 2015.

51. Center for Rural Studies at the University of Vermont. 2011 Vermont sugar-sweetened beverage tax study. http://www.uconnruddcenter.org/files/Pdfs/VT_SSB_Poll_2011.pdf. Updated 2011. Accessed March 23, 2015.

52. Global Strategy Group and The Strategy Group. Survey of DC voters on proposed sugar-sweetened beverage tax. http://www.uconnruddcenter.org/files/Pdfs/DC_SSBTaxSurvey_5_10.pdf. Updated 2010. Accessed March 23, 2015.

53. Citizens' Committee for Children of New York. Voter preferences for closing the New York state budget gap. http://www.uconnruddcenter.org/resources/upload/docs/what/policy/SSBtaxes/NYPoll12.08.pdf. Updated 2008. Accessed March 23, 2015.

54. Global Strategy Group. STC MS statewide soda tax. http://www.uconnruddcenter.org/files/Pdfs/Mississippi_SodaTaxPoll_1_10.pdf. Updated 2010. Accessed March 23, 2015.

55. Quinnipiac University Polling Institute. New Yorkers oppose fat-tax 2–1. http://www.uconnruddcenter.org/files/Pdfs/NY_TaxPoll_4_10.pdf. Updated 2010. Accessed March 23, 2015.

56. Barry CL, Niederdeppe J, Gollust SE. Taxes on sugar-sweetened beverages: results from a 2011 national public opinion survey. *Am J Prev Med.* 2013;44:158–163.

57. Gollust SE, Barry CL, Niederdeppe J. Americans' opinions about policies to reduce consumption of sugar-sweetened beverages. *Prev Med.* 2014;63:52–57.

58. Federal Election Commission. *Federal Elections 2012: Election Results for the U.S. President, the U.S. Senate and the U.S. House of Representatives.* http://www.fec.gov/pubrec/fe2012/federalelections2012.pdf. Updated 2013. Accessed March 23, 2015.

59. Foundation for a Healthy Kentucky. Kentuckians' views on soda and sugary drink policies. http://healthy-ky.org/sites/default/files/KHIP%20soda%20FINAL%2003l015.pdf. Updated 2015. Accessed March 23, 2015.

60. Gollust SE, Niederdeppe J, Barry CL. Framing the consequences of childhood obesity to increase public support for obesity prevention policy. *Am J Public Health.* 2013;103:e96–e102.

61. Barry CL, Brescoll VL, Brownell KD, et al. Obesity metaphors: how beliefs about the causes of obesity affect support for public policy. *Milbank Q.* 2009;87:7–47.

62. Barry CL, Brescoll VL, Gollust SE. Framing childhood obesity: how individualizing the problem affects public support for prevention. *Polit Psych.* 2013;34:327–349.

63. Chokshi DA, Stine NW. Reconsidering the politics of public health. *JAMA: The Journal of the American Medical Association.* 2013;310:1025–1026.

64. Malik VS, Popkin BM, Bray GA, et al. Sugar-sweetened beverages, obesity, type 2 diabetes mellitus, and cardiovascular disease risk. *Circulation.* 2010;121:1356–1364.

65. Malik VS, Pan A, Willett WC, et al. Sugar-sweetened beverages and weight gain in children and adults: a systematic review and meta-analysis. *Am J Clin Nutr.* 2013;98:1084–1102.

66. Chen L, Caballero B, Mitchell DC, et al. Reducing consumption of sugar-sweetened beverages is associated with reduced blood pressure: a prospective study among United States adults. *Circulation.* 2010;121:2398–2406.

67. Fung TT, Malik V, Rexrode KM, et al. Sweetened beverage consumption and risk of coronary heart disease in women. *Am J Clin Nutr.* 2009;89:1037–1042.

68. Duffey KJ, Popkin BM. Shifts in patterns and consumption of beverages between 1965 and 2002. *Obesity (Silver Spring).* 2007;15:2739–2747.

69. United States Department of Agriculture. *Empty Calories: How Many Can I Have?* http://choosemyplate.gov/weight-management-calories/calories/empty-calories-amount.html. Updated 2015. Accessed April 25, 2015.

70. Ogden CL, Kit BK, Carroll MD, et al. Consumption of sugar drinks in the United States, 2005–2008. *NCHS Data Brief.* 2011;71:1–8.

71. Han E, Powell LM. Consumption patterns of sugar-sweetened beverages in the United States. *J Acad Nutr Diet.* 2013;113:43–53.

72. Dodd AH, Briefel R, Cabili C, et al. Disparities in consumption of sugar-sweetened and other beverages by race/ethnicity and obesity status among United States schoolchildren. *J Nutr Educ Behav.* 2013;45:240–249.

73. Brownell KD, Farley T, Willett WC, et al. The public health and economic benefits of taxing sugar-sweetened beverages. *The New England Journal of Medicine.* 2009;361:1599–1605.

74. Chaloupka FJ, Powell LM, Chriqui JF. Sugar-sweetened beverages and obesity: the potential impact of public policies. *J Policy Anal Manage.* 2011;30:645–655.

75. Chriqui JF, Chaloupka FJ, Powell LM, et al. A typology of beverage taxation: multiple approaches for obesity prevention and obesity prevention-related revenue generation. *J Public Health Policy.* 2013;34:403–423.

76. Pomeranz JL. Advanced policy options to regulate sugar-sweetened beverages to support public health. *J Public Health Policy.* 2012;33:75–88.

77. Chaloupka FJ, Powell LM, Chriqui JF. *Sugar-sweetened beverage taxation as public health policy—lessons from tobacco.* http://www.choicesmagazine.org/choices-magazine/policy-issues/sugar-sweetened-beverage-taxation-as-public-health-policylessons-from-tobacco. Updated 2015. Accessed March 23, 2015.

78. Bridging the Gap Research Program. Beverage and snack taxes. http://www.bridgingthegapresearch.org/research/sodasnack_taxes/. Updated 2015. Accessed March 23, 2015.

79. Smith D. Will the soda pop tax go national? Arkansans already pay it. http://www.arktimes.com/arkansas/will-the-soda-pop-tax-go-national/Content?oid=949896. Updated 2009. Accessed March 23, 2015.

80. *Arkansas Soft Drink Tax, Referred Act 1 (1994).* http://ballotpedia.org/Arkansas_Soft_Drink_Tax_Referred_Act_1_(1994). Updated 1994. Accessed March 23, 2015.

81. UCONN Rudd Center for Food Policy & Obesity. *Legislative database.* http://www.uconnruddcenter.org/legislation-database. Updated 2015. Accessed March 23, 2015.

82. Dinkelspiel F. Why Berkeley passed a soda tax while other cities failed. http://www.berkeleyside.com/2014/11/05/why-berkeley-passed-a-soda-tax-where-others-failed/. Updated 2014. Accessed March 23, 2015.

83. Knight H. Why Berkeley passed a soda tax and S.F. didn't. http://www.sfgate.com/bayarea/article/Why-Berkeley-passed-a-soda-tax-and-S-F-didn-t-5879757.php.%20Updated%20November%207. Updated 2014. Accessed March 23, 2015.

84. Dinkelspiel F. Around $3.4m spent on Berkeley soda tax campaign. http://www.berkeleyside.com/2015/02/05/around-3-4m-spent-on-berkeley-soda-tax-campaign/. Updated 2015. Accessed March 23, 2015.

85. Zigas E. Why did Berkeley pass a soda tax and not San Francisco? http://www.spur.org/blog/2014-11-25/why-did-berkeley-pass-soda-tax-and-not-san-francisco. Updated 2014. Accessed March 23, 2015.

86. Oatman M. The soda tax lost. Now what? http://www.motherjones.com/bluemarble/2012/11/soda-taxes-fail-california-richmond-ritterman. Updated 2012. Accessed March 23, 2015.

87. Zingale D. Gulp! The high cost of Big Soda's victory. http://articles.latimes.com/2012/dec/09/opinion/la-oe-zingale-soda-tax-campaign-funding-20121209. Updated 2012. Accessed March 31, 2015.

88. Nixon L, Mejia P, Cheyne A, et al. Big Soda's long shadow: news coverage of local proposals to tax sugar-sweetened beverages in Richmond, El Monte and Telluride. *Crit Public Health.* 2014;25:333–347.

89. Mejia P, Nixon L, Cheyne A, Dorfman L, Quintero F. Issue 21: Two communities, two debates: News coverage of soda tax proposals in Richmond and El Monte. http://www.bmsg.org/resources/publications/news-coverage-soda-tax-proposals-Richmond-El-Monte-California. Updated 2014. Accessed March 23, 2015.

90. Powell LM, Wada R, Persky JJ, et al. Employment impact of sugar-sweetened beverage taxes. *Am J Public Health.* 2014;104:672–677.

91. Simon PA, Chiang C, Lightstone AS, et al. Public opinion on nutrition-related policies to combat child obesity, Los Angeles County, 2011. *Prev Chronic Dis.* 2014;11:E96.

92. Harris Interactive. Many Americans ambivalent over laws aimed at healthy living: poll. http://www.harrisinteractive.com/NewsRoom/PressReleases/tabid/446/mid/1506/articleId/986/ctl/ReadCustom%20Default/Default.aspx. Updated 2012. Accessed March 23, 2015.

93. DiCamillo M, Field M. Unhealthy eating, lack of physical activity seen as greatest health risk facing California kids. http://www.uconnruddcenter.org/files/Pdfs/CA_Field_Poll_4_12.pdf. Updated 2012. Accessed March 23, 2015.

94. DiCamillo M, Field M. Broad voter support for posting a health warning label on sodas and sugary drinks and taxing their sale to provide funds for school nutrition and physical activity programs. http://www.calendow.org/uploadedFiles/Rls2461.pdf. Updated 2014. Accessed March 23, 2015.

95. True M. Poll shows support for carbon, sugary drink taxes. http://vtdigger.org/2015/03/05/poll-shows-support-for-carbon-sugary-drink-taxes/. Updated 2015. Accessed March 23, 2015.

96. Kingdon JW. *Agendas, Alternatives, and Public Policies.* 2nd ed. New York: Addison-Wesley Educational Publishers, Inc.; 2003.

8

Public Policy and Physical Activity

Amy A. Eyler and Marissa Zwald

LEARNING OBJECTIVES

1. Describe the significance of physical inactivity as a public health topic.
2. Explain public policy approaches to increasing population physical activity.
3. Discuss various stakeholders involved with physical activity policy.
4. Describe examples of physical activity policy.

IDENTIFYING THE PROBLEM: PHYSICAL INACTIVITY AND CONSEQUENCES

The importance of physical activity for disease prevention and health promotion is well established. Known health benefits include the prevention of risk factors related to cardiovascular disease, improvements in functional health and mental health, and reduction in premature deaths.[1] Published in 1996, the first U.S. Surgeon General's Report on Physical Activity and Health highlighted the evidence for these important associations and set the stage for subsequent national support for the promotion of physical activity.[2] More recently, an advisory committee was formed to review and analyze existing scientific literature and update the overall physical activity recommendations. This resulted in the 2008 Physical Activity Guidelines for Americans.[3] The authors of these guidelines recommend that for substantial health benefits, adults should participate weekly in at least 150 minutes of moderate intensity activity, 75 minutes of vigorous intensity activity, or an equivalent combination, with additional benefits gained from doubling this amount.[1] Children should participate in 60 minutes or more of physical activity each day, with the majority of these minutes being of moderate-to-vigorous intensity. However, only 36.5% of children and 41.1% of adults met these guidelines in 2009–2010,[4] and rates have shown little improvement over the last decade.[5]

Descriptive Epidemiology

Surveillance data also has shown that physical activity prevalence varies by population subgroup. Being female, older age, Hispanic, having lower levels of education, and having a higher body mass index (BMI) are shown to be associated with being less physically active.[5] Moreover, the prevalence of physical inactivity is also of concern and varies by state. In 33 states, almost one quarter of the population reported not engaging in any leisure-time physical activity. (See Figure 8.1.)

The prevalence of inactivity and increasingly sedentary behaviors comes with additional adverse health effects. Technology coupled with reduced physical activity in occupational work, home/domestic work, and travel have all contributed to an increasingly sedentary population.[6] Current estimates suggest that adults are sedentary for 7.7 hours per day, with screen time (television, video, Internet) being the most common sedentary leisure-time behavior.[7,8] Because living in modern societies

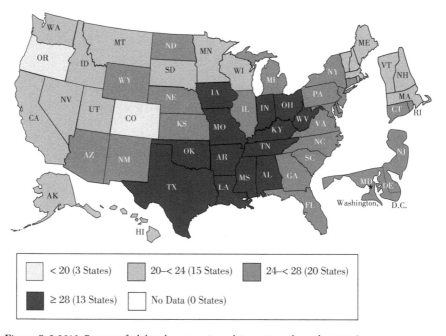

Figure 8.1 2013: Percent of adults who engage in no leisure-time physical activity.*

*Respondents were classified as participating in no leisure-time physical activity if they responded "no" to the following question: "During the past month, other than your regular job, did you participate in any physical activities or exercises such as running, calisthenics, golf, gardening, or walking for exercise?" Adults aged ≥18 years. Respondents with missing data were excluded.

Notes: National includes 50 states and the -District of Columbia.

Data Source: Behavioral Risk Factor Surveillance System.

Suggested Citation: Nutrition, Physical Activity and Obesity Data, Trends and Maps website. United States Department of Health and Human Services, Centers for Disease Control and Prevention (CDC), National Center for Chronic Disease Prevention and Health Promotion, Division of Nutrition, Physical Activity and Obesity, Atlanta, GA; 2015. Available at http://www.cdc.gov/nccdphp/DNPAO/index.html.

requires little daily physical activity and encourages sedentary behavior, direct efforts are needed to promote an increase in "lifestyle" activity or ways to build more physical movement, and less sedentary time, into the daily lives of Americans. Policies can play an important role in promoting lifestyle physical activity by making the choice to be physically active the "easy choice."

PUBLIC POLICY STRATEGIES RELATED TO PHYSICAL ACTIVITY

Motivating people to be physically active can be difficult and is made even more challenging by environments where few opportunities to be physically active exist.[4,9] Traditional strategies that focus on the individual have had limited success in promoting long-term adherence to physical activity, thus emphasizing the need for broader, policy-level approaches.[9,10] Although physical activity is often thought of as a personal choice, rather than something needing policy or governmental influence,[11] policies can impact this behavior in many ways. Effective intervention strategies include policy and environmental changes designed to provide opportunities, support, and cues to help people become more physically active.[12,13] At the public policy level, examples include the initiation and implementation of policies that promote physical activity, policies that enhance opportunities for whole populations to be active, and policies that develop environments for promoting active choices.[14] In the United States, three overarching evidence-based policy and environmental strategies are recommended. These include creating or enhancing safe places for physical activity, enhancing physical education and physical activity in schools, and supporting street and community-scale designs that facilitate physical activity.[15] Intersecting with these policy approaches, a recent Institute of Medicine Committee also recommended enhancing the physical and built environment as an approach to increasing physical activity and reducing obesity.[16] Policies can be particularly relevant in reducing barriers that often inhibit physical activity. These barriers include automobile-oriented transportation systems or community designs that require driving, sedentary jobs, lack of physical education in schools, and lack of or poorly maintained parks and public spaces.[17]

As indicated by the recommended policies for increasing physical activity, the scope for improving this behavior crosses many sectors and policy scales. A key framework on physical activity policy was developed by Schmid and colleagues (2006) and has guided the past decade of physical activity policy research.[18] This conceptual framework illustrates an intersection of scale of policy with settings in which policies are developed or applied. (See Figure 8.2.)

As depicted in Figure 8.2, policy approaches can influence populations at the local, regional, state, or national level and span multiple sectors. Across these varied scales and sectors, policy approaches also can take many different forms, from unwritten social norms that may influence key stakeholders to formal or informal legislation, regulations, codes, or standards, which can be initiated by either governmental

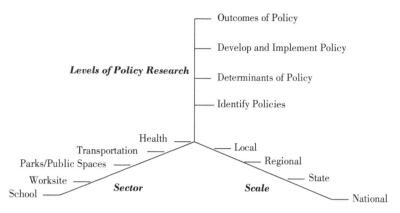

Figure 8.2 Framework for physical activity policy research.
Source: Adapted from Schmid T, Pratt M, Witmer L. A framework for physical activity policy research. *Journal of Physical Activity and Health.* 2006;3(Suppl 1):S20–S29.

or nongovernmental organizations.[9,18,19] Examples of state and local physical activity policies by sector and scale are depicted in Table 8.1.

Because of this broad scope, a policy approach to increasing population physical activity requires collaboration and interaction among a wide variety of stakeholders and policymakers.[9,10,13,18] This often involves sectors outside of health. For example, engagement may be needed from representatives of community organizations, urban planners, transportation specialists, architects, and developers who can provide relevant input in initiating and implementing sustainable strategies for improving the physical environment of communities and making it supportive of physical activity.[20] Transdisciplinary collaboration for these changes, while necessary, can be challenging, because strategies and reasons for desired outcome may differ.[21] Cooperation and a shared vision are key to successful policy initiatives promoting population physical activity.[9,22] Although some stakeholders may have increased physical activity as their primary goal, others see increased physical activity as a conduit to their main purpose. For example, in a study conducted by Eyler et al. on policies related to active transportation to and from school, the authors found that even though increasing the number of children who walk or bicycle to school will inevitably increase the time students spend being physically active, key stakeholders reported a variety of reasons for supporting the policies.[22] They indicated reasons ranging from traffic abatement around the school (public safety officials), reduced bus costs (school administration), to better student attention and focus for lessons (teachers).[22,23] Cooperation and creating a shared vision of varied goals and objectives across stakeholders is key to successful policy initiatives to promote population physical activity.[24]

The complexity of stakeholders and sectors involved in physical activity promotion also is exemplified in the U.S. National Physical Activity Plan.[25,26] This comprehensive plan, established in 2010, provides overall goals for increasing physical activity in the United States. It also offers policy and practice recommendations and epidemiological evidence to support its recommendations across eight different

Table 8.1 Examples of Policy Strategies Related to Physical Activity

Policy Strategy (in alphabetical order)	Example	Typical Jurisdiction(s) Where Policy May Be Adopted	Typical Policy Instrument(s)[a] Employed
Active transportation	Funding for infrastructure improvements and programming for active transport to and from school	Federal State School District	LA, RA, B
Design standards	Require specific design standards such as stairwell placement for public buildings	State Local/Regional	LS, RA
Land use	Zoning ordinance for park development	Local/Regional	RA, B
Parking	Restricting parking near buildings	Local/Regional	RA
Physical activity opportunities in before and after school programs	Specify the percentage of time in programs that must be spent in physical activity	State School District	LS, RA
Physical activity opportunities within the school day	Require daily recess for elementary school students	State School District	LS, RA
Physical education	Specify the required amount and type of physical education in schools	State School District	LS, RA
Public transportation	Providing funding for development or expansion of public transit	Local/Regional	RA, B
Shared use/joint use	Allow for access of school facilities for community physical activity	State School District	LS, RA
Sidewalks/bike lanes	Requiring streets to accommodate all users	State Local/Regional	RA
Trails/active recreation	Providing funding for building and maintenance of recreational trails	State Local/Regional	LS, RA, B

[a]LS=legislative/statutory (includes ordinances and zoning at local levels), RA=regulatory/administrative law, B=ballot initiative.

sectors: public health, business/industry, education, health care, mass media, parks/recreation/fitness/sports, transportation/land use/community design, and volunteer/nonprofit (http://www.physicalactivityplan.org/). Each sector presents strategies aimed at promoting physical activity and outlines specific tactics to address each strategy. Because of the integration of this plan, there are several overarching strategies. One of the overarching strategies states, "Disseminate best practice physical activity models, programs, and policies to the widest extent practical to ensure Americans can access strategies that will enable them to meet federal physical activity guidelines." The models, programs, and policies recommended in the plan will likely cross sectors. And, in order to be effective, they will depend on support from multiple stakeholders at the local, state, and federal level. Transportation funding policy is a good example of this.

Infrastructure that facilitates transportation choices such as walking, bicycling, and transit can affect state systems, communities, schools, and neighborhoods. Funding for transportation infrastructure is allocated from federal transportation money, which is then distributed to the states. Each state then prioritizes projects and allocates funding throughout the state. Advocates, state department personnel, local and regional planning organizations, and policymakers at state and local levels can influence how the allocated funds are spent. Congress, however, develops and approves federal transportation bills, with a specific time parameter. SAFETEA-LU (Safe, Accountable, Flexible, Efficient, Transportation Equity Act—A Legacy for All Users) was the bill signed into law by President George W. Bush in 2005. Provisions of the bill officially ended in 2009, but were extended to 2012. The bill included dedicated funding to support biking and walking activity, through such programs as (1) Transportation Enhancements, (2) Safe Routes to School (SRTS) and (3) Recreational Trails.[27] States were required to use 1.5% of their total transportation fund on Transportation Enhancement programs, which included projects that make active transportation options like biking and walking safer and more convenient. The 2012 federal transportation bill MAP-21 (Moving Ahead for Progress in the 21st century) replaced SAFETEA-LU, but reduced the amount of funds allocated for these programs and consolidated them into one lump sum under a program called Transportation Alternatives. There is no longer a state requirement to spend a percentage of these funds on active transportation, and a broader scope of projects must now compete for a reduced amount of funds. Additionally, there is an option for states to move up to half of their resources in the Transportation Alternatives fund to other unrelated projects. In MAP-21, the reduction in funding amount, change in program structure, and added flexibility for states can be a detriment to bicycle and pedestrian projects.[28] Increased advocacy and collaboration across sectors and policy scales for infrastructure that is conducive to active transportation is vital to successfully competing for these funds.

Physical Activity Policy Examples around the Globe

Several good examples exist of how countries outside the United States are using policy to increase population physical activity. For over a decade, Brazil has recognized the importance of promoting physical activity, and it now has a place on the national agenda. The Brazilian government, along with important nongovernmental organizations and academic institutions, developed The Academia da Cidade Program (loosely translated as "city gyms"), which is a health promotion policy with a focus on physical activity, leisure, and healthy eating. This program, which started in the city of Recife in 2002, now has a participation rate of over 300,000 and includes 19 settings in which activities are offered free of charge.[29-32] To expand this successful program, the Brazilian Ministry of Health has supported the creation of a national network of researchers and practitioners organized around the promotion and development of infrastructure that supports the adoption of healthy lifestyles, including the practice of community-based physical activity. One of the most recent initiatives is the creation of the Academia da Saude, a national program that expands a physical activity intervention to 4,000 new municipalities around the country over the next five years.[33]

Another successful policy example is the Ciclovia Recreativa project, which originated in Bogota, Colombia. The Ciclovia program temporarily closes streets to motorized transport, allowing access only to walkers, runners, and cyclists for recreation and socialization. Between 1974 and 1976, the Ciclovia concept was developed and supported by mayoral decree in Bogota. The Ciclovia movement has sustained turnover within city administration and other challenges throughout the first decades of implementation. It is now implemented every Sunday and holiday throughout the year from 7 AM to 2 PM over a 121-kilometer-long stretch of road in sectors throughout the city. It boasts some 1,000,000 participants per event. Evaluation of Ciclovia in Bogota shows that these events have a positive impact on the community. Participants are likely to meet the recommended amounts of physical activity,[34] and the program has been reported as cost beneficial.[35] The success and popularity of Ciclovia has caused the phenomenon to spread to cities in countries around the globe. In 2014, over 100 cities in the United States hosted a Ciclovia or Open Streets event.[36]

ADVOCACY FOR PHYSICAL ACTIVITY POLICY

Because many policymakers and stakeholders may not think of physical activity as a behavior influenced by a broad scope of policies and environments, education and advocacy is important. Advocacy for physical activity policy through individual and organizational efforts is often the first step in increasing awareness. Communicating effectively with key decision-makers regarding the importance of a physically active population to the health, social well-being, and economic welfare of a region is imperative. (See Chapters 15 and 16 for more information on communication and advocacy.) Additionally, some policies that promote physical activity within communities may cause controversy and adversarial arguments. For example, requiring sidewalks and bike lanes on streets may encourage active transportation, but these policies also may affect automobile travel. Modifications in roads, such as reduced lane size or traffic slowing modifications (e.g., roundabouts or speed bumps) can cause controversy within transportation planning as well as the community. Advocates must provide evidence-based and easy to understand arguments to educate the stakeholders and effectively increase awareness. Several national and international agencies serve as advocates for policies that promote physical activity at the international, federal, state, and local level. Examples of these are listed in Table 8.2.

CASE STUDIES

Some policies explicitly state that increasing physical activity (e.g., requiring daily physical education) is a priority, but others such as those related to transportation or community design may offer increased physical activity as a "byproduct" of the policy. Yet other policies completely unrelated to the goal of increasing physical activity have the potential to impact how physically active we are. The following cases offer some examples.

The Case for Physical Education Policies

Guidance for the requirements for physical education (PE) in schools is a good example of direct policy impact on physical activity. The Institute of Medicine defines PE as "a planned sequential K–12 standards-based program of curricula and instruction designed to develop motor skills, knowledge, and behaviors of healthy active living, physical fitness, sportsmanship, self-efficacy, and emotional intelligence."[37] A review conducted by the U.S. Community Guide taskforce revealed strong evidence connecting improvements in PE with increased amounts of moderate-to-vigorous intensity physical activity and students' physical fitness.[15] Improving PE in schools is also recommended as an equitable strategy to impact child and adolescent health; PE classes reach large numbers of children and adolescents across various geographic regions, income levels, and races/ethnicities. However, national mandates on achievement-related funding for schools have resulted in a reduction in instructional time for subjects such as PE that are deemed "nonessential."[38] In 2013, less than half (48%) of high school students attended PE classes during an average week.[39]

Most states have enacted laws related to PE, but the strength of these policies varies from merely indicating how much PE is required for high school graduation to specifying how many days and minutes of PE schools must offer. The majority (74.5%) of states mandate that students must take PE, but requirements vary by grade level. In 2012, only three states (New Jersey, Louisiana, and Florida) require the nationally recommended 150+ minutes per week/30 minutes per day for elementary schools and 225+ minutes per week/30 minutes per day for middle schools (Montana, West Virginia, Utah).[40,41] Most states also have policies that allow waivers and/or substitutions for PE requirements, thus reducing the strength or impact of the PE requirement policies. In many states, a student's involvement in sports, cheerleading, or military preparation programs can substitute for PE course requirements.[42]

The difference in state governance of schools can influence PE policy development and enactment. Some states establish standards, or very broad guidelines, for curriculum content through state policy but defer to local school districts when it comes time

Table 8.2 Examples of Organizations Involved with Physical Activity Policy Advocacy

Name	Purpose	URL
Smart Growth America	Smart Growth America advocates for building better towns and cities that have housing and transportation options near jobs, shops, and schools.	http://www.smartgrowthamerica.org
America Walks	America Walks advocates for walkable communities to promote physically, mentally, and economically healthy neighborhoods.	http://americawalks.org/a-walkable-america/
National Coalition for Promoting Physical Activity	The National Coalition for Promoting Physical Activity's mission is to unite the strengths of public, private, and industry efforts into collaborative partnerships that empower all Americans to be physically active.	http://www.ncpphysicalactivity.org/about-us
American College of Sports Medicine	This National Association advocates for federal, state, and local policies that are likely to result in healthy lifestyles.	http://www.acsm.org/about-acsm/policy-center
SHAPE America	SHAPE America's mission is to advance professional practice and promote research related to health and physical education, physical activity, dance, and sport.	http://www.shapeamerica.org/about/
Action for Healthy Kids	Action for Healthy Kids fights childhood obesity, undernourishment, and physical inactivity by helping schools become healthier places.	http://www.actionforhealthykids.org/about-us
SPARK	SPARK advocates for quality physical education and physical activity programs in schools.	http://www.sphysicalactivityrkpe.org/physical-education-resources/advocacy/
American Heart Association	The American Heart association advocates for Congress to play a key role in shaping environments and supporting communities in promoting healthy choices.	http://www.heart.org/HEARTORG/Advocate/IssuesandCampaigns/Prevention/Nutrition-and-Physical-Activity_UCM_307737_Article.jsp

(*continued*)

Table 8.2 (Continued)

Name	Purpose	URL
International Society for Physical Activity and Health	ISPAH has an advocacy council aimed at political advocacy, media advocacy, professional and community mobilization, and advocacy within organizations to increase physical activity.	http://www.ispah.org/ispahabout

for specific decisions regarding time, class size, and student assessment.[40] Additionally, enforcement of implementation and evaluation of laws vary.[43,44] A 2010 study by Sanchez-Vaznaugh et al. found that only 50% of school districts studied in California were reported as being in compliance with the state physical education mandate.[45] Without a system for accountability or enforcement of a state PE policy, there is less of a chance the law will achieve its intended outcome of increased physical activity.[42,43,45]

Significant opportunities exist to strengthen PE laws, particularly at the state level. Research shows that district policies are stronger within states that have strong policies.[43,46,47] In a study of district-level PE coordinators, PE was provided more days per week—and had more dedicated minutes in elementary and middle schools—in states with specific PE requirement laws (i.e., specified number of days and minutes of PE) compared with schools in states that lack such requirements.[43] Enacting state PE policies is a way to increase physical activity among children and adolescents, but the success of these policies is dependent upon mechanisms to improve implementation and compliance at both state and district levels.

The Case of *Complete Streets* Policies

Transportation or design policies may have the primary goal of community improvement, but can implicitly affect physical activity. For example, a growing body of evidence suggests that features of the built environment (e.g., infrastructure for walking and bicycling, public transit, street connectivity, mixed land use) influence the likelihood that people will use active transportation for their daily travel.[48] Policies at the state, regional, or local level often guide these design and transportation elements within communities. *Complete Streets* is a concept whereby streets are designed and operated to enable safe access for all users including pedestrians, bicyclists, motorists, and transit riders of all ages and abilities.[28] In 2014, over 665 regional and local jurisdictions, 30 states, the Commonwealth of Puerto Rico, and the District of Columbia have implemented some form of Complete Streets policy.[28]

Complete Streets definitions vary across communities based on local priorities and contexts. Most describe considering multiple modes, accounting for the varying interests of users, and advancing a safer and more accessible transportation system.[49] A "complete" street in a rural area may look different from a "complete" street in a highly urban area, but both are designed to balance the safety and convenience of everyone using the road.[49] In addition to differences in Complete Streets policies across rural and urban settings, these types of policies also come in many shapes and sizes. Complete Streets policies range from laws and ordinances to resolutions, executive orders, and policies adopted by elected boards. Some are merely resolutions passed by city councils, still others are the result of state departments of transportation gaining extensive public input and rewriting their design manuals. Some Complete Streets policies are implemented more formally through state and local legislation or ordinances.[50]

Several good examples of how this policy affects physical activity exist. Boulder, Colorado, for example, has been implementing Complete Streets policy since 1990. The city has made an explicit decision to focus its transportation strategy on multi-modal corridors and networks.[49] Improvements to transportation infrastructure, such as bike lanes, paved shoulders, and a comprehensive transit network, have impacted resident travel patterns.[51] The National Research Center found that between 1990 and 2006, fewer people in the city drove alone, more people walked or bicycled, and transit trips almost doubled.[52] Because trips taken by public transit often begin or end with either walking or bicycling to a bus or rail stop, it is important to note that access to public transit also impacts physical activity. Studies show that transit users participate in an average of 12–19 minutes of physical activity each day walking to and from transit stops.[53,54] Improving access to public transit through Complete Streets policies has the subsequent benefit of increasing physical activity.

Portland, Oregon offers another example of the effect of Complete Streets on physical activity. Between 1991 and 2008, the number of city bikeway miles in Portland increased from 75 miles to 275 miles through Complete Streets policies. Using objective daily counts on four main bridges, the number of bicyclists has exponentially increased.[55]

The Boulder and Portland examples demonstrate policy success and positive physical activity outcomes, but it is important to note that the presence of a policy does not always guarantee resources for implementation. A major obstacle to Complete Streets implementation is that many current transportation policies and planning practices favor mobility over accessibility and automotive travel over alternative modes.[56] A strong Complete Streets policy with adequate funding is ideal, but not the norm. Policies tied to fewer resources still have the potential, however, to influence practices and standards.[10] Guidance on developing and implementing Complete Streets policies is available from national organizations such as Smart Growth America[28] and the American Planning Organization.[50]

The Case of Gas Prices and Physical Activity

Sometimes policies completely unrelated to public health or physical activity can influence health behavior. Such is the case with policies related to increased gasoline prices. Economic theory suggests that higher gasoline prices may alter individual behavior both via a "substitution effect" whereby people seek alternatives to motorized transportation, and an "income effect" whereby the effects of higher gasoline prices on a family's disposable income leads to adjustments in how money is spent.[57] In a 2011 study, Courtemanche et al. found a significant association between lower gasoline prices and increased risk of obesity over 1979–2004. Specifically, the findings suggest that lower gasoline prices are associated with less frequent walking and bicycling.[58] These findings were the impetus of another study by Sen (2012) that investigated the association between higher gasoline prices and time spent in various physical activities among the U.S. population aged 15 years and older, over a period from 2003 to 2008. When Sen compared gasoline price fluctuations to pooled cross-sectional time-series data from the American Time Use Survey (an annual survey sponsored by the Bureau of Labor Statistics) from 2003 to 2008, the results indicated that higher gasoline prices are associated with increased participation in and increased time spent on certain physical activities. Increases were noted in recreational walking, bicycling, and running, and in walking and bicycling to do errands, as well as in "moderate intensity housework." These associations were weaker for minorities and individuals with low socioeconomic status.[57]

Hou et al. conducted another study relating physical activity to gasoline prices using longitudinal data from the Coronary Artery Risk Development in Young Adults (CARDIA) study.[59] An aggregate physical activity score at three time points for over 5,000 people was matched with their home location using Geographical Information System data. Their data were linked with county-level inflation adjusted gasoline prices. After controlling for relevant variables, the authors found that a 25-cent increase in inflation-adjusted gasoline price was significantly associated with an increase in physical activity score.[59]

Although an increase in gas prices (e.g., increased gasoline tax) may be a policy with the added benefit of increasing physical activity in some segments of the population, there may be better tax alternatives for a more equitable effect. Courtemanche suggests an income-adjusted tax credit as an alternative to purposefully increasing taxes,[58] and other options may exist. The studies on the association of gasoline prices and behavior are novel, but they have limitations inherent in cross-sectional analyses. These associations do bring to light, however, how there may be unforeseen benefits, such as increased physical activity, even in policies that are not explicitly related to health. Other benefits can occur with policies such as increased gas prices. Estimates of gas-tax increases also reveal safety benefits in the form of reduced traffic fatalities[60] and per-mile crash rates.[61] Advocates and stakeholders with a vested interest in promoting policies supportive of physical activity should consider framing other benefits (e.g., reduced traffic injury and fatality) to potentially leverage change in this behavior.[62]

CONCLUSION

In spite of decades of evidence on the importance of physical activity to health promotion and disease prevention, many Americans are not physically active enough to meet the national guidelines.[1,4,5,39] Broad-scale policies are a promising strategy to facilitate a change in physical activity prevalence. Opportunities exist to strengthen the influence of policy on this important health behavior. One opportunity involves enhancing cross-sector and cross-scale policies that foster physically active defaults. Policy approaches supportive of "lifestyle" physical activity, many of which were discussed throughout this chapter, can be challenging to develop, adopt, and implement. Complex, but necessary, collaborations often span multiple sectors and policy scales. For instance, while PE policies can directly impact physical activity behaviors of youth, school personnel may be more concerned with addressing federal and state educational mandates. In such cases, public health professionals should consider leveraging alternative and more appropriate policy points, such as the link between physical education and academic performance.[37]

Additionally, increasing physical activity through policy requires collaboration among varied stakeholders. As highlighted in our Complete Streets policy example, agencies and stakeholders with very diverse roles, responsibilities, and perspectives approach the activities associated with a Complete Streets policy differently. Public health advocates and decision-makers need to become aware of these priorities and adjust their policy strategies and messages to foster the necessary collaborations with stakeholders across disciplines and sectors.

Lastly, direct physical activity outcomes as the result of policy changes are difficult to measure without very specific and rigorous evaluation designs and often, longitudinal analysis. Because the policy environment can likely be unpredictable, the study of "natural experiments" such as changes in the environment (e.g., extension of trails or transit routes) or policies (e.g., state mandate for daily PE) are good ways to identify outcomes. Baseline data is necessary, however, and needs to exist or be quickly assessed prior to the policy change. Funding mechanisms and facilitation of study partnerships are needed in order to gain more evidence of physical activity outcomes that result from policy changes.

REFERENCES

1. US Department of Health and Human Services (USDHHS). *Physical Activity Guidelines Advisory Committee Report, 2008.* Washington, DC: USDHHS; 2008.
2. United States Department of Health and Human Services. *Physical Activity and Health. A Report of the Surgeon General.* Atlanta, GA: Centers for Disease Control and Prevention; 1996.
3. US Department of Health and Human Services (USDHHS). *2008 Physical Activity Guidelines for Americans.* Washington, DC: USDHHS; 2008. http://www.health.gov/paguidelines/default/aspx. Accessed April 15, 2015.
4. Centers for Disease Control and Prevention. *State Indicator Report on Physical Activity, 2014.* Atlanta, GA: Author; 2014.
5. Carlson SA, Fulton JE, Schoenborn CA, Loustalot F. Trend and prevalence estimates based on the 2008 Physical Activity Guidelines for Americans. *Am J Prev Med.* Oct 2010;39(4):305–313.
6. Ng SW, Popkin BM. Time use and physical activity: a shift away from movement across the globe. *Obes Rev.* Aug 2012;13(8):659–680.
7. Matthews CE, Chen KY, Freedson PS, et al. Amount of time spent in sedentary behaviors in the United States, 2003–2004. *Am J Epidemiol.* Apr 2008;167(7):875–881.

8. Wijndaele K, Brage S, Besson H, et al. Television viewing time independently predicts all-cause and cardiovascular mortality: the EPIC Norfolk study. *Int J Epidemiol.* Feb 2011;40(1):150–159.

9. Eyler A, Brownson R, Schmid T, Pratt M. Understanding policies and physical activity: frontiers of knowledge to improve population health. *J Phys Act Health.* Mar 2010;7(Suppl 1):S9–S12.

10. Woods CB, Mutrie N. Putting physical activity on the policy agenda. *Quest.* Apr 2012;64(2):92–104.

11. Jones E, Eyler AA, Nguyen L, Kong J, Brownson RC, Bailey JH. It's all in the lens: differences in views on obesity prevention between advocates and policy makers. *Child Obes.* Jun 2012;8(3):243–250.

12. Brownson RC, Haire-Joshu D, Luke DA. Shaping the context of health: a review of environmental and policy approaches in the prevention of chronic diseases. *Annu Rev Public Health.* 2006;27:341–370.

13. Brownson RC, Kelly CM, Eyler AA, et al. Environmental and policy approaches for promoting physical activity in the United States: a research agenda. *J Phys Act Health.* Jul 2008;5(4):488–503.

14. Bull FC, Bellew B, Schoppe S, Bauman AE. Developments in National Physical Activity Policy: an international review and recommendations towards better practice. *J Sci Med Sport.* Apr 2004;7(1 Suppl):93–104.

15. Centers for Disease Control and Prevention. Guide to Community Preventive Services: Promoting physical activity, environmental and policy approaches. 2003; http://www.thecommunityguide.org/pa/environmental-policy/index.html. Accessed June 10, 2014.

16. Institute of Medicine. *Accelerating Progress in Obesity Prevention.* Washington, DC: The National Academies Press; 2012.

17. King AC, Sallis JF. Why and how to improve physical activity promotion: lessons from behavioral science and related fields. *Prev Med.* Oct 2009;49(4):286–288.

18. Schmid T, Pratt M, Witmer L. A framework for physical activity policy research. *J Phys Act Health.* 2006;3(Suppl 1):S20–S29.

19. Bauman AE, Reis RS, Sallis JF, et al. Correlates of physical activity: why are some people physically active and others not? *Lancet.* Jul 2012;380(9838):258–271.

20. Institute of Medicine. Transportation Research Board. National Research Council, Committee on Physical Activity, Transportation and Land Use. *Does the Built Environment Influence Physical Activity?: Examining the Evidence—Special Report 282.* Washington DC; 2005.

21. Borner K, Contractor N, Falk-Krzesinski HJ, et al. A multi-level systems perspective for the science of team science. *Sci Transl Med.* Sep 2010;2(49):49cm24.

22. Eyler AA, Brownson RC, Doescher MP, et al. Policies related to active transport to and from school: a multisite case study. *Health Educ Res.* Oct 2007;23(6):963–975.

23. Eyler A, Baldwin J, Carnoske C, et al. Parental involvement in active transport to school initiatives: A multi-site case study. *Am J Health Educ.* 2008;39(3):138–147.

24. Allender S, Cavill N, Parker M, Foster C. 'Tell us something we don't already know or do!'—The response of planning and transport professionals to public health guidance on the built environment and physical activity. *J Pub Health Policy.* Apr 2009;30(1):102–116.

25. Pate R. A national physical activity plan for the United States. *J Phys Act Health.* 2009;6 Suppl(2):S157–S158.

26. Pate R. Inside the National Physical Activity Plan. *J Phys Act Health.* 2014;11(3):461–462.

27. United States Department of Transportation. SAFETEA-LU. 2014; http://www.fhwa.dot. gov/safetealu/. Accessed March 24, 2015.

28. Smart Growth America. National Complete Streets Coalition. 2015; http://www.smart-growthamerica.org/complete-streets. Accessed March 24, 2015.

29. Hoehner C, Soares J, Parra DC, et al. Physical activity interventions in Latin America: what value might be added by including conference abstracts in a literature review? *J Phys Act Health.* Jul 2010;7(Suppl 2):S265–S278.

30. Parra DC, Hoehner CM, Hallal PC, et al. Perceived environmental correlates of physical activity for leisure and transportation in Curitiba, Brazil. *Prev Med.* Mar–Apr 2011;52(3–4):234–238.

31. Reis RS, Hallal PC, Parra DC, et al. Promoting physical activity through community-wide policies and planning: findings from Curitiba, Brazil. *J Phys Act Health.* Jul 2010;7(Suppl 2):S137–S145.

32. Simoes EJ, Hallal P, Pratt M, et al. Effects of a community-based, professionally supervised intervention on physical activity levels among residents of Recife, Brazil. *Am J Public Health.* Jan 2009;99(1):68–75.

33. Network G. *Guide for Useful Interventions for Physical Activity in Brazil and Latin America: Academia De Cidade.* 2015; http://www.projectguia.org/en/projects/academia-de-cidade/. Accessed April 30, 2015.

34. Torres A, Sarmiento OL, Stauber C, Zarama R. The Ciclovia and Cicloruta programs: promising interventions to promote physical activity and social capital in Bogota, Colombia. *Am J Public Health.* Feb 2013,103(2):e23–e30.

35. Montes F, Sarmiento OL, Zarama R, et al. Do health benefits outweigh the costs of mass recreational programs? An economic analysis of four Ciclovia programs. *J Urban Health.* Feb 2012;89(1):153–170.

36. Alliance for Biking and Walking. Open Streets Project. 2015. http://www.bikewalkalliance. org/resources/reports/open-streets-guide. Accessed April 30, 2015.

37. Institute of Medicine. *Educating the Student Body: Taking Physical Education and Physical Activity to School.* Washington, DC: The National Academies Press; 2013.

38. Sallis JF, McKenzie TL, Beets MW, Beighle A, Erwin H, Lee S. Physical education's role in public health: Steps forward and backward over 20 years and HOPE for the future. *Res Q Exerc Sport.* 2012;83(2):125–135.

39. Centers for Disease Control and Prevention. Youth Risk Behavior Surveillance—United States, 2013. *MMWR.* 2014;63:SS-4.

40. National Association for Sport and Physical Education & American Heart Association. *2012 Shape of the Nation Report: Status of Physical Education in the USA.* Reston, VA: American Alliance for Health, Physical Education, Recreation and Dance; 2012.

41. Perna FM, Oh A, Chriqui JF, et al. The association of state law to physical education time allocation in U.S. public schools. *Am J Public Health.* Aug 2012;102(8):1594–1599.

42. Carlson JA, Sallis JF, Chriqui JF, Schneider L, McDermid LC, Agron P. State policies about physical activity minutes in physical education or during school. *J School Health.* 2013;83(3):150–156.

43. Chriqui JF, Eyler A, Carnoske C, Slater S. State and district policy influences on district-wide elementary and middle school physical education practices. *J Public Health Manag Pract.* 2013;19:S41–S48.

44. Eyler AA, Brownson RC, Aytur SA, et al. Examination of trends and evidence-based elements in state physical education legislation: a content analysis. *J School Health.* Jul 2010;80(7):326–332.

45. Sanchez-Vaznaugh EV, Sánchez BN, Rosas LG, Baek J, Egerter S. Physical education policy compliance and children's physical fitness. *Am J Prev Med*. 2012;42(5):452–459.

46. Chriqui J, Resnick E, Schneider L, et al. School district wellness policies: evaluating progress and potential for improving children's health five years after the Federal mandate. *Robert Wood Johnson Foundation. Brief Report*. 2013;3:19–20.

47. Slater SJ, Nicholson L, Chriqui J, Turner L, Chaloupka F. The impact of state laws and district policies on physical education and recess practices in a nationally representative sample of U.S. public elementary schools. *Arch Pediatr Adolesc Med*. 2012;166(4):311–316.

48. Saelens BE, Sallis JF, Frank LD, et al. Neighborhood environment and psychosocial correlates of adults' physical activity. *Med Sci Sports Exerc*. 2012;44(4):637–646.

49. Slotterback CS, Zerger C. Complete Streets from Policy to Project: The Planning and Implementation of Complete Streets at Multiple Scales. 2013. http://www.dot.state.mn.us/research/TS/2013/201330.pdf. Accessed May 1, 2015.

50. American Planning Association. *Complete Streets: Best Policy and Implementation Practices*. American Planning Association Chicago, IL; 2010.

51. Henao A, Piatkowski D, Luckey KS, Nordback K, Marshall WE, Krizek KJ. Sustainable transportation infrastructure investments and mode share changes: A 20-year background of Boulder, Colorado. *Transport Policy*. 2015;37:64–71.

52. National Research Center. *Modal Shift in the Boulder Valley 1990–2006*. National Research Center, Inc. Boulder, CO; 2006.

53. Freeland AL, Banerjee SN, Dannenberg AL, Wendel AM. Walking associated with public transit: moving toward increased physical activity in the United States. *Am J Public Health*. 2013;103(3):536–542.

54. Saelens BE, Vernez Moudon A, Kang B, Hurvitz PM, Zhou C. Relation between higher physical activity and public transit use. *Am J Public Health*. 2014;104(5):854–859.

55. Protland Office of Transportation. *Portland Bicycle Counts: 2008*. Portland, OR; 2008.

56. Litman T. *Toward More Comprehensive and Multi-modal Transport Evaluation*. Victoria Transport Policy Institute; Victoria, BC, Canada; 2012.

57. Sen B. Is there an association between gasoline prices and physical activity? Evidence from American time use data. *Journal of Policy Analysis and Management*. 2012;31(2):338–366.

58. Courtemanche C. A silver lining? The connection between gasoline prices and obesity. *Economic Inquiry*. 2011;49(3):935–957.

59. Hou N, Popkin BM, Jacobs DR, et al. Longitudinal trends in gasoline price and physical activity: the CARDIA study. *Prev Med*. 2011;52(5):365–369.

60. Grabowski DC, Morrisey MA. Do higher gasoline taxes save lives? *Economics Letters*. 2006;90(1, (1)):51–55.

61. Chi G, Cosby AG, Quddus MA, Gilbert PA, Levinson D. Gasoline prices and traffic safety in Mississippi. *Journal of Safety Research*. 2010;41(6):493–500.

62. Litman T. Transportation and public health. *Annu Rev Public Health*. 2013;34:217–233.

9

Public Policy and Alcohol Use

Richard A. Grucza and Andrew D. Plunk

LEARNING OBJECTIVES

1. Describe the problem of alcohol misuse.
2. Explain public policy approaches to decreasing alcohol misuse.
3. Discuss how politics impacts alcohol policy.
4. Describe the evolution and impact of minimum legal drinking age laws.

IDENTIFYING THE PROBLEM: ALCOHOL MISUSE AND CONSEQUENCES

It is estimated that alcohol misuse is the third leading cause of preventable mortality in the United States and among the top two contributors to years of healthy life lost in high-and middle-income countries.[1,2] In addition to causing health problems for heavy drinkers, the behavioral effects of alcohol result in health risks for moderate drinkers and nondrinkers through alcohol-related accidents, alcohol-induced violence, sexual assault, and other consequences.[3,4] Accordingly, the health effects of alcohol can be parsed into internal and external consequences; the former are experienced by those who use alcohol to excess, whereas the latter are borne by society at large. Recognizing that some of the consequences of drinking affect nondrinkers is key to advocating for just and effective alcohol policy. Even those who favor a limited role of government involvement in protecting individuals from the consequences of their own actions should recognize the potential for some drinking behavior to impinge on the rights of nondrinkers (e.g., drunk driving). The social costs of unregulated alcohol availability, which are not always immediately apparent or intuited, are also high. For example, high rates of alcohol use are associated with direct economic costs such as those incurred by the justice system and indirect economic costs such as decreased workforce productivity.[5]

In the United States, risk for alcohol dependence and alcohol-related health consequences is nearly universal—over 80% of people drink alcohol at some point in their lives. However, heritability and family environment play significant roles in determining this risk, as do other environmental risk factors, meaning that this risk is not evenly distributed across the population.[6] There are also significant sociodemographic differences in risk for alcohol dependence. Some of these differences are described in Table 9.1, which provides the estimated prevalence of alcohol dependence for various groups in 2013. Not all risk factors for alcohol problems are fixed over time. Some demographic shifts in the distribution of alcohol problems have occurred. For example, men are at higher risk for alcohol dependence than women, but this gap has been narrowing in recent years.[7,8] The role of educational attainment is also complex; college graduates are at similar risk for alcohol dependence compared to those with less education, but this may be a recent phenomenon: older studies suggested that education was a protective factor.[9,10] In fact, current college students are more likely to drink to excess than their non-college peers, while the reverse was true two decades ago.[11]

Risk for alcohol dependence is fairly evenly distributed among the most populous racial/ethnic groups, but risk for the internal and external health consequences of alcohol use falls disproportionately on poor and disadvantaged populations.[12,13] National surveys have shown that higher income groups are more likely to drink, but lower income groups exhibit higher risk for alcohol dependence.[9,10] These observations

Table 9.1 Estimated Prevalence of Past-Year DSM-IV Alcohol Dependence by Select Demographic Groups (Data from the 2013 National Survey on Drug Use and Health)

	Prevalence	*95% CI*
Sex		
Women	2.4	(2.1, 2.7)
Men	4.1	(3.7, 4.5)
Race		
Non-Hispanic White	3.2	(3.0, 2.6)
Non-Hispanic Black	3.2	(2.5, 3.9)
Hispanic	3.4	(2.7, 4.3)
Asian/Hawaiian/Pacific Islander	1.5	(1.1, 2.2)
Native American	7.3	(4.5, 11.6)
Biracial or multiracial	5.1	(3.1, 8.3)
Age		
18–25 years	5.5	(5.0, 6.0)
26–34 years	5.1	(4.4, 5.9)
35–49 years	3.5	(3.0, 3.9)
50 years and older	1.7	(1.7, 2.1)
Educational Attainment		
No diploma or GED	3.6	(3.2, 4.2)
Highschool only	2.9	(2.4, 3.4)
Some college	3.1	(2.7, 3.6)
College degree	3.2	(2.7, 3.9)

suggest that while those with relative social advantage still exhibit significant risk for alcohol problems, the most serious consequences of alcohol misuse and abuse are strongly correlated with social disadvantage. Given the relationship between alcohol-related morbidity and mortality, and socioeconomic factors associated with poorer health outcomes, sound alcohol control policy could play an important role in limiting and mitigating health disparities.

Outcomes Relevant for Policy Studies

Alcohol policy researchers study a variety of outcomes to examine whether a policy is effective. Examples include alcohol-related traffic fatalities, alcohol use disorder prevalence, frequency of heavy drinking (usually defined as five or more drinks on one occasion for men or four for women), and overall alcohol consumption in the population or among subpopulations of interest. Given that most people who drink do so without serious consequences, it might seem unusual that policy researchers would place much emphasis on overall alcohol consumption, rather than focusing on more serious consequences of alcohol use. The importance of consumption measures can be understood by examining the distribution of alcohol consumption in the population, which is shown in Figure 9.1. The Figure plots the cumulative distribution of drinks consumed over the past 30 days, using data from a large, nationally representative sample of legal age drinkers (solid black line). The solid gray line shows the new

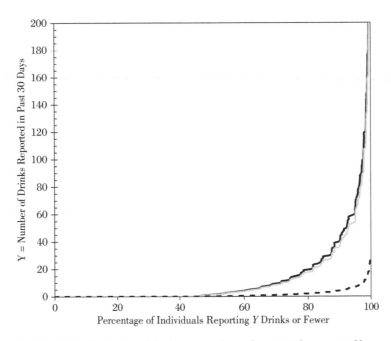

Figure 9.1 Cumulative distribution of drinks consumed over the past 30 days, reported by participants aged 21 years and older from the 2002–2010 National Surveys on Drug Use and Health. (solid black line). The solid gray line represents the distribution after a 10% reduction in consumption by all drinkers. The dashed line shows the difference between the two solid curves.

distribution after a hypothetical intervention that results in an across-the-board 10% reduction in consumption, and the dashed line shows the difference between the two solid curves. The figure illustrates that a large majority of people in the United States are light-to-moderate drinkers, if they drink at all. For example, 40% of the population reported no alcohol use over the prior 30 days, 60% of the population reported fewer than four drinks, and 90% reported fewer than 40 drinks (averaging just over 1.3 drinks per day). Examination of the area under the curve suggests that the 7% of the population that drinks the most accounts for about half of the alcohol consumed. The hypothetical intervention curve shows that if an intervention causes all drinkers to reduce their consumption by a fixed proportion, it can result in large absolute reductions among the heaviest drinkers, which would likely result in reductions in some of the most harmful consequences of alcohol, while having minimal effect on most of the population. For these reasons, it is reasonable to assume that reductions in overall population consumption have significant public health benefits.

PUBLIC POLICY STRATEGIES

Most public policies designed to limit alcohol use can be thought of as attempts to regulate the total cost of alcohol. The total cost includes the total monetary price (i.e., including taxation) as well as factors that influence the availability, convenience, and legal consequences associated with use or misuse of alcohol.[14] Examples of factors that contribute to these costs include taxation, regulation of outlet density, restrictions on hours of sale, and legal limits on blood-alcohol content for driving. Policy strategies that influence these factors are described in more detail below.

Policies that Influence Price

One of the most well-studied policy strategies is the regulation of the price of alcoholic beverages through the imposition of excise taxes.[15] Excise taxes are imposed on alcoholic beverages prior to retail sale and are, therefore, included in the consumed product and are usually set on a volume basis (e.g., the per-barrel federal tax on beer). Taxes are typically established separately for beer, wine, and spirits, and both federal and state governments in the United States impose volume-based excise taxes. Increases in taxes result in increases in prices.[16] Economists use the concept known as *price elasticity of demand* as a tool to understand the impact of price changes. It quantifies the responsiveness ("elasticity") of demand for a good in relation to changes in its price, operationalized as the percentage change in demand in response to a 1% change in price. For example, a price elasticity of the demand for a product of −1.0 indicates that a 1% increase in price leads to a 1% decrease in consumption of that product. Such a product would be considered "unit elastic." Like tobacco and illicit drugs, the demand for alcohol is considered to be "relatively inelastic," meaning that the elasticity coefficient is negative, but its absolute value is less than 1. Recent reviews and meta-analyses confirm this; mean elasticities from 112 studies were −0.46 for beer, −0.69 for wine and −0.80 for spirits.[17,18]

An ideal alcohol control policy might target specific groups or behaviors, such as underage drinkers or heavy drinking at any age, without penalizing moderate, responsible drinkers. At first glance, tax and price increases might seem like an indiscriminate approach that would impose costs on all drinkers without regard to age or quantity of drinking. However, economic theory would predict that taxes would be especially effective in changing the behavior of underage drinkers who tend to have less discretionary income than adults, and of heavy drinkers, who tend to spend a larger portion of their income on alcohol. Empirical research confirms that young people, particularly those who drink heavily, are more sensitive to price increases than adult drinkers.[19] On the other hand, studies focusing on heavier-drinking adults have found that the price elasticity of demand is less negative among this group.[19] However, even though the *relative* reductions in consumption among problem drinkers might be small in response to a tax, the harm reduction could be significant (e.g., if a small number of heavy drinkers stops drinking altogether). Furthermore, the imposition of tax or price increases may prevent moderate drinkers from escalating their alcohol use. Consistent with this notion, studies have found that the population frequency of heavy drinking decreases in response to increases in excise taxes: A meta-analysis of 10 studies estimated that a 10% increase in alcohol prices would lead to a 2.8% reduction in the population frequency of heavy drinking days.[18] A similar analysis suggested that a 10% increase in beverage prices would reduce alcohol related morbidity and mortality in relation to alcohol price by 3.5%, suggesting that price increases do lead to decreases in consumption among heavier drinkers and/or prevent people from becoming chronic heavy drinkers.[20] Numerous studies also affirm that increases in alcohol prices lead to reductions in the external consequences of alcohol use, such as motor vehicle accidents, violent crimes, and sexually transmitted diseases.[20,21] Taken together, recent literature reviews and meta-analyses support the idea that taxation and price increases are effective means of reducing not only alcohol consumption but also the negative consequences associated with it.

An alternative or complementary strategy to the use of excise taxes is minimum unit pricing policies for alcohol. These policies set minimum prices for given quantities and types of alcohol and have the effect of setting a lower limit to the price of a standard drink (i.e., a volume of beverage containing a quantity of ethanol specified by the standard). Because heavy drinkers are thought to minimize their costs by choosing less expensive brands, these policies could be particularly effective at reducing consumption among heavier drinkers and could prevent drinkers from substituting lower-price beverages in response to excise tax increases.[22,23] Minimum prices might also mitigate hazards associated with "happy hour" and other discounted-price promotions.[24] A handful of studies on the effects of minimum unit pricing on alcohol consumption have been conducted in Canada, where all 10 provinces have such policies. Studies based in Saskatchewan and British Columbia found that total alcohol consumption declined by 0.3% and 0.8% for each 1% increase in the minimum unit price.[23,25] Although these studies did not examine whether heavy drinking was impacted by the policies, reductions in alcohol-attributable deaths and hospital admissions also have been documented in response to increased minimum prices, suggesting that such policies are effective means of reducing alcohol-related harms.[26,27]

Policies that Influence Availability and Convenience

Other factors that might influence the "total cost" of obtaining alcohol include physical availability, convenience, and time spent driving to an outlet where alcohol is sold. For example, an individual may be inclined to forgo drinking on a given day if he or she has to drive a long distance to a bar or liquor store. Limiting the number of alcohol outlets in a given state would set a lower limit to the average distance needed to travel to obtain alcohol. Many studies have shown that alcohol consumption and the prevalence of related problems are consistently associated higher outlet densities.[28,29] The density of outlets can be limited by the state's licensing arrangements or by direct state ownership of retail outlets (known as state monopolies). Likewise, the alcohol consumer incurs an "inconvenience cost" of sorts if bars or liquor stores are closed at the time she or he wishes to make the purchase. Restrictions on hours and days during which sales are permitted also reduce alcohol-related external consequences, such as assaults and injuries, though the evidence that such policies result in reduced consumption is limited.[30]

The most stringent way of limiting access to alcohol is to prohibit commercial sales altogether. This is not a viable policy option in the United States or in most developed nations, but it is the approach in a handful of nations and some states in India today, and famously was once the law of the land in the United States.[5] Prohibition in the United States did not criminalize the possession or use of alcohol (though local laws did in some cases),[31] but instead made the sale of alcohol illegal. The popular view of this policy experiment in the United States is that it was a failure. A more nuanced and empirically informed view is that the policy was partially successful in its intent to reduce alcohol consumption, but that the unintended consequences of prohibition were too burdensome. Infringements on individual liberty and the rise of black markets and organized crime are seen as having outweighed any public health benefits, but there is solid evidence that alcohol consumption was reduced, at least temporarily.[32,33] The rate of liver cirrhosis dropped by 50% during Prohibition and the preceding years, when many individual states adopted prohibition policies.[34] Because liver cirrhosis rates are highly correlated with per-capita alcohol consumption, this indicates that alcohol consumption and the prevalence of one of its most serious internal consequences were reduced by the prohibition of commercial sales.

Traffic Policies

As a licit drug, there are no legal risks associated with drinking per se for those above the legal drinking age. Policies regulating driving under the influence of alcohol, however, present the possibility of legal consequences for heavy alcohol use when coupled with driving a motor vehicle. As of 2006, all 50 states and the District of Columbia penalize drivers who are shown to have a blood alcohol concentration (BAC) of 0.08 g/deciliter or 0.08% (mass/volume), though many states had higher limits in prior years, typically 0.10%. These are generally "per se" laws, which establish that individuals shown to have that amount of alcohol in their blood are legally intoxicated by definition. To reach this blood alcohol level, on average, a 170-pound man would have to consume about four standard drinks in the course of an hour. A meta-analysis of data from the United States suggests that lowering the BAC from 0.10% to 0.08% corresponded with a 14.8% decrease in the number of intoxicated drivers involved in fatal crashes.[35] Furthermore, at least one study indicates that the reduction in BAC limits did lead to an overall reduction in alcohol consumption among men of about 5%.[36] Thus, BAC limits are an effective means of reducing one of the primary external consequences of alcohol use, as well as perhaps reducing alcohol consumption in general. (See case study in Chapter 15 on BAC and injury prevention). Notably, the median BAC limit among countries with a national policy is 0.05%, significantly lower than the limits in the United States. Sweden, Norway, and several other countries have even lower limits of 0.02%, while Russia and many Eastern European countries have "zero tolerance" policies. The National Transportation Safety Board has recommended a reduction in the BAC limit to 0.05%, an issue that will likely be the subject of public debate in the near future.[5,37]

Many countries also set lower BAC limits for youth. Notably, in the United States, every state has adopted a zero tolerance BAC policy for drivers under the legal drinking age. These policies were implemented state-by-state throughout the 1990s[38] and establish BAC limits at 0.01%–0.02% for young drivers—the lowest levels that can be reliably detected by breath testing equipment.[14] The adoption of these policies appears to have conferred significant benefits to public health, as literature reviews conclude that they have resulted in reductions in crashes, injuries, and the percentage of young drivers with detectable BAC levels.[39,40] At least one study has indicated zero tolerance policies may result in lower rates of heavy drinking among underage men.[41]

Youth Access Policies

The minimum legal drinking age (MLDA) in the United States is the focus of our case study below, and its history and overall effectiveness are described in more detail there. The "drinking age" is shorthand for a suite of policies that vary across states, but all serve the purpose of reducing the legal availability of alcohol to those younger than 21 years. Federal policy, described below, requires that states prohibit the purchase and possession of alcohol by those under 21. In most states, there are legal penalties for consumption, although exceptions may be allowed, such as for consumption in the presence of parents/guardians and/or in private homes.[42,43] A key feature of all MLDA policies, however, is that the total cost of alcohol to youth under age 21 is increased—due to limiting the convenient availability of alcohol as well as increasing the legal risks associated with its use.

Other means of restricting access include policies governing the age of those who work in establishments that sell or serve alcohol, laws imposing liability on adults who host underage drinking parties, laws prohibiting the use or sale of false identification documents (IDs), and laws that make it easier to examine the veracity of IDs presented by purchasers.[42,43] There is no question that youth access policies, including the MLDA of 21 years, have had a positive impact on public health,[44,45] but it is difficult to say which specific policies are the most effective because many of them were adopted simultaneously. Nonetheless, there is an emerging body of primary literature in this area. For example, several studies suggest that policies facilitating the checking of identification, or policies making it illegal to present false identification, are effective at reducing underage drinking and driving while drinking.[43,46,47]

Many of the policies aimed at limiting underage drinking are targeted toward the supply side of alcohol transactions; for example, by prohibiting adults from furnishing alcohol to minors, and requiring that retailers ensure that the purchaser is of legal age. However, the federal policy effectively criminalizes the purchase and possession of alcohol by minors, which can result in considerable penalties for youth who illicitly purchase or use alcohol. For example, "use and lose" laws can result in administrative license revocation for young people using or possessing alcohol, even if they are not driving.[48] Not having access to transportation affects employability, and is likely to disproportionately impact poor and minority populations, raising questions about whether such demand-side policies are just and proportionate.[49]

It might also be debated whether harsh penalties for underage users are the most effective policies aimed at deterring use. Recent research on the psychology of deterrence suggests that the certainty of sanctions may have a larger deterrent effect than the severity of penalties.[50] Although there is little doubt that the uniform minimum legal drinking age has had public health benefits, it may be possible to attain these same results by regulating availability of alcohol to minors (supply-side restrictions) while ensuring that sanctions against youth who possess or attempt to purchase alcohol are proportionate and fair. Thus, more effective and just policy could be developed by taking care to distinguish between policies that limit access to alcohol by youth and those that punish underage drinkers.

Other Policies and Other Considerations

The discussion above focused primarily on state and federal/national policies that have a significant evidence base, but is by no means a comprehensive review of the policy levers available for the purpose of alcohol control. The evidence suggests that reduced population consumption and decreased prevalence of alcohol-related problems at the population level can be achieved through policies that limit alcohol availability, decrease the price or convenience associated with alcohol consumption, or result in legal risks when alcohol is misused. Another set of policies that might be seen as limiting the convenience of alcohol use are those that place restrictions on where alcohol can be consumed; for example, laws against consumption in public places or in motor vehicles.[5] Health warning labels on alcohol can be seen as increasing the "total cost" by attempting to make the user aware of health risks entailed by consuming alcohol in excess.

The "total cost" framework is a useful heuristic for discussing policy, but it is not a comprehensive theory of the determinants of alcohol use. For example, perceived norms are likely to influence an individual's alcohol consumption (i.e., whether one thinks of his or her level of consumption as "normal"), and many campus-based interventions are aimed at correcting misperceptions surrounding the normativity of heavy alcohol use.[51] Policies that place limits on advertising and marketing[s] might also be conceptualized as attempts to reframe the social norms surrounding alcohol use.

The Role of Political Will

Alcohol policy presents something of a paradox: Most people in developed nations drink and most drinkers do not experience significant harms from drinking. Yet, alcohol causes more external harms than any other drug.[52] Thus, significant public health benefits could be realized by stronger alcohol control policies, but popular political resistance to such policies can be expected to be quite strong. More importantly, the lobbying power of the alcoholic beverage industry is formidable: The largest beverage industries spend more on lobbying than the tobacco industry.[53]

Taxation and Minimum Pricing

An examination of state and federal volume-based excise taxes for beer in the United States between the years 1950 and 2012 illustrates that increases in these taxes, which arc neces sary in order to maintain pace with inflation, are incremental and rare. As seen in Figure 9.2, the federal beer excise tax declined by more than 75% between 1950 and 1990. In 1991, the beer excise tax was doubled from $9 to $18 per barrel—along with comparable

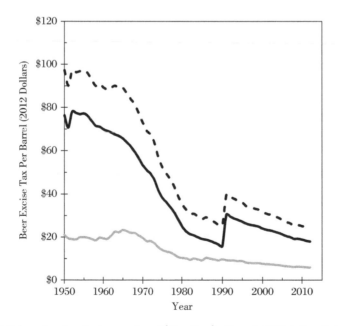

Figure 9.2 Volume-based excise taxes per barrel (31 gallons) of beer, in 2012 dollars. Federal tax (solid black), median state tax (solid gray), and their sum (dashed).

increases in taxes on wine and distilled spirits—resulting in a noticeable spike, but one which only set the tax to 1980 levels. The post-1991 tax was still less than half of its level after the previous adjustment in 1951. The median state beer excise tax is also shown in Figure 9.2; the median combined state and federal beer excise tax is about $24 per 31 gallon barrel, or about 7 cents per 12 ounces of beer. Although the state median did not decline as precipitously as the federal tax, the general trend is toward lower taxes after adjustment for inflation. In fact, the 1991 federal excise tax increase might be viewed as a rare exception to the rule. Passed as part of the 1990 federal budget,[54] it is likely that its passage had little to do with alcohol control, but was instead motivated by high deficits at the time and the necessity for political compromise in a divided government.[55]

Although taxation is not the sole determinant of beverage price, declines in taxes have paralleled declines in the real (inflation-adjusted) price of alcoholic beverages.[21] Arguments against such taxes include the fact that they are regressive and impinge on the ability of people of limited means to choose their lifestyle.[56] It also could be argued, however, that taxes on alcohol should be sufficient to cover the costs imposed on society as a result of the external consequences of alcohol use. Such an argument is based on the concept of "Pigovian taxation," articulated by British economist Arthur Pigou in the early 20th century.[57] Simply put, this is a tax imposed on transactions that have external consequences that result in social costs. This premise was implicit in an analysis conducted by health economist Willard Manning and his colleagues that calculated the costs associated with alcohol-related externalities, including costs passed on through health and life insurance. They concluded that taxes on alcohol covered only about half of these costs. This analysis was conducted in 1989, prior to the federal increases of 1991, but today's taxes are roughly comparable to those of 1989 (Figure 9.2).

Academic studies of the passage of a yet-to-be implemented minimum pricing policy in Scotland, as well as debate over similar measures throughout the United Kingdom, shed light on the significant barriers to such evidence-based policies.[58] McCambridge and his colleagues note that actors from the transnational beverage industry have utilized relationships with policymakers at all levels of government to insert themselves into the policymaking process. A Scottish government study in 2008 recommended a number of population-based measures to reduce the high levels of heavy drinking in the country, including a minimum unit pricing policy.[59] Following this report, the industry used media campaigns to rally opinion of both policymakers and the general public against such a measure. Despite these efforts, changes in the political environment led to passage of the minimum pricing policy by the Scottish parliament in 2012. The industry then took a more aggressive stance, initiating legal challenges under both domestic law and with the European Union and World Trade organization. These challenges will likely prevent implementation of the minimum pricing policy for many years.[58]

Drinking Age Policies

Because only a relatively small proportion of the drinking population is affected by drinking-age policies, they are not subject to the same level of political opposition as alcohol excise taxes and minimum pricing policies. In the United States, the minimum drinking age of 21 years continues to enjoy broad political support.[60] In fact, segments of the beverage industry have devoted money to campaigns to discourage underage drinking,[61] and it seems likely that a shift against the status quo would lead to negative public perceptions of the industry. It is likely, however, that industry will resist any attempts to increase the drinking age in other countries. Research from New Zealand revealed united and unanimous opposition from hospitality and beverage industry groups to proposals to raise the drinking age there from 18 years to 20 years in 2006 (the age had been lowered from 20 just seven years earlier).[62] Despite broad public support, the bill was defeated in parliament; a similar proposal was again defeated in 2012.[63]

In summary, increases in alcohol excise taxes are likely to be unpopular with the general public and to face major opposition from a powerful industry with much to lose. Minimum pricing strategies face less grass-roots opposition—perhaps because they effect only the poorest and heaviest of drinkers. The experience of the United Kingdom, however, shows that these policies also face major barriers to implementation because of the power of the beverage industry to sway public opinion and, failing that, to finance litigation. Other policy options discussed in this chapter, such as limiting outlet density, are also likely to face challenges, given that there is a strong trend towards privatization of beverage sales and away from state-run retail sales.[64] Drinking-age policies in the United States still enjoy broad political support, and commercial interests are content with the status quo but are unlikely to support higher drinking ages in countries with more permissive drinking age policies.

CASE STUDY: MINIMUM LEGAL DRINKING AGE LAWS

The Twenty-first Amendment to the U.S. Constitution repealed the federal prohibition on alcohol, explicitly giving control over alcohol regulation back to the states. Some states remained dry—with state-mandated prohibition still in effect—long after the repeal of prohibition (the last, Mississippi, remained dry until 1966).

In 1970, the minimum legal drinking age (MLDA) was 21 years in most states. Only two states allowed liquor sales to those under 21 years of age and 13 states allowed beer sales to those younger than 21.[65] This would soon change in response to a broad social movement questioning the appropriate age of majority in light of the Vietnam War. When the Twenty-sixth Amendment lowered the voting age to 18 years, many states also lowered the drinking age; by 1976 only 12 states retained the MLDA of 21 years.

However, lowering the MLDA proved to be dangerous. Researchers at the time linked lower MLDA to higher consumption,[66] but the most striking consequence was increased traffic fatalities for 15-to-20-year-olds.[67] This motivated organizations like Mothers Against Drunk Driving and the National Parent Teacher Association to lobby for the passage of the National 21 Uniform Minimum Drinking Age Act of 1984, which required states to have a MLDA of 21 or lose a portion of federal highway funds.[44]

The effects of permissive MLDA (i.e., < 21 years) have been widely studied[5] and linked to a range of adverse consequences, both for those who gained the ability to legally purchase alcohol (i.e., ages 18–20) and their underage peers (e.g., age 17 years when the MLDA was 18).[15,67–69] Increasing the MLDA to 21 has been consistently linked to reductions in alcohol consumption and traffic crashes/drunk driving.[15,19,70–76] Lower MLDA also has been linked to increased sexually transmitted disease rates,[77] increased suicide risk,[78,79] and lower educational attainment.[68,69]

Research also suggests that exposure to permissive MLDA can have persistent, life-long effects; this work has been motivated by the theory that the teenage years are a critical period for developing addiction vulnerability.[80] Legal access to alcohol during adolescence has been linked to increased alcohol consumption during young adulthood,[81] and seems to affect drinking behavior even decades later by promoting heavier drinking patterns and increasing risk for developing alcohol use disorders.[82,83] Higher lifelong rates for several consequences of risky drinking are also associated with permissive MLDA exposure during adolescence; for example, violence against women, female suicide,[84] and poorer birth outcomes.[85,86] These observations are consistent with the critical-period hypothesis for addiction vulnerability;[80] they suggest that reducing alcohol involvement among adolescents could result in healthier alcohol use patterns in adulthood.

Several factors have influenced the effectiveness of the 21 MLDA. Enforcement has been an issue, especially directly after the MLDA was increased.[87] The impact of MLDA also is reduced when there are alternate means of accessing alcohol. For example, of-age individuals are the most common source of alcohol for underage drinkers,[87] and most legal-aged college students report providing alcohol to underage peers.[88] These factors likely contribute to an environment on college campuses that insulates underage students from the effects of policies aimed at curbing underage drinking, including the MLDA.[11,82,89] This has made the 21 MLDA a contentious issue to some, who have supported lowering the MLDA because of unhealthy drinking on college campuses.[44] However, while rates of underage drinking, especially binge drinking, are of concern, there have been steady declines overall since the MLDA was increased.[11] Even though the U.S. drinking age is higher than many countries (most notably all of Europe), rates of problematic youth drinking are lower in the United States than most European countries.[90] Further, although some might resent that the federal government circumvented the Twenty-first Amendment by using denial of funding to force states to adopt the 21 MLDA,[91] public support for the 21 MLDA remains strong.[5,44] It is unlikely that the MLDA will be lowered again in the United States; therefore, future alcohol policy should focus on evidence-based prevention and stricter enforcement for high-risk underage drinkers.[44]

CONCLUSION

Substantial evidence suggests that alcohol policy can have a positive impact on public health. Challenges still exist, most notably with regard to how certain populations react to policy or disproportionately shoulder the burden of alcohol-related morbidity and mortality. Further research is needed on the insulating effect of the college campus environment, which blunts the impact of policy efforts to restrict underage access to alcohol. We also must ensure that social disadvantage, which already is a marker for more severe alcohol-related health outcomes, does not also lead to disproportionate legal consequences when running afoul of policies that were designed ultimately to promote health. Finally, the failure and repeal of Prohibition carries with it some historical baggage but also offers valuable insight on the appropriate limits of policy. Quite simply, the public is willing to accept many of the harms associated with widely available alcohol because people enjoy drinking. Furthermore, the lobbying power of industry can marshal public opposition to certain policies, such as taxation and minimum pricing, even though the majority of drinkers would only be minimally affected. Policies aimed at reducing risky drinking behaviors, such as those that focus on drunk driving and restricting underage access—two areas with strong public support—will have a greater chance of being successful.

ACKNOWLEDGMENTS

Preparation of this chapter was supported in part by the National Institute on Drug Abuse, of the National Institutes of Health under award numberR01DA031288. The funding source had no role in influencing the content of the chapter.

REFERENCES

1. Mokdad AH, Marks JS, Stroup DF, Gerberding JL. Actual causes of death in the United States, 2000. *JAMA: The Journal of the American Medical Association*. 2004;291(10):1238–1245.
2. World Health Organization. *Global Health Risks: Mortality and Burden of Disease Attributable to Selected Major Risks*. Geneva, Switzerland: Author; 2009.
3. Abbey A, Zawacki T, Buck PO, Clinton AM, McAuslan P. Alcohol and sexual assault. *Alcohol Res Health*. 2001;25(1):43–51.
4. Hingson RW, Heeren T, Zakocs RC, Kopstein A, Wechsler H. Magnitude of alcohol-related mortality and morbidity among U.S. college students ages 18–24. *J Stud Alcohol Drugs*. 2002;63(2):136.
5. World Health Organization. *Global Status Report on Alcohol and Health 2014*. 2014; http://www.who.int/substance_abuse/publications/global_alcohol_report/en/. Accessed August 8, 2014.
6. Rhee SH, Waldman ID. Genetic and environmental influences on antisocial behavior: a meta-analysis of twin and adoption studies. *Psychol Bull*. 2002;128(3):490.
7. Grucza RA, Bucholz KK, Rice JP, Bierut LJ. Secular trends in the lifetime prevalence of alcohol dependence in the United States: a re-evaluation. *Alcohol Clin Exp Res*. 2008;32(5):763–770. doi:10.1111/j.1530-0277.2008.00635.x.
8. Keyes KM, Grant BF, Hasin DS. Evidence for a closing gender gap in alcohol use, abuse, and dependence in the United States population. *Drug Alcohol Depend*. 2008;93(1-2):21–29. doi:10.1016/j.drugalcdep.2007.08.017.
9. Chen CM. *Alcohol Use and Alcohol Use Disorders in the United States: Main Findings from the 2001–2002 National Epidemiologic Survey on Alcohol and Related Conditions (NESARC)*. National Institute on Alcohol and Alcoholism, Rockville, MD; 2006.

10. Grant BF. Prevalence and correlates of alcohol use and DSM-IV alcohol dependence in the United States: results of the National Longitudinal Alcohol Epidemiologic Survey. *J Stud Alcohol*. 1997;58(5):464–473.

11. Grucza RA, Norberg KE, Bierut LJ. Binge drinking among youths and young adults in the United States: 1979–2006. *J Am Acad Child Adolesc Psychiatry*. 2009;48(7):692–702. doi:10.1097/CHI.0b013e3181a2b32f.

12. Caetano R. Alcohol-related health disparities and treatment-related epidemiological findings among Whites, Blacks, and Hispanics in the United States. *Alcohol Clin Exp Res*. 2003;27(8):1337–1339.

13. Singh GK, Hoyert DL. Social epidemiology of chronic liver disease and cirrhosis mortality in the United States, 1935–1997: trends and differentials by ethnicity, socioeconomic status, and alcohol consumption. *Hum Biol*. 2000;75(5):801–820.

14. Thomas Babor. *Alcohol: No Ordinary Commodity: Research and Public Policy*. Oxford University Press, New York; 2010.

15. Wagenaar AC, Toomey TL. Alcohol policy: gaps between legislative action and current research. *Contemp Drug Probs*. 2000;27(4):681.

16. Kenkel DS. Are alcohol tax hikes fully passed through to prices? Evidence from Alaska. *Am Econ Rev*. 2005;95(2):273–277.

17. Elder RW, Lawrence B, Ferguson A, et al. The effectiveness of tax policy interventions for reducing excessive alcohol consumption and related harms. *Am J Prev Med*. 2010;38(2):217–229.

18. Wagenaar AC, Salois MJ, Komro KA. Effects of beverage alcohol price and tax levels on drinking: a meta-analysis of 1,003 estimates from 112 studies. *Addiction*. 2009;104(2):179–190.

19. Chaloupka FJ, Grossman M, Saffer H. The effects of price on alcohol consumption and alcohol-related problems. *Alcohol Res Health*. 2002;26(1):22–34.

20. Wagenaar AC, Tobler AL, Komro KA. Effects of alcohol tax and price policies on morbidity and mortality: a systematic review. *Am J Public Health*. 2010;100(11):2270–2278.

21. Chaloupka FJ, Straif K, Leon ME. Effectiveness of tax and price policies in tobacco control. *Tob Control*. 2011;20(3):235–238. doi:10.1136/tc.2010.039982.

22. Kerr WC, Greenfield TK. Distribution of alcohol consumption and expenditures and the impact of improved measurement on coverage of alcohol sales in the 2000 National Alcohol Survey. *Alcohol Clin Exp Res*. 2007;31(10):1714–1722.

23. Stockwell T, Auld MC, Zhao J, Martin G. Does minimum pricing reduce alcohol consumption? The experience of a Canadian province. *Addiction*. 2012;107(5):912–920.

24. Thombs DL, O'Mara R, Dodd VJ, et al. A field study of bar-sponsored drink specials and their associations with patron intoxication. *J Stud Alcohol Drugs*. 2009;70(2):206.

25. Stockwell T, Zhao J, Giesbrecht N, Macdonald S, Thomas G, Wettlaufer A. The raising of minimum alcohol prices in Saskatchewan, Canada: impacts on consumption and implications for public health. *Am J Public Health*. 2012;102(12):e103–e110.

26. Zhao J, Stockwell T, Martin G, et al. The relationship between minimum alcohol prices, outlet densities and alcohol-attributable deaths in British Columbia, 2002–2009. *Addiction*. 2013;108(6):1059–1069.

27. Stockwell T, Zhao J, Martin G, et al. Minimum alcohol prices and outlet densities in British Columbia, Canada: estimated impacts on alcohol-attributable hospital admissions. *Am J Public Health*. 2013;103(11):2014–2020.

28. Treno AJ, Marzell M, Gruenewald PJ, Holder H. A review of alcohol and other drug control policy research. *J Stud Alcohol Drugs*. 2014;(17):98.

29. Campbell CA, Hahn RA, Elder R, et al. The effectiveness of limiting alcohol outlet density as a means of reducing excessive alcohol consumption and alcohol-related harms. *Am J Prev Med.* 2009;37(6):556–569.

30. Popova S, Giesbrecht N, Bekmuradov D, Patra J. Hours and days of sale and density of alcohol outlets: impacts on alcohol consumption and damage: a systematic review. *Alcohol Alcohol.* 2009;44(5):500–516.

31. Okrent D. *Last Call: The Rise and Fall of Prohibition.* Simon and Schuster, New York; 2010.

32. Miron JA, Zwiebel J. *Alcohol Consumption during Prohibition.* Cambridge, MA: National Bureau of Economic Research; 1991.

33. Blocker JS. Did Prohibition really work? Alcohol prohibition as a public health innovation. *Am J Public Health.* 2006;96(2):233–243. doi:10.2105/AJPH.2005.065409.

34. Mann RE, Smart RG, Govoni R. The epidemiology of alcoholic liver disease. *Alcohol Res Health.* 2003;27:209–219.

35. Tippetts AS, Voas RB, Fell JC, Nichols JL. A meta-analysis of .08 BAC laws in 19 jurisdictions in the United States. *Accid Anal Prev.* 2005;37(1):149–161.

36. Carpenter C, Harris K. How do "Point Oh-Eight" (.08) BAC laws work? *Top Econ Anal Policy.* 2005;5(1):2194–6108. doi:10.1515/1538-0653.1381.

37. 0.05 urged as standard for drunken driving. *The Washington Post.* May 15, 2013; A03.

38. Ponicki W. Statewide Availability Data System II: 1933–2003. National Institute on Alcohol Abuse and Alcoholism. Research Center Grant P60-AA006282-23. Berkeley, CA: Pacific Institute for Research and Evaluation, Prevention Research Center. 2004.

39. Zwerling C, Jones MP. Evaluation of the effectiveness of low blood alcohol concentration laws for younger drivers. *Am J Prev Med.* 1999;16(1):76–80.

40. Voas RB, Tippetts AS, Fell JC. Assessing the effectiveness of minimum legal drinking age and zero tolerance laws in the United States. *Accid Anal Prev.* 2003;35(4):579–587.

41. Carpenter C. How do zero tolerance drunk driving laws work? *J Health Econ.* 2004;23(1):61–83.

42. National Institute on Alcohol Abuse and Alcoholism. Alcohol Policy Information System. Bethesda, MD: National Institutes of Health, United States Department of Health and Human Services http://alcoholpolicy.niaaa.nih.gov. Accessed February 5, 2015.

43. Fell JC, Fisher DA, Voas RB, Blackman K, Tippetts AS. The relationship of 16 underage drinking laws to reductions in underage drinking drivers in fatal crashes in the United States. *Annu Proc Assoc Adv Automot Med Assoc Adv Automot Med.* 2007;51:537–557.

44. DeJong W, Blanchette J. Case closed: research evidence on the positive public health impact of the age 21 minimum legal drinking age in the United States. *J Stud Alcohol Drugs Suppl.* 2014;75(Suppl 17):108–115.

45. Wagenaar AC, Toomey TL. Effects of minimum drinking age laws: review and analyses of the literature from 1960 to 2000. *J Stud Alcohol Suppl.* 2002;(14):206–225.

46. Bellou A, Bhatt R. Reducing underage alcohol and tobacco use: Evidence from the introduction of vertical identification cards. *J Health Econ.* 2013;32(2):353–366.

47. Yörük BK. Can technology help to reduce underage drinking? Evidence from the false ID laws with scanner provision. *J Health Econ.* 2014;36:33–46.

48. Ulmer RG, Shabanova V, Preusser DF. *Evaluation of Use and Lose Laws.* Washington, D.C. U.S. Department of Trasnportation, National Highway Traffic Safety Administration; 2001. http://www.nhtsa.gov/people/injury/research/pub/alcohol-laws/eval-of-law/pagei.html

49. Marcus AJ. Are the roads a safer place because drug offenders aren't on them: an analysis of punishing drug offenders with license suspensions. *Kan JL Pub Pol*. 2003;13:557.

50. Nagin DS, Pogarsky G. Integrating celerity, impulsivity, and extralegal sanction threats into a model of general deterrence: theory and evidence. *Criminology*. 2001;39(4):865–892.

51. Moreira MT, Smith LA, Foxcroft D. Social norms interventions to reduce alcohol misuse in university or college students. *Cochrane Database Syst Rev*. 2009;(3):CD006748. doi:10.1002/14651858.CD006748.pub2.

52. Nutt DJ, King LA, Phillips LD. Drug harms in the UK: a multicriteria decision analysis. *The Lancet*. 2010;376(9752):1558–1565.

53. Moodie R, Stuckler D, Monteiro C, et al. Profits and pandemics: prevention of harmful effects of tobacco, alcohol, and ultra-processed food and drink industries. *The Lancet*. 2013;381(9867):670–679.

54. Grossman M, Sindelar JL, Mullahy J, Anderson R. Policy watch: alcohol and cigarette taxes. *J Econ Perspect*. 1993;7(4):211–222.

55. All taxes are on the budget bargaining table; Reining in the deficit is priority. *USA Today*. May 8, 1990. Jessica Lee; 1990.

56. Reiter JB. Citizens or sinners—the economic and political inequity of sin taxes on tobacco and alcohol products. *Colum JL Soc Probs*. 1995;29:443.

57. Pigou AC. *The Economics of Welfare*. London: McMillan and Co; 1920; 1932.

58. McCambridge J, Hawkins B, Holden C. Vested interests in addiction research and policy. The challenge corporate lobbying poses to reducing society's alcohol problems: Insights from UK evidence on minimum unit pricing. *Addiction*. 2014;109(2):199–205.

59. Scottish Government. *Changing Scotland's Relationship with Alcohol: A Discussion Paper on Our Strategic Approach*. 2008.

60. Jones JM. Americans Still Oppose Lowering the Drinking Age. *Gallup Poll Brief*. 2014:2–2. http://www.gallup.com/poll/174077/lowering-drinking-age.aspx?utm_source=tagrss&utm_medium=rss&utm_campaign=syndication

61. Bonnie RJ. *Reducing Underage Drinking: A Collective Responsibility*. Washington, DC: The National Academies Press; 2004.

62. Kypri K, Wolfenden L, Hutchesson M, Langley J, Voas R. Public, official, and industry submissions on a bill to increase the alcohol minimum purchasing age: a critical analysis. *Int J Drug Policy*. 2014;25(4):709–716.

63. Young A. MPs vote to keep drinking age at 18. *New Zealand Herald*. August 30, 2012; http://www.nzherald.co.nz/nz/news/article.cfm?c_id=1&objectid=10830588. Accessed August 8, 2014.

64. Hahn RA, Middleton JC, Elder R, et al. Effects of alcohol retail privatization on excessive alcohol consumption and related harms: a Community Guide systematic review. *Am J Prev Med*. 2012;42(4):418–427.

65. Males MA. The minimum purchase age for alcohol and young-driver fatal crashes: a long-term view. *J Leg Stud*. 1986;15(1):181–211.

66. Smart RG, Suurvali HM, Mann RE. Do changes in per capita consumption mirror changes in drinking patterns? *J Stud Alcohol*. 2000;61(4):622–625.

67. Cook PJ, Tauchen G. The effect of minimum drinking age legislation on youthful auto fatalities, 1970–1977. *J Leg Stud*. 1984;XIII(1), January, 169–190.

68. Plunk AD, Agrawal A, Tate WF, Cavazos-Rehg PA, Bierut LJ, Grucza RA. Did the 18 Drinking Age Promote High School Dropout? Implications for Current Policy. 2014. *J Stud Alcohol Drugs*. 2015;76(5):XX–XX.

69. Dee TS, Evans WN. Teen drinking and educational attainment: evidence from two-sample instrumental variables estimates. *J Labor Econ.* 2003;21(1):178–209. doi:10.1086/344127.

70. Coate D, Grossman M. Change in alcoholic beverage prices and legal drinking ages: effects on youth alcohol use and motor vehicle mortality. *Alcohol Health Res World.* 1987;12(1):22–25.

71. Coate D, Grossman M. Effects of alcoholic beverage prices and legal drinking ages on youth alcohol use. *NBER Working Paper No. 1852.* 1986 Cambridge, MA: National Bureau of Economic Research. http://www.nber.org/papers/w1852. Accessed February 11, 2015.

72. Cook PJ. *Paying the Tab: The Costs and Benefits of Alcohol Control.* Princeton, NJ: Princeton University Press; 2007.

73. Dee TS. State alcohol policies, teen drinking and traffic fatalities. *J Public Econ.* 1999;72(2):289–315. doi:10.1016/S0047-2727(98)00093-0.

74. Wilkinson JT. Reducing drunken driving: Which policies are most effective? *South Econ J.* 1987;54(2):322–334. doi:10.2307/1059317.

75. Laixuthai A, Chaloupka FJ. Youth alcohol use and public policy. *Contemp Econ Policy.* 1993;11(4):70–81. doi:10.1111/j.1465-7287.1993.tb00402.x.

76. Ornstein SI. A survey of findings on the economic and regulatory determinants of the demand for alcoholic beverages. *Subst Alcohol Actions Misuse.* 1984;5(1):39–44.

77. Chesson H, Harrison P, Kassler WJ. Sex under the influence: the effect of alcohol policy on sexually transmitted disease rates in the United States. *J Law Econ.* 2000;43(1):215–238.

78. Carpenter C. Heavy alcohol use and youth suicide: Evidence from tougher drunk driving laws. *J Policy Anal Manag.* 2004;23(4):831–842. doi:10.1002/pam.20049.

79. Birckmayer J, Hemenway D. Minimum-age drinking laws and youth suicide, 1970–1990. *Am J Public Health.* 1999;89(9):1365–1368. doi:10.2105/AJPH.89.9.1365.

80. Chambers RA, Taylor JR, Potenza MN. Developmental neurocircuitry of motivation in adolescence: a critical period of addiction vulnerability. *Am J Psychiatry.* 2003;160(6):1041–1052.

81. O'Malley PM, Wagenaar AC. Effects of minimum drinking age laws on alcohol use, related behaviors and traffic crash involvement among American youth: 1976–1987. *J Stud Alcohol.* 1991;52(5):478–491.

82. Plunk AD, Cavazaos-Rehg PA, Bierut LJ, Grucza RA. The persistent effects of minimum legal drinking age laws on drinking patterns later in life. *Alcohol Clin Exp Res.* 2013;37(3):463–469. doi:10.1111/j.1530-0277.2012.01945.x.

83. Norberg KE, Bierut LJ, Grucza RA. Long term effects of minimum drinking age laws on past-year alcohol and drug use disorders. *Alcohol Clin Exp Res.* 2009;33(12):2180–2190. doi:10.1111/j.1530-0277.2009.01056.x.

84. Grucza RA, Hipp PR, Norberg KE, et al. The legacy of minimum legal drinking age law changes: long-term effects on suicide and homicide deaths among women. *Alcohol Clin Exp Res.* 2012;36(2):377–384. doi:10.1111/j.1530-0277.2011.01608.x.

85. Fertig AR, Watson T. Minimum drinking age laws and infant health outcomes. *J Health Econ.* 2009;28(3):737–747. doi:10.1016/j.jhealeco.2009.02.006.

86. Zhang N, Caine E. Alcohol policy, social context, and infant health: the impact of minimum legal drinking age. *Int J Environ Res Public Health.* 2011;8(9):3796–3809. doi:10.3390/ijerph8093796.

87. Wagenaar AC, Wolfson M. Enforcement of the legal minimum drinking age in the United States. *J Public Health Policy.* 1994;15(1):37–53. doi:10.2307/3342606.

88. Brown RL, Matousek TA, Radue MB. Legal-age students' provision of alcohol to underage college students: an exploratory study. *J Am Coll Health*. 2009;57(6):611–618.

89. Johnston LD, Bachman JG, Schulenberg JE. *Monitoring the Future: National Survey Results on Drug Use, 1975–2004. Volume II: College Students and Adults Ages 19–45*. Bethesda, MD: National Institute on Drug Abuse; 2008.

90. Toomey TL, Nelson TF, Lenk KM. The age-21 minimum legal drinking age: a case study linking past and current debates. *Addiction*. 2009;104(12):1958–1965.

91. King RF. The politics of denial: the use of funding penalties as an implementation device for social policy. *Policy Sci*. 1987;20(4):307–337. doi:10.1007/BF00135869.

10

Public Policy and Infectious Disease Prevention and Control

William G. Powderly

LEARNING OBJECTIVES

1. Describe the importance and health impact of infectious diseases.
2. Explain the main ways in which policy is used in prevention and control of infectious disease.
3. Explain the importance of vaccines in prevention and control of infectious disease.
4. Describe the importance of policy in reducing Health Care Acquired Infections and HIV transmission.

IDENTIFYING THE PROBLEM: INFECTIOUS DISEASES AND CONSEQUENCES

Historically, prevention of infectious diseases provided one of the cornerstones of public health. Many of the approaches that the public health community uses to tackle ongoing problems stem from the policies used to deal with major infectious-disease challenges in the late 19th and early 20th century. These include careful epidemiology, interventions grounded in scientific understanding of causality, sound public policy, and strong public support based on clear messaging and a public understanding of the benefit of prevention.

It is important to note, however, that in spite of many significant advances, infectious diseases still account for about one quarter of annual deaths worldwide.[1] (Table 10.1). The burden of these diseases varies greatly by geography, with the greatest impact being seen in low-income countries. Although the Western world, including the United States is much less affected by the infectious diseases of childhood (such as pneumonia, diarrhea, and malaria), it remains vulnerable to and affected by emerging infections and other infectious-disease problems, and these continue to present significant challenges to the developed world.

In the United States, chronic viral infections, such as HIV[2] and hepatitis B and C[3], are readily transmitted and contribute to ongoing morbidity. Outbreaks of

Table 10.1 Major Causes of Global Premature Death: 2010

	Major Causes of Premature Death: 2010
1	Ischemic Heart Disease
2	Lower Respiratory Infections*
3	Stroke
4	Diarrhea*
5	Malaria*
6	HIV/AIDS*
7	Preterm Birth Complications
8	Road Injury
9	Chronic Obstructive Pulmonary Disease (COPD)
10	Neonatal Encephalopathy
11	Tuberculosis*
12	Neonatal Sepsis*

* = infectious disease.

Adapted from: Lozano R, Naghavi M, Foreman K, et al. Global and regional mortality from 235 causes of death for 20 age groups in 1990 and 2010: a systematic analysis for the Global Burden of Disease Study 2010. *Lancet.* 2012;380:2095–2128.

food-borne infections are extremely common with both health and economic consequences. Health-care associated infections have been identified as an important preventable cause of death in modern health care. Outbreaks of vaccine-preventable infections have increasingly been seen, reflecting public complacency, misinformation (sometimes deliberate), and, in some communities, distrust of government.

Increasing global connectivity is a reason why antimicrobial resistance has now become a global public health crisis, whose solution will require multinational, transdisciplinary, and policy approaches. The world as a whole is also vulnerable to changes in vector-borne and zoonotic infections, which often reflect changes in land use (whereby humans come into contact with previously un-encountered animal pathogens) and/or changes in climate (which facilitates survival of vectors of infection). In these cases, the increasing connectivity of the world with rapid and global transportation enhances the risk of localized infections becoming pandemic problems. The recent outbreak of Ebola virus infection in West Africa provides an object lesson in global vulnerability.[4] Infection, caused by a filovirus, is a zoonosis where the primary host is probably a fruit bat. Incidental contact between humans and the mammalian host led to slow but progressive transmission among humans—with lethal effect. Spread of the epidemic was facilitated by the fact that the initial infection occurred in a part of the world where there has been significant breakdown of public governance (after many years of civil war) and where public health infrastructure was essentially nonexistent. Increasing urbanization in resource-poor countries also added to more rapid transmission of this virus than had been seen in many prior outbreak situations.

Prevention policy as it pertains to infectious diseases has a long history; one which has brought together the clinical, research, and public health communities to develop policies that have been implemented at local, state, and national levels. A prevention policy strategy can be planned for virtually every infectious disease, given that prevention usually means disrupting transmission from an affected individual or source to other vulnerable individuals (or communities). Appropriate and scientifically based prevention policy approaches for infectious disease must involve an understanding of pathogenesis and transmission dynamics and must be designed to address the multifactorial aspect inherent to this topic. Specifically, infectious disease prevention policy must include the following components: tracking methods, transmission and control protocols, prevention strategies, and treatment regimens.

Public policy is driven in part by public attitudes, which, in turn, affect policy makers' readiness to take action. Public acceptance of approaches to prevent and control infectious diseases is generally high, in spite of the fact that the laws and regulations that underpin these approaches generally involve some invasion of privacy and personal rights. Control and prevention of infectious diseases can involve mandatory reporting of cases (with identification of individuals) to public authorities, tracing of contacts (with attendant loss of privacy and occasional embarrassment and/or public disclosure), compulsory quarantine, mandatory treatment, mandatory vaccination, and in some extreme cases even incarceration. Pets or other animals that are regarded as potential sources of human infection can be seized, quarantined, and even destroyed. Businesses, such as restaurants, can be closed. In all of these scenarios, there has been little or no public debate as to the appropriateness of the public health measures. This may reflect a general acceptance of the reasons for these measures; although in many cases it also may reflect the general fear (whether reasonable or groundless) that the public has regarding contagious diseases. It is perhaps striking to observe that the area in which we have had the greatest effect in controlling infection, (i.e., vaccination), has become an area in which there is now greater public skepticism and debate. In addition, there are newer areas of infectious disease, where new and different strategies may need to be adopted, which will offer new challenges and opportunities in terms of public health policy.

Importance of Tracking Infectious Diseases

A critical need exists for communities at all levels to have the capacity to track infections and identify potential outbreaks. This requires appropriate epidemiologic infrastructure that collects data on important communicable diseases, has the ability to analyze such data to identify outbreaks or potential sources of new infection, and has the capacity to intervene where appropriate. Policies in which processes and resources for tracking are outlined are extremely important. Examples of infectious diseases where such data gathering is critical in prevention include sexually transmissible infections (e.g., HIV), hospital-associated infections, tuberculosis, and foodborne illnesses. Tracking and data gathering are also vital in understanding emerging infectious diseases that might have pandemic potential. (See Box 10.1.) In ideal circumstances,

> **Box 10.1** 2012 Outbreak of MERS-CoV
>
> - In 2012, the first cases of an acute syndrome of respiratory failure described in hospitalized patients in Saudi Arabia: Middle East Respiratory Syndrome (MERS) [5]
> - Evidence of nosocomial transmission in hospitals and outbreaks in families
> - Novel coronavirus isolated—Middle East respiratory syndrome coronavirus (MERS-CoV)
> - Multiple cases throughout the Arabian Peninsula with some secondary cases spread from infected individuals
> - No clear epidemiologic connection between human cases; because coronaviruses are often also animal viruses, search for animal source begun
> - Ninety percent of adult dromedary camels in the Middle East and Africa seropositive for MERS-CoV[6]
> - MERS-CoV detected in camels that were in close contact with patients with MERS.
> - Seroprevalence of antibodies to MERS-CoV twentyfold greater in camel-exposed individuals than in general population.[7]
> - Current hypothesis is that camels are primary hosts for MERS-CoV and that asymptomatic infection in individuals in close contact with camels can then serve as route of transmission within humans. How humans become infected from camels remains unclear.

this infrastructure should have a local focus, but also should be linked into state and national public health structures so that emerging outbreaks that have epidemic or pandemic potential can be rapidly identified and effective prevention policy solutions determined.

The role of surveillance and identification of possible infections is so critical to public health that most states (and/or other jurisdictions) have a list of reportable infectious diseases, the incidence of which must be reported to the local or state public health department. Box 10.2 illustrates some of the infections that require mandatory reporting to the Missouri Department of Health and Senior Services. Full details of all the many reporting requirements can be found online[8]. Reporting requirements vary depending on the seriousness of the infection and the urgency with which a public health response must be deployed. The onus for such reporting falls on diagnostic laboratories, individual physicians, or others; and, the penalties for failing to report can be significant.

Preventing Transmission of Infectious Diseases

Vector-borne Infections

Having identified potential infectious diseases that threaten public health, prevention policies must then address control measures that interrupt transmission. The type of intervention needed will depend on the mode of transmission of the infection. For vector-borne disease, attempts to control vectors (i.e., use of insecticides and control

Box 10.2 Examples of Reportable Infectious Diseases*

Immediately Reportable Diseases or Findings that Suggest High Priority Diseases (including possible bioterrorism events)

- Anthrax
- Botulism
- Plague
- Rabies (Human)
- Severe Acute Respiratory Syndrome (SARS)-associated Coronavirus Disease
- Smallpox (variola)
- Tularemia (pneumonic)
- Viral hemorrhagic fevers (e.g., Ebola, Lassa)

Diseases Reportable Within One Day

- Brucellosis
- Cholera
- Dengue fever
- Diphtheria
- Hepatitis A
- Measles (rubeola)
- Meningococcal disease, invasive
- Pertussis
- Poliomyelitis
- Shigellosis
- Syphilis, including congenital syphilis
- Tuberculosis
- Typhoid fever (Salmonella typhi)

Diseases Reportable Within Three Days

- Acquired immunodeficiency syndrome (AIDS) and/or HIV infection
- Campylobacteriosis
- Chancroid
- *Chlamydia trachomatis* infections
- Gonorrhea
- Hepatitis B
- Hepatitis C
- Legionellosis
- Leptospirosis
- Rocky Mountain spotted fever
- Salmonellosis
- Toxic shock syndrome,
- Varicella (chickenpox)
- West Nile virus

of stagnant water) are important public-health measures, especially in resource-poor settings. However, vector control also remains important in the United States, as mosquito-borne infections have increased in importance over the last 15 years. This was first noted with the arrival of West Nile virus in the early part of the 21st century.[9] Dengue fever[10] and Chikungunya fever[11] are moving into the southern United States from the Caribbean and Central America. Prevention of acquisition (by preventing insect bites in particular) is also an important public health strategy. These strategies include wide-scale provision of bed netting, as well as the use of medication to prevent parasites from establishing infection when individuals are bitten by the vector, such as malaria prophylaxis for travel to endemic areas. Prevention of tick bites is also important in parts of the United States, where tick-borne illnesses such as New England and Lyme disease are prevalent.[12]

For significant zoonotic infections, policy prevention approaches largely involve coordination with animal control regulations. For example, to prevent rabies in both domestic animals and incidental human transmission, most jurisdictions have developed laws or regulations to require rabies vaccination for dogs, with penalties for those who do not comply. For countries such as the United Kingdom or Ireland where rabies is not endemic in local animals, these regulations have been extended to require either evidence of immunity or quarantine for up to six months before dogs can be imported.

Food-borne Infections

Prevention of food-borne infections is another area where prevention policies overlap with regulations governing other industries (i.e., agriculture and food). Most food-borne outbreaks are local, making local and state epidemiology critical in identifying such outbreaks. Epidemiologic investigation may identify a source, which would then necessitate involvement of other regulators (e.g., those involved in licensing restaurants) to determine whether breaches in existing laws and regulations have occurred. However, with the industrialization and centralization of food production and supply, multistate and multinational outbreaks have become more frequent. By necessity, investigation of such outbreaks involves agencies with broader remits, such as the U.S. Centers for Disease Control and Prevention (CDC), state health departments, the Food and Drug Administration (FDA), and the U.S. Department of Agriculture, along with equivalent regulators in Europe and elsewhere. This has led to stronger regulations in the United States, such as efforts by the FDA to regulate egg safety in order to better control Salmonella contamination, and efforts by the CDC to increase population-based surveillance of common food-borne pathogens.

Human-to-Human Transmission

Serious infections that involve human-to-human transmission require prevention policies based on the risk and timing of acquisition of infection by vulnerable hosts. A very important public health strategy, which often requires the law to enforce it, is quarantine. Although quarantine is often raised as an emotive public response to new or emerging infections (especially those with lethal consequences), it is only an effective public health strategy when individuals with infection can be identified before they become contagious, and, therefore, have the ability to infect others. The recent outbreak of Ebola virus infection provided an object lesson in the effectiveness of quarantine. Individuals with Ebola virus infection are only infectious after they become symptomatic, and indeed, the likelihood of transmission increases with the duration of symptoms and severity of illness.[4] Thus, quarantining symptomatic individuals is a very effective way of interrupting transmission and halting an epidemic. It is notable that (with the occasional exception of healthcare workers) there have been no secondary cases among the imported cases of Ebola virus in the recent epidemic. In contrast, quarantine is a less effective strategy to adopt in cases where individuals are highly infectious before they become symptomatic, such as influenza[13] or measles.[14] However, a form of quarantine, namely, selective isolation of symptomatic individuals until they are no longer infectious, is often used for these viral illnesses. As an example, policies within healthcare organizations require that healthcare workers who develop influenza do not return to work until symptoms resolve.

Another important public health strategy to deal with infections transmitted from one human to another involves identifying contacts of infected individuals and providing them with either treatment or prophylaxis. Contact tracing (identification and diagnosis of persons who may have come into contact with an infected individual) is an important element of public health prevention strategies for sexually transmitted diseases and tuberculosis (TB). TB is a bacterial disease transmitted through the air, and although rare in developed countries, is most often associated with infection in immigrants.[15] The public health approach to prevention of TB starts with identifying infected individuals. In the case of persons with active infection, contacts are identified and screened to determine if they have infection (latent disease) or active disease from TB. Such cases are then offered either treatment (for active disease) or chemoprophylaxis (for latent infection).

Policies exist to allow public health authorities to use an extreme form of control (albeit one that is rarely exercised) to curb the spread of TB. Patients with active TB are quite contagious, but the risk to others is eliminated with effective therapy. In some cases, individuals with infectious TB refuse treatment. In such cases, public health departments have the ability to forcibly incarcerate individuals and mandate treatment. Such draconian laws stem from an earlier era when effective control measures were often not available; however, these laws are still valid in many jurisdictions and have rarely been successfully challenged. In such cases, the courts have accepted that protection of the public outweighs the rights of an individual.

Vaccination as a Prevention Strategy

The public health measure that has had the greatest success in controlling infectious diseases has been the development of vaccination. Indeed, many would regard vaccination as the greatest advance in human medicine ever. Many lethal infections (especially viral infections of childhood) are now merely memories in the developed world, and an effective worldwide vaccination campaign has led to the eradication of smallpox, one of the great killers in human history.[16] In the United States, for example, it is estimated that for each birth cohort, childhood immunization prevents 40,000 deaths and as many as 20 million infections.[17] Vaccinations involve the administration of an antigen (a living attenuated pathogen, a killed pathogen, or a reactive component of a pathogen), which then stimulates an immune response in the human host. If the host is then exposed to the pathogen, the immune response generated by the vaccine usually prevents infection from being established. In some circumstances, vaccines do not prevent infection but do prevent disease. Vaccinations usually are administered starting in early childhood but can continue throughout life. Enforcement of the use of vaccinations as a public health strategy usually involves demonstrating immune status at various points in an individual's life. U.S. public health policy now recommends early childhood vaccination against polio, measles, mumps, rubella, pertussis, rotavirus, hemophilus influenza pneumococcus, and varicella.[18] Most school districts require evidence of immunity to common childhood infections prior to school admission. Thus, while early childhood vaccination may remain voluntary, the requirement for school admission has been a very important component of public uptake of vaccines.[19] Vaccination against hepatitis B and human papilloma virus is also recommended during childhood. Interestingly, these vaccines also prevent cancer because of the role of viral infection in the development of hepatic cancer and cancer of the cervix, respectively. It is recommended that college students and military recruits be vaccinated against meningococcal infection because of the higher risk of exposure associated with these jobs and settings.[20]

Certain occupations require additional vaccinations as mandatory employment stipulations. Most healthcare workers are required to demonstrate evidence of immunity to hepatitis B (which usually means prior vaccination), and healthcare facilities increasingly are mandating that employees with patient contact undergo annual influenza vaccination. Many jurisdictions require food handlers to present evidence of immunity to hepatitis A (which again usually mandates vaccination) because of evidence that most outbreaks of hepatitis A are a result of fecal contamination from infected hosts. There are also recommendations for other population subgroups. For example, a vaccine against herpes zoster virus is recommended for older adults to boost preexisting immunity and prevent shingles.

There has been tremendous progress in the development of new vaccines over the last 20 years, through both improved vaccines for previously controlled diseases as well as new vaccines for emerging pathogens. This progress has been paralleled, however, by an increasing loss of public confidence for vaccines in general. It is critically important that public health professionals understand and effectively address this public reaction to ensure that vaccination remains a vital part of infectious-disease prevention policy.

The public's increasing skepticism regarding the effectiveness and use of vaccinations is complex. An individual's acceptance or rejection of vaccination for herself, or more importantly for her children, may be based on many factors. One of the critical issues with vaccines is that the public health benefit is derived when a large number of healthy individuals are vaccinated. Thus, unlike many other health interventions, vaccination is given to a healthy person and the immediate benefit to that individual may not be apparent. For some infections, there must be widespread immunization of the population to create "herd immunity"—that is, immunity at a population level, and the actual major benefit is not to the vaccinated individual but to unvaccinated members of the community (usually infants too young to be vaccinated themselves). When devastating infections such as polio, measles, and diphtheria were part of "normal" childhood development, parents and families rushed to vaccinate their children to protect them from the fatal or chronically debilitating effects of such infections. In the developed world, however, several generations separate the era when these infections were common from the present day. Today, parents (and even grandparents) have no personal recollection of the potentially catastrophic effects of early childhood infections. This can lead to complacency, which is often coupled with a misplaced confidence that modern medicine can deal with an infection if it does occur. More importantly, the very fact that these vaccines have been so effective means that possible risks of the vaccines (and/or the schedules by which the vaccines are given) have gained greater prominence than they might have gained in an era when the diseases were more common and greatly feared.

A number of interlinking factors have resulted in this false sense of security. Some people are skeptical of the vaccine industry and question the financial motives of large corporations; others are skeptical of science in general and concerned that scientists might minimize risk because of conflicts of interest. A lack of understanding of the scientific process can lead to doubts about science in general. Recommendations are based on emerging data, yet changing vaccination recommendations can be perceived by the public as scientific uncertainty. As scientifically based guidelines and advice changes, confidence in the science can paradoxically decrease. Adverse events may occur by coincidence but are often attributed by individual parents to vaccination because the adverse event coincided with a vaccination. This particular phenomenon has been exacerbated by scientific fraud (as in the case of a putative, but false, link between autism and the measles vaccine[22]) and by celebrity endorsement.[23] Indeed, the entire antivaccination movement has been greatly enhanced by the Internet and social media, which allow for the rapid exchange of information, along with misinformation, and can fuel a self-perpetuating community of doubters.

One additional and disturbing element of decreased vaccination rates among children reflects a form of social elitism, more often seen in affluent and, presumably, more informed communities. In this situation, nonvaccination of children is a conscious decision based on the notion that such parents do not need to vaccinate their children if enough other people are continuing to vaccinate to maintain a community herd immunity.[24]

Another factor that has added to public concern is the addition of more vaccines to what was already perceived as a robust immunization schedule for children. Some of these are novel vaccines against illnesses for which there was not previously an available preventive strategy. Many others are variations of vaccines that have been available for years, with technical improvements and changes that add to complexity. Furthermore, as new vaccines are introduced, the schedule by which children receive them changes. This increasing complexity of products and scheduling has undoubtedly led to more public questioning of vaccine choices. Furthermore, individual countries have recommended different schedules for childhood vaccination, again raising legitimate questions among the public as to the rationale behind the policy recommendation.[25] Public confidence also is challenged when various authorities take different stances on vaccination. This is particularly true in the current Internet and social media era, wherein a government's decision in one jurisdiction is rapidly disseminated globally. For example, the Japanese government decided in 2011 to temporarily suspend use of the pneumococcal conjugate vaccine and the hemophilus influenzae vaccine while investigating possible adverse events. Although the suspension was short-lived, the event was rapidly disseminated worldwide through social media, leading to widespread disquiet in many communities.

Increased reluctance to vaccinate children has resulted in the re-emergence of dangerous childhood infections. The United States continues to see outbreaks of vaccine-preventable infections that are often linked to initial cases in individuals coming from countries where the diseases are endemic. After initial contact with the infected individual, the outbreak spreads among unvaccinated U.S. residents. About 50–100 cases of measles occur annually in the United States.[26] In 2015, a significant multistate outbreak of measles occurred following an index case in a visitor to Disneyland in California.[27] (See Box 10.3.) Although most of the cases of measles have been uncomplicated and self-limited, there have been fatalities and complications. Furthermore, ongoing transmission provides substantial risk to the small population of children (e.g., those too young to receive vaccination or with abnormal immune systems) who cannot be immunized and who have a higher risk of dying with infection. In addition to the health consequences of such outbreaks, there are also financial costs to the public health system. For example, two outbreaks of measles in Utah in 2011 involved only 13 cases but were estimated to cost the public health system over $300,000 in additional resources.[28] Outbreaks of mumps[29] and a steady rise in the cases of pertussis[30] (whooping cough) also have been documented in the United States over the last 10 years. It should be emphasized, however, that in both of these diseases, factors other than failure to vaccinate might be playing a role. For example, infections that may be caused by strains not well covered by vaccination, and a lack of complete protection in every recipient, are additional issues that may contribute to these outbreaks.

There is substantial variation among different populations or communities in terms of belief in vaccine efficacy or risk and in terms of trust in government and authority. Success in safeguarding vaccination as a trusted and effective strategy in the prevention of infectious diseases requires an understanding of local factors such as religious beliefs, political will, historical context, and sociodemographics. Understanding these factors can aid in the development of effective strategies to address the issue. For example, the outbreak of measles in California in 2015 has brought much attention to the rights and responsibilities of parents with regard to vaccination. Policies have been seen as a potential solution to address the issue of "rights." Schools in some areas have considered policies allowing refusal of attendance for unvaccinated children. In 2015, several states introduced legislation to limit or abolish religious exemptions to mandatory vaccination.

Case Study: Policies Related to Health Care-associated Infections

In the United States, it is estimated that 100,000 people die of health care associated infections (HCAIs) in hospitals each year.[31] This estimate does not include mortality in nonhospital settings (e.g., outpatient clinics, long-term care facilities, or dialysis centers) that are increasingly a standard part of American health care. These infections are estimated to add at least $30 billion in additional direct medical costs and probably have an even greater economic consequence. [32] In spite of these astounding numbers, it is only recently that HCAIs have come to be regarded as a public health problem, and as an issue where policy approaches factor into the solution.[33]

Traditional public health approaches to control infectious diseases in the community are also applicable in the healthcare setting. Surveillance for sentinel infection rates (e.g., line-associated blood stream infection, postoperative wound infection, and catheter-associated urinary tract infection) has allowed infection control professionals and epidemiologists to identify important preventable risk factors for such infections and to investigate interventions that can decrease rates. Investigation of outbreaks also adds to identification of risk behaviors or practices that can be ameliorated or prevented, quite often via policy. Isolation of patients (a form of quarantine) has decreased transmission of antimicrobial resistant infection. Behavior changes among healthcare professionals, particularly better adherence to handwashing requirements, are also critical components of infection prevention in the healthcare setting. Increasingly, it has been recognized that a series of policies and practices, bundled together, can significantly decrease, if not eliminate, some of these infections.

From a policy perspective, the most important advance has been the development of federal and state measures to enforce the necessary behavioral responses. All 50 states in the United States have HCAI prevention plans.[34] Many states have developed mandatory reporting of certain HCAIs to increase accountability and transparency in hospital settings. From the federal perspective, the Centers for Medicare and Medicaid Services (CMS) have introduced financial incentives to increase adherence to the CDC's infection control guidance. The CDC has developed a national tracking system, the National Healthcare Safety Network (NHSN), which tracks data on rates of infection with antimicrobial resistant organisms, use of antimicrobials, adherence rates to certain infection control measures, and vaccination rates among healthcare workers.[35] The NHSN includes over 12,000 facilities (hospital and other facilities) in all states and has been able to demonstrate encouraging trends toward a decreasing burden of HCAIs in the country. But complacency is not warranted. Certain infections, such as Clostridium difficile infection and multi-drug resistant gram-negative infections have not decreased, and in the case of the latter may be increasing in prevalence.[36] In late 2014, legislation was introduced to address the threat of antimicrobial resistant organisms and additional policy changes are being considered. For example, it is likely that the CMS will require all hospitals to implement antibiotic stewardship programs intended to restrict the use of certain drugs so that resistance to them is less likely to emerge and their effectiveness can be maintained for more serious infections and appropriate indications.

Case Study: Policies Relating to Human Immunodeficiency Virus (HIV) Infection

Infection with HIV has been one of the greatest global public health challenges of the last 30 years. Since 1981, there have been over 20 million deaths from HIV infection, and even now, nearly 20 years after the development of effective treatment for HIV, there are 2.5 million new cases of HIV each year across the world and at least 1.5 million people die annually from HIV disease.[37] Prevention of HIV infection is without doubt one of the most critical public health challenges of the 21st century.

Transmission of HIV infection is well understood. The major route of infection is sexual and most infection occurs in the setting where neither party is aware of their HIV status. The likelihood of infection occurring during sexual transmission is most strongly correlated with the amount of HIV in the blood of an infected person (viral load). This is highest during acute infection and, therefore, transmission during acute infection is a major driver of epidemic HIV. Transmission also occurs from mother to child during pregnancy (especially in the third trimester), during childbirth, and with breastfeeding. Transmission occurs when individuals have direct inoculation with blood or blood products, as has occurred with blood transfusions and continues to occur with intravenous drug users sharing needles or syringes.

As with other viral infections, the ideal prevention strategy would be an effective vaccine. However, in spite of over 25 years of concerted and well-financed research, a vaccine for HIV has proven elusive. Unlike some other viral infections, live attenuated virus is never likely to be felt a safe proposition for HIV immunization. Current challenges include uncertainty as to what would constitute protective immunity, the genetic diversity of the virus, and great difficulty in finding antigens that can provoke sustained immune responses that might be effective. Therefore, prevention strategies other than an HIV vaccine should be considered.

As indicated previously in this chapter, knowledge of the transmission characteristics can guide effective public health prevention strategies. One of the success stories in HIV prevention has been in the prevention of mother-to-child transmission of the virus. Early clinical trials demonstrated that treating mothers during pregnancy and labor, and treating infants for a short period after birth, could greatly reduce the rate of childhood infection. These studies rapidly led to public health policies of screening all mothers for HIV during pregnancy and offering treatment to infected pregnant women. Initially, all mothers were asked to give consent for HIV testing. Screening policies were further refined to an opt-out approach whereby mothers were assumed to consent unless they formally declined. This policy approach has led to a situation where neonatal and pediatric HIV infection is extraordinarily rare in the developed world, and usually occurs in situations where mothers have had little or no prenatal care. Not surprisingly, the situation is different in the developing world, where availability of effective antiretroviral therapy is much more variable and where antenatal care is less organized. One important policy difference between developed and developing countries concerns breastfeeding. In the Western world, it is recommended that HIV-infected women not breastfeed. However, in the developing world, formula feeding is associated with higher mortality and not breastfeeding may stigmatize the HIV-infected mother. Consequently, prevention policies in the developing world have had to be refined to reflect this reality, and where it is available, current guidelines recommend that the mother continue to receive antiretroviral therapy throughout the period of breastfeeding. This approach is based on evidence that such a policy has the best outcomes for both mother and child.[38,39]

Prevention of HIV infection by transfusion was rapidly achieved after the development of diagnostic tests for HIV and screening of donors and blood products. Because there remained a small window whereby an infected donor could transmit HIV without testing positive, screening of donors was accompanied by a policy of a lifetime ban on blood donation by individuals, particularly homosexual men, who engaged in high-risk sexual practices. (See Chapter 13 case study for more information on transfusion policy.) As testing technology improved and knowledge of transmission risk increased, this approach made less scientific sense. Nonetheless, it was not until late 2014 that the FDA changed its policy to one that banned individuals who had engaged in high-risk sexual practices during the previous 12 months. Relevant scientific groups, such as the Infectious Diseases Society of America, continue to advocate for a more scientifically based policy that would reduce the window to high-risk behavior in the previous 6 months.

Both behavioral and biomedical approaches have their place in preventing sexual transmission of HIV. Condom use has been known to be effective in reducing HIV risk for many years. However, advocacy of condom use as public policy and education approaches to increase both use and acceptability of condoms have often been hampered by political considerations that ignored scientific evidence. For example, between 2001 and 2008, the CDC was unable to fully advocate for condom use as a strategy in HIV prevention. Instead, public policy focused on abstinence as a strategy, in spite of minimal evidence that such an approach was effective. This is an area where public policy (driven by political and/or religious considerations rather than science) can actually have detrimental effects. Discrimination against male homosexuals is likely to keep such activity hidden, and an abstinence-based approach to prevention actually increases the risk of heterosexual transmission of HIV, as gay men conceal their sexuality.

One of the most critical scientific advances in prevention of HIV infection has been the demonstration that treatment of infected individuals can significantly decrease (and possibly completely eliminate) their risk of infecting uninfected sexual partners.[40] There are lower transmission rates in the community when there is a higher proportion of treated HIV-positive individuals in that community. This has given rise to the concept of community viral load. For example, if more HIV-infected people in a community are being treated, there will be less HIV available to infect new patients. Given that most current infections occur via individuals who do not know they are HIV positive, the public policy approach that is now being tested around the world is known as "test and treat." This would imply developing strategies to increase HIV testing and then increase access to treatment for infected persons. The current CDC recommendations for HIV testing suggest that all patients in healthcare settings should be tested for HIV.

Parallel to the clinical studies that show that treating HIV-infected persons decreases their infectivity, are studies that indicate that giving uninfected high-risk individuals (especially men who have sex with men) antiretroviral drugs can protect them from acquiring HIV infection in spite of continued high-risk behavior.[41] This approach is known as *pre-exposure prophylaxis* or PrEP and is being increasingly used. Opponents to this strategy believe that it will increase the possibility of generating treatment-resistant HIV strains and that it also will increase high-risk behavior, because recipients of PrEP may minimize other protective strategies, such as condom use. Nevertheless, in 2014, the U.S. Public Health Service issued guidelines suggesting that PrEP be considered as an option for individuals at substantial risk for HIV acquisition.

It is important to emphasize that in spite of all the program and policy strategies being implemented, HIV infection remains an important public health challenge. In the United States, the CDC estimates that 50,000 new cases of HIV are acquired each year and that this number has not changed in over 10 years.[42] So clearly, better public health approaches, especially ones targeting the communities at greatest risk are needed.

CONCLUSION

Prevention of infectious diseases has been one of the great public health success stories of the last 150 years. Policies based on sound scientific principles, including understanding of pathogenesis and transmission of infection have been developed and implemented. Most jurisdictions have a public health infrastructure that monitors important infections and has policies to control and/or to prevent many of the important risks to the population. Vaccination policies have led to the virtual elimination of many important infections (especially those of early childhood) in the developed world. However, the risk of infection has not been eliminated. There has been a decrease in funding for public health over the last 30 years, with consequent inadequate responses to emerging or new infections. Trends in globalization and travel have increased the risk of many infections, including vector-borne, food-borne, and zoonotic infections. Antimicrobial resistance and hospital-associated infections are now global problems that will require a multinational and multidisciplinary response.

The policy implications for prevention of infectious diseases are many. Currently, public health professionals at state and local levels have many powers to prevent infectious diseases, as the balance between individual rights and community health needs has played out historically. For certain infections, public health authorities have the right to mandate testing of individuals or communities for communicable illnesses. They can enforce mandatory quarantine or isolation. They can mandate treatment and provide legal sanction against those who refuse therapy. In extreme cases, they can even force individuals to be treated for infectious diseases without their consent.

Development of scientific knowledge may offer novel possibilities for prevention and control with subsequent new or evolved policy implications. However, as we become more precise in determining risk from an infected individual to others in the community, the tension between the rights of individuals and the rights of the general public are likely to become heightened, leading to even more debate about policies appropriate for adoption.

REFERENCES

1. Lozano R, Naghavi M, Foreman K, et al. Global and regional mortality from 235 causes of death for 20 age groups in 1990 and 2010: a systematic analysis for the Global Burden of Disease Study 2010. *Lancet.* 2012;380:2095–2128.

2. Centers for Disease Control and Prevention. Monitoring selected national HIV prevention and care objectives by using HIV surveillance data—United States and 6 dependent areas—2012. HIV Surveillance Supplemental Report 2014;19 (No. 3). http://www.cdc.gov/hiv/library/reports/surveillance/. Published November 2014. Accessed Sept 13, 2015.

3. Centers for Disease Control and Prevention. Disease burden from viral hepatitis A, B, and C in the United States, 2012. http://www.cdc.gov/hepatitis/pdfs/disease_burden.pdf Accessed April 25, 2015.

4. Farrar JJ, Piot P. The Ebola emergency—immediate action, ongoing strategy. *N Engl J Med.* 2014;371:1545–1546.

5. Zaki AM, van Boheemen S, Bestebroer TM, Osterhaus AD, Fouchier RA. Isolation of a novel coronavirus from a man with pneumonia in Saudi Arabia. *N Engl J Med.* 2012;367:1814–1820.

6. Chu DK, Poon LL, Gomaa MR, et al. MERS coronaviruses in dromedary camels, Egypt. *Emerg Infect Dis.* 2014;20:1049–1053.

7. Muller MA, Meyer B, Corman VM, et al. Presence of Middle East respiratory syndrome coronavirus antibodies in Saudi Arabia: a nationwide, cross-sectional serological study. *Lancet Infect Dis.* 2015;15:559–564

8. Missouri Department of Health and Senior Services. Diseases and Conditions Reportable in Missouri (19 CSR 20-20.020) http://health.mo.gov/living/healthcondiseases/communicable/communicabledisease/pdf/reportablediseaselist1.pdf Accessed April 25, 2015.

9. Petersen LR, Brault AC, Nasci RS. West Nile virus: review of the literature. *JAMA: Journal of the American Medical Association.* 2013;310:308–315.

10. Messina JP, Brady OJ, Pigott DM, et al. The many projected futures of dengue. *Nat Rev Microbiol.* 2015;13:230–239.

11. Powers AM. Risks to the Americas associated with the continued expansion of chikungunya virus. *J Gen Virol.* 2015;96:1–5.

12. Centers for Disease Control and Prevention. Diagnosis and management of tickborne rickettsial diseases: Rocky Mountain spotted fever, ehrlichiosis, and anaplasmosis—U.S.: A practical guide for physicians and other health-care and public health professionals. *MMWR.* 2006;55 (No.RR-4).

13. Canini L, Carrat F. Population modeling of influenza A/H1N1 virus kinetics and symptom dynamics. *J Virol.* 2011;85:2764–2770.

14. Lau LL, Cowling BJ, Fang VJ, et al. Viral shedding and clinical illness in naturally acquired influenza virus infections. *J Infect Dis.* 2010;201:1509–1516.

15. Cain KP, Benoit SR, Winston CA, MacKenzie WR. Tuberculosis among foreign-born persons in the United States. *JAMA: Journal of the American Medical Association.* 2008;300:405–412.

16. Henderson DA. Principles and lessons from the smallpox eradication programme. *Bull World Health Organ.* 1987;65:535–546.

17. Whitney CG, Zhou F, Singleton J, Schuchat A. Benefits from immunization during the vaccines for children program era—United States, 1994–2013. *MMWR.* 2014;63:352–355.

18. Advisory Committee for Immunization Practices (ACIP). Vaccine Recommendations of the ACIP. http://www.cdc.gov/vaccines/hcp/acip-recs/index.html. Accessed April 25, 2015.

19. Briss PA, Rodewald LE, Hinman AR, et al. Reviews of evidence regarding interventions to improve vaccination coverage in children, adolescents, and adults. *Am J Prev Med.* 2000;18:97–140.

20. Stephens DS, Greenwood B, Brandtzaeg P. Epidemic meningitis, meningococcaemia, and Neisseria meningitidis. *Lancet.* 2007;369:2196–2210.

21. Gershon AA, Gershon MD. Pathogenesis and current approaches to control of varicella-zoster virus infections. *Clin Microbiol Rev.* 2013;26:728–743.

22. Murch SH, Anthony A, Casson DH, et al. Retraction of an interpretation. *Lancet.* 2004;363:750.

23. Conis E. Jenny McCarthy's new war on science: Vaccines, autism and the media's shame. http://www.salon.com/2014/11/08/jenny_mccarthys_new_war_on_science_vaccines_autism_and_the_medias_shame/ Accessed April 2015.

24. Offit PA. *Deadly Choices: How the Anti-vaccine Movement Threatens Us All.* New York, NY: Basic Books; 2011.

25. World Health Organization. WHO vaccine preventable diseases monitoring system. http://apps.who.int/immunization_monitoring/en/globalsummary/scheduleselect.cfm Accessed April 25, 2015.

26. Gastanaduy PA, Redd SB, Parker Fiebelkorn A, et al. Measles—United States, January 1–May 23, 2014. *MMWR.* 2014;63:496–499.

27. Zipprich J, Winter K, Hacker J, Xia D, Watt J, Harriman K. Measles outbreak, California. December 2014–February 2015. *MMWR.* 2015;64:153–154.

28. Centers for Disease Control and Prevention. Two measles outbreaks after importation—Utah, March–June 2011. *MMWR.* 2013; 62:222–225.

29. Dayan GH, Quinlisk MP, Parker AA, et al. Recent resurgence of mumps in the United States. *N Engl J Med.* 2008;358:1580–1589.

30. Winter K, Harriman K, Zipprich J, et al. California pertussis epidemic, 2010. *J Pediatrics.* 2012:161:1091–1096.

31. Klevens RM, Edwards J, Richards C, et al. Estimating health care-associated infections and deaths in U.S. hospitals, 2002. *Public Health Rep.* 2007;122:160–166.

32. Scott RD. *The Direct Medical Costs of Healthcare-associated Infections in U.S. Hospitals and the Benefits of Prevention.* Atlanta, GA: Centers for Disease Control and Prevention; 2009.

33. Srinivasan A. Influential outbreaks of healthcare-associated infections in the past decade. *Infect Control Hosp Epidemiol.* 2010:31:S70–S72.

34. United States Department of Health and Human Services. Action plan to prevent healthcare-associated infections: road map to elimination. June 2009. http://www.hhs.gov/ash/initiatives/hai/actionplan/hhs_hai_action_plan_final_06222009.pdf Accessed April 25, 2015.

35. Malpiedi PJ, Peterson KD, Soe MM, et al. 2011 National and state healthcare-associated infection standardized infection ratio report: using data reported to the National Healthcare Safety Network as of September 4, 2012. Atlanta, GA: Centers for Disease Control and Prevention. http://www.cdc.gov/hai/pdfs/SIR/SIR-Report_02_07_2013.pdf Accessed April 25, 2015.

36. Centers for Disease Control and Prevention. Vital signs: carbapenem-resistant Enterobacteriaceae. *MMWR.* 2013;62:165–170.

37. UNAIDS. *2014 Progress Report on the Global Plan.* http://www.unaids.org/en/resources/documents/2014/JC2681_2014-Global-Plan-progress Accessed April 25, 2015.

38. Chasela CS, Hudgens MG, Jamieson DJ, et al. BAN Study Group. Maternal or infant antiretroviral drugs to reduce HIV-1 transmission. *N Engl J Med.* 2010; 362:2271–2281.

39. Thomas TK, Masaba R, Borkowf CB, et al, and the KiBS Study Team. Triple-antiretroviral prophylaxis to prevent mother-to-child HIV transmission through breastfeeding—the Kisumu Breastfeeding Study, Kenya: a clinical trial. *PLoS Med.* 2011;8:e1001015.

40. Cohen MS, Chen YQ, McCauley M, et al. Prevention of HIV-1 infection with early antiretroviral therapy. *N Engl J Med.* 2011;365:493–505.
41. Grant RM, Lama JR, Anderson PL, et al, and the iPrEx Study Team. Preexposure chemoprophylaxis for HIV prevention in men who have sex with men. *N Engl J Med.* 2010;363:2587–2599.
42. Centers for Disease Control and Prevention. *HIV in the United States: At a Glance.* http://www.cdc.gov/hiv/statistics/basics/ataglance.html Accessed May 5, 2015.

11

Law, Policy, and Injury Prevention*

David A. Sleet and Frederic E. Shaw

"IOM urges ... agencies to familiarize themselves with the public health and policy interventions at their disposal that can influence behavior and more importantly change conditions—social, economic and environmental—to improve health."
Institute of Medicine. *For the Public's Health: Revitalizing Law and Policy to Meet New Challenges.* Washington DC, National Academy of Sciences, 2011.

LEARNING OBJECTIVES

1. Describe how policies can impact injury prevention.
2. Describe types of policies related to injury prevention.
3. Provide examples of policy success in injury prevention.

IDENTIFYING THE PROBLEM: INJURIES

Injuries are a tremendous public health problem, killing more people during the first four decades of life than any other cause.[1] Injuries are not accidents—like many other diseases, they are predictable and preventable. Because the word "accident" implies an unexpected and unintended event that happens by chance or fate, it should not be used when referring to an injury, which is the medical outcome of an unintended event like a crash or a fall. The word, *injury,* itself is derived from the Latin *in-juris,* which literally means "unjust," "not lawful," or "not right." Policies, which can be defined broadly as statutes, ordinances, or other measures adopted by democratic lawmaking bodies, regulations adopted by government agencies, and procedures, incentives, voluntary practices, or other sub-regulatory policies taken up by government or non-government institutions, can be among the most important tools to reduce injuries and the events that predispose them. Whether by changing behavior, modifying the

---

* Adapted from: Shaw FE, Sleet DA, Ogolla C, Dorigo L. Law and injury prevention. In: Gullotta TP, Bloom M (Eds.), *Encyclopedia of Primary Prevention and Health Promotion* (2nd ed.), New York: Springer; 2014.

physical environment, or improving product safety, policies have had a significant impact on saving lives and reducing injuries.[2,3] Policies function in a variety of ways in primary, secondary, and tertiary prevention. For primary prevention, policies can help prevent an injury before it happens (e.g., deterring drunk driving by defining the legal limit for blood alcohol concentration while operating a vehicle). They can also reduce or eliminate the injury damage from an event once it occurs (e.g., installation of airbags and requirements to use seatbelts), or they can improve the likelihood that a person will survive an injury (e.g., policies that assure qualified emergency medical services (EMS) responders and community emergency response capability to deliver pre-hospital care to the injured).

In motor vehicle safety, policies (in this case statuses), requiring drivers and passengers to wear seat belts, requiring parents to put children in child safety seats, and prohibiting blood alcohol levels at or above .08% have helped reduce traffic fatalities by 25% since 2005, and have lowered the fatality rate per 100,000 population to one of the lowest rates in history, despite a significant increase in the number of vehicle miles driven.[4] Policies requiring helmet use while riding motorcycles and bicycles have effectively reduced death rates and traumatic brain injuries.[5]

Most every evidence-based policy introduced, implemented and enforced to reduce motor vehicle injuries have led to reductions in both deaths and death rates. (See Figure 11.1.) Not all of these policies produced immediate results, however, and many efforts experienced significant lag time from passage to public health outcome due to variations in how they were implemented and enforced, as well as in how the

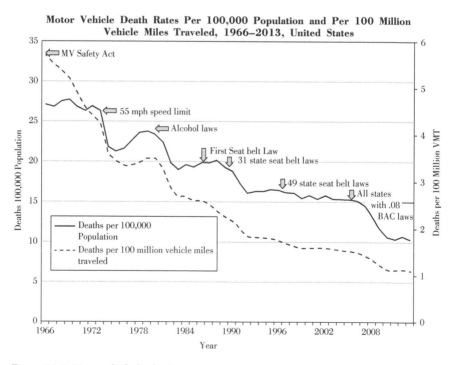

Figure 11.1 Motor vehicle death rates.

public accepted and complied with them. At times, passage of the legislation or policy had a "phase-in" element that allowed states several years to come into compliance before penalties were assessed. For example, the federal .08% BAC legislation was signed into law in 2000, but it allowed states until 2004 to be in full compliance before reductions in highway construction funds took effect.[6]

One good example of the effectiveness of policy adoption are laws and regulations to prevent drowning, such as swimming pool regulations requiring four-sided pool fencing, mandated life jacket use while boating, and environmental changes such as anti-entrapment drain covers on pools and spas.[7] These have saved lives and prevented injuries. In part because of their demonstrated effectiveness, at least 12 states now have laws related to swimming pool safety, including requirements for certified lifeguards, fencing, pool alarms, and pool drain standards.[8]

LAWS AND LEGAL TOOLS FOR ADDRESSING INJURY PREVENTION

Policies, including legislation (i.e. statutes and ordinances) and regulations, and policies that do not carry the force of law, all have been effective approaches to saving lives from injury.[2] Examples of various types of policies that can influence injuries include organizational policies, regulatory policies, and legislative policies.

Organizational Policies

- School districts (e.g., antibullying or violence prevention)
- Hospitals (e.g., requiring car seats at discharge for newborns)
- Community-based organizations (e.g., ensuring safe sporting environments)
- Business, industry, or corporations (e.g., workplace hard-hat and safety-goggle requirements)
- Professional associations (e.g., policies against serving alcohol at association events).

Regulatory Policies

- At the State level (e.g., regulations pertaining to child day-care facilities);
- At the Federal level (e.g., consumer product safety regulations; vehicle safety regulations)
- At the local level (e.g., building and fire codes)

Legislative Policies

- Local government policies (e.g., speed limits on local roads; limitations on bar and liquor-store hours; local enforcement of bicycle helmet use)
- State government policies (e.g., seat belt, child-safety seat, and motorcycle helmet laws; vehicle inspection requirements; speed limits on state roads; Blood Alcohol Concentration [BAC] laws)

- Federal government policies (e.g., the Occupational Safety and Health Act of 1970 to protect America's workers; Public Health Service Act; maternal and child health block grants; highway construction and road building standards; airbag warning labels).

INJURY PREVENTION AND THE ROLE OF POLICY

Laws and policies can affect the occurrence of injuries in at least three ways: (1) modifying the physical and social environment; (2) changing the social meaning of risk behavior; and (3) changing individual behaviors by requiring persons to either refrain from a behavior (e.g., driving too fast) or to undertake a preventive action (e.g., wearing a seat belt).[9] Of these, changing behavior might be the most difficult to achieve, in part because noncompliance may result from misjudging one's own risk of injury.[10] For example, the chances that a U.S. resident who traveled in a motor vehicle would die in a car crash on any individual trip in 2005 is on the order of 1 in 19,000,[11] low enough that the everyday experience of many people might not prompt a perception of risk or preventive action. However, under the legal requirement to wear seat belts, perception of risk may shift from the risk of being injured in a crash to the risk of being punished for breaking the law—a far more relevant and immediate threat. Similarly, a regulation requiring that all workers in a factory wear eye and ear protection may be effective, in part, because of expected sanctions against the worker for noncompliance, but also because of repercussions from other workers and management for violating a social norm.

Policies that Modify the Physical and Social Environment

Polices that make the physical environment safer can benefit all of society. For example, schools that modify playground equipment by installing soft surfaces under equipment will protect many children from injuries equipment. Municipalities that require regular safety and hazard assessments of playing fields, parks, and public spaces to identify and remediate dangerous play environments will protect all users. None of these changes require behavior change on the part of children or playground users. However, success in changing the physical environment often requires large-scale institutional changes that are costly and may compete with other municipal priorities. For example, progressively reducing the number of lanes on a highway to reduce the speed of vehicles entering a city might lower the severity of traffic injuries, but also may be a lower priority than reinforcing bridges or conducting asphalt paving. Frieden has emphasized the importance of making physical and social environment changes that can alter the context for behavior, making the healthy (or safe) choices the easy choices. Policy is an important strategy for accomplishing this.[12]

Using Policy to Change the Social Meaning of Risk Behavior

Changing the social meaning of risk behavior can also affect injury behavior. When compliance with a law or policy is seen as an official or widely accepted view, compliance is more likely.[13] According to Bonnie (1986), "Expressions of the law, over time, may affect attitudes about right or wrong and about desirable and undesirable conduct and ultimately—in this indirect way—may influence behavior" (p. 183). Thus, people may obey the law not only because they fear detection and punishment, but also because they wish to comply with stated social norms. A child safety seat law that is viewed by the culture as acceptable because it is something that protects children, who cannot protect themselves, is one example. Another example is Mothers Against Drunk Driving (MADD), which promulgated the social norm that driving while alcohol impaired is socially unacceptable. Variations in compliance with laws and policies, therefore, may reflect cultural ideals that favor (or disfavor) compliance with the rule of law.

Using Law and Policy to Change Individual Behavior

Public health laws have played a fundamental role in advancing health through their role in encouraging behavior and environmental change.[14] Just because a policy is in place, however, does not guarantee compliance. The public may be unaware of a law, or enforcement of a law may be inadequate or imperceptible. Laws sometimes accomplish individual behavior change by removing a person's ability to offend in the first place (e.g., by installing ignition interlock devices in cars to prevent alcohol-impaired driving) or through general or specific deterraence, as in the influence of criminal laws.

Oftentimes the public is aware of a law but does not perceive any benefit from it, or perceives the law to be rarely enforced or sanctions to be minimal or tolerable, or sees it to be too harsh, burdensome, or an excessive infringement on personal liberty (e.g., motorcycle helmets). Despite these limitations, laws can be an effective mechanism for inducing individuals to adopt safer behaviors,[15] provided the laws are:

- Widely known
- Fair and acceptable to the public
- Designed so that the probability of being caught is appreciable
- Enforced so that punishment is perceptibly swift and certain; and
- Perceived to be of more benefit than harm (e.g., social benefits vs. harm; health benefit vs. costs).

Public education is an important adjunct to implementation of the law. It assures that the public is prepared and persuaded, and that it accepts the law or policy as meaningful and contributing to the public good, or sees it as a way to improve population health.[16] Even before the 1980s, the injury prevention field already had recognized that individual behavior change to prevent injuries was more successful when the behavior was easily observable and required by law.[17] On the other hand, some authors have proposed that mandating a protective behavior can lead to an increase in risk taking, resulting in a nullification of the preventive effects of the law. For example, when drivers perceive that cars are built safer or that bicycling is safer while wearing a helmet, they might respond by taking more chances, such as speeding in a car or bicycling in a more reckless way. This phenomenon is referred to as risk compensation or risk homeostasis.[18] Experts differ on the extent to which risk compensation actually operates,[19] and its effects seem to be specific to each risk behavior.

Legal challenges to laws that regulate individual behavior are not uncommon. When courts make decisions on these challenges, they often must balance the public health interests of the state against the constitutional rights of individuals. The Iowa case of State v. Hartog (1989) is often cited as a classic judicial explanation of this principle. The defendant, John Hartog, received a citation for failing to use his seat belt while driving an automobile, as required by Iowa law. He was found guilty and appealed his conviction on grounds that the Iowa seat belt law was unconstitutional because it violated his Fourteenth Amendment right to autonomy and that the state had no authority to require him to wear a seat belt. In disagreeing with Hartog, the court explained that the state's exercise of the power to restrict freedom is valid as long as a "reasonable relation to the public welfare exists." Furthermore, the court said, because the costs of car crash injuries are shared by all of society, Hartog was not entitled to decide for himself whether to wear a seat belt.[20] In similar legal challenges in Canada to the right by police to randomly stop drivers and test for alcohol impairment,[21] courts ruled the ". . . the right to circulate in a motor vehicle on the public highway (i)s a "liberty . . . however . . . the right is not a fundamental liberty like the ordinary right of movement of the individual, but a licensed activity that is subject to regulation and control for the protection of life . . . ." (para 68).

The Importance of Enforcement

The effectiveness of a law is directly related to its enforceability. Recent examples are the state-level policies to enhance the use of prescription drug monitoring programs (PDMPs) for controlling the prescription drug overdose (PDO) and abuse epidemic.[27] The rate of fatal PDO involving opioids almost quadrupled from 1999 to 2011. Forty-nine states have responded by developing PDMPs, which are state-run electronic databases used to track the prescribing and dispensing of controlled prescription drugs to patients. Prescriber utilization of this information, however, is low, in part due to the fact that "only 22 of the 49 states with PDMPs now legally mandate prescribers to query the system before writing (a prescription) for a controlled substance with potential for abuse or dependence"[28] (p. 891). Without mandated registration or even mandated use, PDMPs have limited potential for impacting public health outcomes.

Enforcing state-level policies that regulate pain clinics or "pill mills" have shown promising results. In Florida, for example, a policy was implemented in 2010 to regulate pain clinics and stop healthcare providers from dispensing prescription painkillers from their offices. By 2012, more than a 50% decrease in oxycodone overdose deaths was documented.[29] Similarly, in New York, a 2012 regulation requiring prescribers to check the state's PDMP before prescribing painkillers resulted in a 75% drop in patients seeing multiple prescribers for the same drugs.[30]

Increasing the level of enforcement or increasing the penalty for violations can have a positive effect on behavior. High visibility well-enforced seat belt laws work because most people would rather buckle up than pay a fine. But in many states, fines for violating seat belt laws are so small that they do not motivate people to comply. For instance, a $40 fine for nonuse of seat belts may not get people to buckle up, but a $200 fine might. Even a modest increase can make a difference; an increase from $25 to $60 can increase belt use by 3 to 4 percentage points, while an increase from $5 to $100 can increase seat belt use by more than 10 percentage points.[31]

A local ordinance in a rural town in Georgia requiring children to wear a bicycle helmet, had virtually no effect on helmet use because enforcement was either low or nonexistent. When police began vigorously enforcing the ordinance by confiscating bicycles from any child who was not wearing a helmet, rates of helmet use increased dramatically.[32] Confiscation was a visible, dramatic, and well-publicized outcome of violating the law. In this case, it resulted in a 70% helmet-use compliance rate after targeted enforcement. When a, policy is insufficiently enforced, compliance rates will be predictably low, and safety will be compromised.

Using a Combination of Regulation and Tort Law to Make Consumer Products Safer

A good example of the use of law for public health is in the realm of product safety. Law has made an important contribution to making consumer products safer[22], and this has been accomplished through a combination of state regulation and private lawsuits (i.e., tort law). In the regulatory realm, the Consumer Product Safety Commission, a federal regulatory agency, has repeatedly illustrated the power of compiling data on injury risks from unsafe products, developing and enforcing mandatory standards to improve safety, and reducing risks to consumers by recalling dangerous products. The effort to enact sleepwear-flammability standards to reduce burns is a prime example.[23] These standards, intended to protect children from burns by requiring that children's sleepwear be flame resistant, exemplify (1) the benefits of regulating commonly used products; (2) the difficulty of keeping pace with changes in family customs, fashions, and changes in industry; (3) the interplay among government agencies, technical experts, industry, and advocacy groups; and (4) the public's frequent confusion over highly technical terms used for standard-setting.[24]

Another example of regulation to make products safer is the prevention of scald injuries in children from hot tap water. In the past, many children were scalded each year by overheated tap water. The thermostat dial setting of hot water heaters often was pre-set at the factory to 140 or 150 degrees, a temperature that can cause burns. The solution was to adopt regulations requiring the hot water heater manufacturers to reduce the factory setting to 120 degrees[23,25] and provide education regarding the risks of tap water flow at higher temperatures. Scald injuries from tap water were reduced.

Another example involves burns in children from disposable cigarette lighters. Prior to the mid-1990s, more than 200 deaths per year had been attributed to children igniting disposable cigarette lighters by using them as "sparking toys" on rugs and beds. In 1994, the Consumer Product Safety Commission mandated that lighter manufacturers develop and install child-resistant features on every lighter sold. The cost of this engineering change was about .07 cents per lighter. Although it took 10 years to pass and be fully implemented, in the years after the rule took effect, fires caused by disposable lighters were reduced by 58 percent. Over 100 lives were saved and 680 burn injuries prevented annually from this action.[26] Many countries, including those in the European Union have since adopted similar regulations.

Product Liability and Litigation

The role of law in creating safety consumer products, however, is not only about regulation. Litigation also has played a major role. Tort law (lawsuits for civil wrongs) is, in effect, another form of regulation, and can be effective where no legislation exists, or where consumer safety agencies have chosen not to regulate a particular hazard.[33] One way that tort law can reduce injuries is by holding manufacturers liable for making and selling dangerous products. Lawsuits against product manufacturer can yield compensation for damages to the injured party, but they can also deter manufacturers from producing unsafe products.[34] For example, lawsuits against manufacturers have been successful in deterring manufacturers from making dangerous toys. In a recent case, children were ingesting Buckyballs (marble-shaped powerful rare earth magnets used as a novelty toy to create a variety of shapes) and experiencing severe intestinal problems. Some of the ingested magnets resided in different loops of intestine and attracted each other through intestinal walls, causing pressure necrosis, perforation, fistula formation, or intestinal obstruction, including death.[36,37] In one case, doctors surgically removed 37 Buckyballs from the abdomen of a 3-year-old girl during a 2 hour surgery.[35] The creator of Buckyballs was forced out of business because of pending law suits, product recalls, and Consumer Product Safety Commission actions.[35]

Product liability lawsuits have been especially important in advancing motor vehicle safety by forcing recalls and improvements in engineering, manufacturing, and production after defects were found in brakes, tires, airbags, accelerators, and child safety seats. Modern product liability actions are based on the presence of and harm from a product defect, and do not require a finding of negligence by the manufacturer. The injured party must prove that the product was defective in its manufacture or design, that it was the cause of the plaintiff's injuries, and that the defect existed when it left the hands of the manufacturer. The legal consequences can be especially great if the manufacturer knew about the defect, but did not reveal it, or purposely withheld the defect information from regulators, as alleged in the recent case of a major producer of airbags, Takata, and its defective airbags. The overall effect of product liability lawsuits has been to heighten manufacturers' awareness of the importance of building safety into products, monitoring safety claims, and reporting defects in their products.

Effectiveness of Laws and Policies
Related to Injury Prevention

With the right policies, effective implementation, and strong enforcement, injuries can be prevented and lives can be saved by, for example, getting drunk drivers off the road, monitoring prescription drug use for overdose potential, getting helmets on every cyclist, reducing the blood alcohol concentration of drivers, removing dangerous products from the market, reducing vehicle speeds and many other interventions. However, in order to do this, laws must be effective. Ineffective laws are of no (or even negative) utility to public health and, in some cases, might even be unconstitutional. Many public health laws intrude upon the autonomy of individuals. For example, laws requiring motorcyclists to wear a helmet are unquestionably an impingement on the liberty of the rider.

Under the 14th Amendment due process principles, set out in the 1905 decision by the U.S. Supreme Court in *Jacobson v. Massachusetts* and subsequent cases, the government is permitted to intrude upon the autonomy of individuals for public health purposes, but the intrusion must have a real or substantial relation to the public health threat. A law that was known to have no substantial effectiveness likely would not pass that test. More importantly, though, effectiveness has important economic connotations. Governments always work with limited resources, and to affect public health optimally they must favor laws that are the effective per unit of cost. Cost is relatively easy to measure but effectiveness can be difficult.[38]

The Community Preventive Services Task Force, the Cochrane Collaboration, and the Public Health Law Research initiative of the Robert Wood Johnson Foundation have systematically evaluated the effectiveness of some injury prevention policies. The Task Force, for example, found strong evidence that 0.08% blood alcohol levels for drivers are effective in reducing alcohol-impaired driving. But it recommended against further privatization of alcohol sales in settings with current government control of retail sales based on strong evidence of increased per capita alcohol consumption.[40] The Cochrane Collaboration found that bicycle helmet legislation appears to be effective in increasing helmet use and decreasing head injury; however, there were very few high-quality studies that measured these outcomes, and none that reported data on declines in bicycling as a result of helmet legislation.[41]

Although measuring the effectiveness of laws and policies is not easy, it is an important element in enforcing and preserving the law. Research shows, for instance, that a primary seat belt law works better than a secondary law to reduce injuries[39] and that universal motorcycle helmet laws work better than partial helmet laws.[5,42]

If people know that a particular law is effective, the knowledge alone can improve enforcement. Ineffective laws can breed cynicism among lawmakers and the public about the effectiveness of all laws aimed at injury prevention. Ineffective laws also may drain scarce enforcement or advocacy resources away from more fruitful pursuits.[43] Ideally, the evaluation of laws should be planned at the time the laws are adopted, with careful attention to the most appropriate research methodology.[44]

Even when evidence is abundant that an intervention or policy could save lives, however, the evidence does not always lead to action. For example, bicycle helmets are 85% effective in preventing head injury—yet only 25% of Americans use helmets. Cell phone use while driving results in four times as many crashes, yet cell phone use while driving is increasing. Reducing BAC to .05% saves lives, but less than half of all countries in the world have implemented it.[6]

Research, no matter how compelling, will never fully contribute to improved health unless new findings are translated into products, practices, and policy.[45,46] One such effort was the translation of evidence on the effectiveness of reducing the blood alcohol content of drivers from 0.10% to 0.08%, which led to a new national BAC standard. (See Box 11.1). Another example is the Prioritizing Interventions and Cost Calculator for States (MV PICCS), an interactive calculator and tool that will help state decision-makers prioritize and select from a suite of 12 effective motor vehicle injury prevention interventions. Developed by RAND Corporation with funding from the CDC, MV PICCS is designed to calculate the expected number of injuries prevented and lives saved at the state level, as well as the costs of implementation, while taking into account available resources.[47]

FUTURE DIRECTIONS

Evidence-based laws and policies can be effective tools in efforts to reduce injuries and save lives and health care dollars. Public health can provide the scientific evidence that is so important to making good policy choices; this scientific evidence can complement information brought from other sectors such as justice, law enforcement, and social services.[49] An urgent need exists to evaluate the effectiveness of policy approaches to injury prevention to ensure that they are making an impact.[50]

The future role of policy in injury prevention will depend on the extent to which policies are successful in changing injury-related behaviors, environments, and products in ways that improve public health, and on the extent to which those successes are carefully documented and made known to policy makers.

Some of the remaining challenges include:

- Raising public awareness of existing policies designed to prevent injuries
- Evaluating the effectiveness of existing or proposed laws
- Assessing public and political support for injury prevention policies
- Documenting characteristics and costs of effective policy implementation, including enforcement strategies
- Disseminating success stories in which policies have led to reduced injuries and healthcare costs

Box 11.1 Case Study

Evidence to Policy: Reducing the Blood Alcohol Limit for
Drivers to .08% in the United States: 1998–2000[48]

Alcohol is a significant factor in fatal motor vehicle crashes. Reducing the alcohol concentration limit for drivers is believed to be an effective means to reduce alcohol-impaired driving fatalities. The U.S. Centers for Disease Control and Prevention (CDC), and the Taskforce for Community Preventive Services conducted a systematic review of the effectiveness of 0.08% blood alcohol concentration laws in reducing deaths and injuries. In 1997, 32 states had BAC laws of 0.10% and only 16 states had .08% laws. At .10%, the United States had one of the highest BAC limits in the world.

The Research Team conducted a systematic literature review of the evidence of effectiveness of state laws that lowered the allowable blood alcohol concentration (BAC) for motor vehicle drivers from 0.10% to 0.08%, using protocols for reviewing and evaluating evidence according to standards set by the Task Force and the Guide to Community Preventive Services.

Nine studies of sufficient design quality and execution qualified for the review. Of those, seven studies reported percent change values in fatal alcohol-related crashes following implementation of a 0.08% BAC law. The median reduction in fatal alcohol-related crashes was 7%, with an interquartile range of −15% to −4%. Results were generally consistent in direction and size across the studies. The Task Force on Community Preventive Services considered the evidence and quickly issued a strong recommendation that state policy makers consider implementing 0.08% BAC laws, based on the findings.

Shortly after the Task Force made its recommendation, Congressional hearings were held on lowering the BAC limit. During their deliberations, members of the subcommittee requested information about the effectiveness of 0.08% BAC laws from the CDC. In response to these requests, the Task Force summarized its findings in the recommendation that 0.08% BAC laws be implemented.

The House and Senate approved the Transportation Appropriations bill with the .08% provision as a result of testimony using the CDC evidence. If states did not enact the .08% legislation by 2004, they would lose 2%–8% of federal highway construction funds. The bill was sent to the White House and signed into law by President Clinton on October 23, 2000. Because of the lower BAC standard, it is estimated that 400–600 alcohol-related crash deaths may be prevented annually.

The case study suggests the value of: (1) clearly outlining the relationships among health problems, interventions, and outcomes; (2) systematically assessing and synthesizing the evidence; (3) using a credible group and rigorous process to assess the evidence; (4) having an impartial body make specific policy recommendations on the basis of the evidence; (5) being ready to capitalize on briefly open policy windows; (6) engaging key partners and stakeholders in the production and dissemination of the evidence; (7) undertaking personalized and targeted dissemination; (8) involving multiple stakeholders in encouraging uptake and adherence of policy recommendations; and (9) addressing sustainability.

CONCLUSION

Using a policy framework can often provide structure and a theoretical base when designing public health interventions to prevent injuries.[51] Policy also can set the stage for changes in the social and physical environment, making the safest choices the easiest choices.[12] As the Institute of Medicine, in its book on revitalizing law and policy in public health, states, "Healthy public policy is particularly important in a time of scarce resources, because it can diminish or preclude the need for other, more costly and potentially less effective interventions . . ."[3] This is particularly relevant for injury prevention and control where the use of policies and laws has resulted in a measurable impact on health.

DISCLAIMER

The views in this paper are those of the authors, and do not necessarily represent the official views of the Centers for Disease Control and Prevention.

ACKNOWLEDGMENT

We acknowledge the help of Ann Dellinger, Tamara Haegerich, Joann Yoon, and Leslie Dorigo, from the Injury Center at CDC and Chris Ogolla for commenting on various sections of this chapter, particularly the relevance of policy and law to injury prevention.

REFERENCES

1. Centers for Disease Control and Prevention. *Injury Prevention and Control: Data & Statistics (WISQARS)*. 2015; http://www.cdc.gov/injury/wisqars/. Accessed April 1, 2015.
2. Goodman R, Hoffman R, Lopez W, et al. *Law in Public Health Practice*. New York: Oxford University Press; 2007.
3. Institute of Medicine. *For the Public's Health: Revitalizing Law and Policy to Meet New Challenges*. Washington, DC: The National Academies Press; 2011.
4. National Highway Traffic Safety Administration. Traffic fatalities in 2010 drop to lowest level in recorded history. 2011; Accessed May 25, 2015. http://www.nhtsa.gov/PR/NHTSA-05-11.
5. Centers for Disease Control and Prevention. Guide to Community Preventive Services. Use of motorcycle helmets: universal helmet laws. Atlanta, GA: Author; 2013.
6. Sleet DA, Mercer SL, Cole KH, Shults RA, Elder RW, Nichols JL. Scientific evidence and policy change: lowering the legal blood alcohol limit for drivers to 0.08% in the USA. *Global Health Promotion*. Mar 2011;18(1):23–26.
7. United States House of Representatives. Virginia Graeme Baker Pool and Spa Act. *House Report 100-365, HR 1721*. Washington, DC; 2007.
8. Children's Safety Network. Drowning prevention. 2015. http://www.childrens-safetynetwork.org/injury-topics/drowning-prevention. Accessed April 1, 2015.

9. Bailey TM, Caulfield TA, Ries NM. *Public Health Law and Policy in Canada.* LexisNexis Butterworths; Markham, Ontario, Canada, 2005.

10. Tversky A, Kahneman D. Judgment under uncertainty: Heuristics and biases. *Science.* Sep 27 1974;185(4157):1124–1131.

11. National Safety Council. What are the odds of dying? 2005; http://www.nsc.org/learn/safety-knowledge/Pages/injury-facts-odds-of-dying.aspx. Accessed April 1, 2015.

12. Frieden TR. A framework for public health action: the health impact pyramid. *Am J Public Health.* Apr 2010;100(4):590–595.

13. Bonnie RJ. The efficacy of law as a paternalistic instrument. *Nebraska Symposium on Motivation.* 33: 1985 pg 131–211. Lincoln: University of Nebraska Press; 1986.

14. Mensah GA, Goodman RA, Zaza S, et al. Law as a tool for preventing chronic diseases: expanding the range of effective public health strategies. *Prev Chron Dis.* Jan 2004;1(1):A13.

15. Sleet D. Injury prevention. In: Arnold J, Gorin S, Eds. *Health Promotion Handbook.* St. Louis, MO: Mosby; 1998.

16. Kahan S, Gielen A, Fagan P, Green L, (Eds.). *Health Behavior Change in Populations.* Baltimore, MD: Johns Hopkins University Press; 2014.

17. Institute of Medicine. *Injury in America: A Continuing Public Health Problem.* Washington, DC: The National Academies Press; 1985.

18. Adams J, Hillman M. The risk compensation theory and bicycle helmets. *Inj Prev.* Dec 2001;7(4):343.

19. Hedlund J. Risky business: safety regulations, risks compensation, and individual behavior. *Inj Prev.* Jun 2000;6(2):82–90.

20. Supreme Court of Iowa. *State v. Hartog.* 440 N. W. 2d 8521989.

21. *R. vs. Dedman.* 1985; S.C.J. No 45, (1985), 2 at para. 68 (cited by Bailey, Caulfield, Reiss (2005), p 255. http://www.lawyers.ca/cases/results.asp?ID=201. Accessed May 25, 2015.

22. Porter BE, Bliss JP, Sleet DA. Human factors in injury control. *Am J Lifestyle Med.* 2010;4(1):90–97.

23. Schieber R, Gilchrist J, Sleet DA. Legislative and regulatory strategies to reduce childhood unintentional injuries. *Future of Children.* 2000;10:111–136.

24. Consumer Product Safety Commission. Standards for the flammability of Children's Sleepwear. *Federal Register.* 2000;65(48):12924–12929.

25. Katcher ML. Tap water scald prevention: it's time for a worldwide effort. *Inj Prev.* Sep 1998;4(3):167–168.

26. Smith LE, Greene MA, Singh HA. Study of the effectiveness of the U.S. safety standard for child resistant cigarette lighters. *Inj Prev.* Sep 2002;8(3):192–196.

27. Centers for Disease Control and Prevention. *Injury Prevention & Control: Prescription Drug Overdose.* 2015; http://www.cdc.gov/drugoverdose/. Accessed May 15, 2015.

28. Haffajee RL, Jena AB, Weiner SG. Mandatory use of prescription drug monitoring programs. *JAMA: The Journal of the American Medical Association.* Mar 3 2015;313(9):891–892.

29. Johnson H, Paulozzi L, Porucznik C, Mack K, Herter B. Decline in drug overdose deaths after state policy changes—Florida, 2010–2012. *MMWR.* 2014;63(26):569–574.

30. Prescription Drug Monitoring Program (PDMP) Center of Excellence. *Mandating Medical Provider Participation in PDMPs.* 2015; http://www.pdmpexcellence.org/content/mandating-medical-provider-participation-pdmps. Accessed May 20, 2015.

31. United States Department of Transportation. Primary laws and fine levels are associated with increases in seat belt use, 1997–2008. *Traffic Tech: Technology Transfer Series.* 2010;400.

32. Gilchrist J, Schieber RA, Leadbetter S, Davidson SC. Police enforcement as part of a comprehensive bicycle helmet program. *Pediatrics.* Jul 2000;106(1 Pt 1):6–9.

33. Christoffel T, Gallagher SS. *Injury Prevention and Public Health: Practical Knowledge, Skills, and Strategies.* Burlington, MA: Jones & Bartlett Learning; 2006.

34. Shaw FE, Ogolla CP, Sleet DA, Dorigo L. Law and injury prevention. *Encyclopedia of Primary Prevention and Health Promotion* (2nd Ed). New York, Springer; 2014:328–334.

35. Helm B. Buckyballs vs. The United States of America. *Inc.,* May 9, 2014.

36. Cox S, Brown R, Millar A, Numanoglu A, Alexander A, Theron A. The risks of gastrointestinal injury due to ingested magnetic beads. *South African Medical Journal (Suid-Afrikaanse tydskrif vir geneeskunde).* Apr 2014;104(4):277–278.

37. Hernandez Anselmi E, Gutierrez San Roman C, Barrios Fontoba JE, et al. Intestinal perforation caused by magnetic toys. *J Pediatric Surg.* Mar 2007;42(3):E13–E16.

38. Shaw F, Ogolla C. Law, behavior and injury prevention. In: Gielen A, Sleet D, DiClemente R (Eds), *Injury and Violence Prevention: Behavioral Science Theories, Methods, and Applications.* San Francisco, CA: Jossey-Bass; 2006:442–466.

39. Shults RA, Nichols JL, Dinh-Zarr TB, Sleet DA, Elder RW. Effectiveness of primary enforcement safety belt laws and enhanced enforcement of safety belt laws: a summary of the Guide to Community Preventive Services systematic reviews. *J Safety Res.* 2004;35(2):189–196.

40. Hahn RA, Middleton JC, Elder R, et al. Effects of alcohol retail privatization on excessive alcohol consumption and related harms: a community guide systematic review. *Am J Prev Med.* Apr 2012;42(4):418–427.

41. Macpherson A, A. Spinks. Bicycle helmet legislation for the uptake of helmet use and prevention of head injuries. *Cochrane Database of Systematic Reviews.* 2008(3): CD005401. doi: 005410.001002/14651858.CD14005401.pub14651853.

42. National Center for Injury Prevention and Control. Helmet use among motorcyclists who died in crashes and economic cost savings associated with state motorcycle helmet laws—United States, 2008–2010. *MMWR.* 2012;61(23):425.

43. Sederburg W. Perspectives of the legislator: Allocating resources. *MMWR.* 1992;41(Suppl): 37–48.

44. Weisbuch JB. The prevention of injury from motorcycle use: epidemiologic success, legislative failure. *Accid Anal Prev.* Feb 1987;19(1):21–28.

45. Hanson D, Allegrante JP, Sleet DA, Finch CF. Research alone is not sufficient to prevent sports injury. *Br J Sports Med.* Apr 2014;48(8):682–684.

46. Canadian Institutes of Health Research Knowledge Translation Strategy 2004–2009. 2004;. http://www.cihr-irsc.gc.ca/e/26574.html. Ottawa, Canada, Accessed April 1, 2015.

47. Centers for Disease Control and Prevention. *Motor Vehicle Prioritizing Interventions and Cost Calculator for States (MV PICCS).* 2015; http://www.cdc.gov/motorvehiclesafety/calculator/index.html. Accessed May 20, 2015.

48. Mercer SL, Sleet DA, Elder RW, Cole KH, Shults RA, Nichols JL. Translating evidence into policy: lessons learned from the case of lowering the legal blood alcohol limit for drivers. *Ann Epidemiol.* Jun 2010;20(6):412–420.

49. Kone RG, Zurick E, Patterson S, Peeples A. Injury and violence prevention policy: celebrating our successes, protecting our future. *J Safety Res.* Sep 2012;43(4):265–270.

50. Brownson RC, Chriqui JF, Stamatakis KA. Understanding evidence-based public health policy. *Am J Public Health.* Sep 2009;99(9):1576–1583.

51. Degutis LC. Approaching injury and violence prevention through public health policy: a window of opportunity to renew our focus. *West J Emerg Med.* Jul 2011;12(3):271–272.

12

Public Policy and Prevention of Violence Against Women

Melissa Jonson-Reid, Janet L. Lauritsen,
Tonya Edmond, and F. David Schneider

LEARNING OBJECTIVES

1. Describe the health impact of violence against women.
2. Describe past and current policy strategies to prevent violence against women.
3. Define key stakeholders in the use of policy to prevent violence against women.

IDENTIFYING THE PROBLEM: VIOLENCE AGAINST WOMEN

Despite increasing attention to the overlap among forms of violence,[1,2] policy associated with violence prevention, where it exists, is quite siloed. Approaches differ for education, criminal justice, social services, and health care and tend to vary by age as well (e.g., child maltreatment, youth violence, violence against women, and elder abuse). This poses a dilemma when attempting to review how policy intersects with violence prevention. Further, although studies of violence suggest that there may be "root" structural and cultural causes of violence, these types of factors, such as entrenched poverty, present more challenges for policy development than do attempts to alter more proximate causal factors. It is not possible within a single chapter to detail how the various forms of violence are addressed in policy across systems. We have, therefore, narrowed the focus of this chapter to violence against women, because of the current interest in issues such as sexual assault on college campuses, the impact of the Affordable Care Act on healthcare approaches, and some recent empirical evidence for criminal justice approaches. That being said, there is no good empirical evidence, thus far, that any specific public policies significantly impact large-scale trends in violence.

Generally, violence against women refers to both domestic violence, also called intimate partner violence (IPV), and sexual assault. We begin with a brief overview of the prevalence and costs related to sexual assault and domestic violence. We then briefly discuss the problems inherent in moving from early intervention approaches in response to a violent event or serious risk of violence to actual primary prevention because of the multidetermined nature of violence. We outline the major veins of policy guiding current programming and conclude with a review of current practices.

Sexual Assault and Intimate Partner Violence

Sexual violence is characterized as completed rape, attempted rape, child sexual abuse, or any other kind of coerced, completed, or attempted unwanted sexual contact.[3] Sexual assault is a pervasive public health problem affecting millions of people every year and inflicting significant emotional, mental, physical, and social consequences on survivors and their loved ones.[4,5] According to the most recent Centers for Disease Control and Prevention National Intimate Partner and Sexual Violence Survey (2011), 19.3% of women and 1.7% of men experience rape in their lifetime and most typically at the hands of someone they know. Nearly 9% of women report experiencing rape perpetrated by an intimate partner during their lifetime, and 43.9% of the women surveyed had experienced other forms of sexual violence that did not include rape.[4] In 2010 the National Crime Victimization Survey estimated roughly 200,000 cases of rape, attempted rape, or sexual assault yearly—there has been a drop in violent crime generally over the last decade prior. It is estimated that roughly one third of cases are reported.[6] Sexual violence can result in emotional and physical injury as well as the transmission of sexually transmitted diseases (STDs).[7] Research also has found an association between maternal history of sexual victimization and negative impacts on next generation victimization.[8] Financial costs per rape are estimated to range from $87,000 to $240,776.[9]

Intimate partner violence, also called domestic violence, is defined by the Centers for Disease Control and Prevention (CDC) as physical, sexual, or psychological/emotional violence (or any threat thereof) directed to a current or former partner or spouse.[10] It is unclear whether the recent recession may have partially reversed the downward trend in known cases[11] or whether this trend includes populations like American Indian and Alaska Native women, who have been found to be at higher risk.[12] Excess healthcare and medical costs due to intimate partner violence are approximately $19.3 million per year for every 100,000 women aged 18–64 years.[13] Intimate partner violence increases the likelihood of unwanted pregnancy—most likely through partner control of reproductive practices[14]; and intimate partner violence rates have been found to be higher during pregnancy,[15] placing both mother and child at significant risk of harm.

Although the focus of this chapter is on policy in the United States, it is important to point out that violence against women is a global phenomenon. The specific acts included as violence may vary by country, but the remarkable similarity in prevalence rates reported led to the "1 in 3" graphic (see Figure 12.1), which was used in the campaign specific to addressing violence toward Native American women during the effort to reauthorize the federal Violence Against Women Act in 2013.

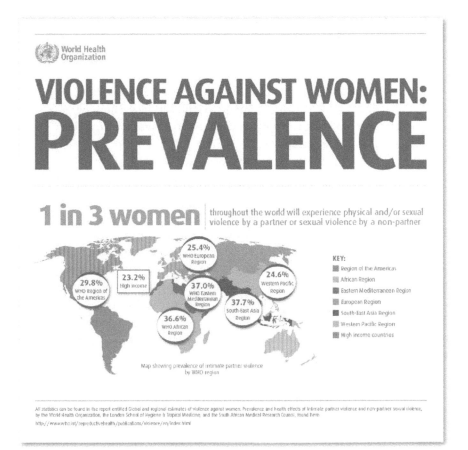

Figure 12.1 Violence against women is a global phenomenon.

PUBLIC POLICY STRATEGIES IN PREVENTION OF VIOLENCE AGAINST WOMEN

National Policy Approaches

Readers will notice that the policies highlighted herein tend to involve detection and response rather than any alteration of underlying risks related to the onset of violence. Although primary prevention approaches such as school-based prevention programming related to child sexual abuse, sexual assault, and dating violence exist, these have not been the focus of most policy-driven approaches. Major policy approaches are briefly presented here and then discussed further in segments specific to campus sexual assault, criminal justice approaches to intimate partner violence, intimate partner violence prevention, in-home visitation, and screening for intimate partner violence in health care. Policies are presented in order of scale, with overall federal guidance first, followed by system-specific policies.

The Violence Against Women Reauthorization Act (VAWRA) of 2013 (PL 111-4) addresses domestic violence, sexual violence, and stalking. The newest version includes provisions that:

- Improve protections for Native women when offenders are non-Native
- Expand housing protection for victims in federally subsidized housing
- Add additional reporting and programming requirements for IPV, dating violence, and stalking on college campuses
- Maintain program grants to states and coalitions
- Prohibit discrimination for Gay Lesbian Bisexual Transgender survivors, and
- Improve protections for immigrant survivors.

Provisions for LGBT and Native Americans were among the most controversial, as illustrated in this infographic used in the campaign to pass the Act (see Figure 12.2).

Core grant programs of the Act include Services, Training, Officers, and Prosecutors (STOP; formula grants to states to support enforcement and advocates); Sexual Assault Services Program; Civil Legal Assistance for Victims; Transitional Housing Grants; Grants to Encourage Arrest; and grants that support services for rural victims, tribal communities, underserved communities, and prevention and youth programs.

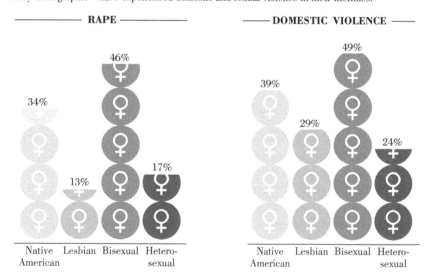

Why The House's Version Of VAWA Isn't Good Enough
The House unveiled a new version of the Violence Against Woman Act on Friday, stripping provisions from the Senate bill that would have protected LGBT woman and making it harder for Native American victims to seek justice. Too many woman in these groups—and every demographic—have experienced domestic and sexual violence in their lifetimes.

———— RAPE ————   —— DOMESTIC VIOLENCE ——

46%   49%
34%   39%
                                       29%
                    17%   24%
13%

Native   Lesbian Bisexual Hetero-   Native   Lesbian Bisexual Hetero-
American   sexual   American   sexual

THE HUFFINGTON POST

Figure 12.2 Violence Against Women Act.

System-specific Policy

Although federal policy sets the stage for addressing violence against women, system-specific policies can make additional impact. Education, criminal justice, and health care are examples of such systems. In education, Title IX is a civil rights law within the Education Amendments of 1972 that expressly prohibits discrimination on the basis of sex in institutions of education that receive federal financial assistance. Title IX prohibits any such institution from discriminating against persons based on their sex across a broad spectrum of institutional contexts and policies. Over the course of time, guidance documents have been developed by the Office of Civil Rights (OCR), which evolved in part from case law that led to expressly identifying sexual harassment and sexual assault as forms of sex discrimination. The criminal justice system also has relevant system-related policies. Intimate partner violence and sexual assault are crimes. (See 42 U.S. Code Chapter 136, Subchapter III.) All 50 states have criminal justice statutes related to the arrest and consequences associated with domestic violence and sexual assault. However, the means by and degree to which such statutes are enforced vary. For example, about half of all states have mandatory arrest policies in place, while in other states, arrests may be at the officer's discretion.[16]

Within the healthcare system, the Affordable Care Act of 2010 (Health Resources and Services Administration, 2012; The Patient Protection and Affordable Care Act) provided for two health-related avenues for addressing domestic violence: screening and services. While not required, per se, several major national health associations have recommended screening among women of childbearing age as a part of routine medical care.[17] The Maternal, Infant, and Early Childhood Home Visiting Program, established under the Patient Protection and Affordable Care Act of 2010, provided $1.5 billion in mandatory funds over five years for states to implement and expand home-visiting models. The final legislation allows states to use 25% of the funds to invest in promising models that may overcome the many research and practice gaps in well-researched programs. This has become a resource within states for encouraging program development related to issues like addressing domestic violence. More in-depth discussion of these three systems, including specific policy-examples from them, appears in the next section.

Examples of Policy Initiatives: Education, Criminal Justice and Health Care

Although the VAWRA provides an overarching framework for federal policy related to violence against women, programmatic and policy approaches vary by system. Further, the availability of research to inform understanding of the effectiveness of these approaches varies dramatically. Because of the recent increased federal attention to the issue, we begin by discussing the issue of sexual assault on college campuses.

The vast majority (78.7%) of completed rapes experienced by girls/women first occur before they reach the age of 25 years. A particularly vulnerable time period for women is between the ages of 18 and 24 years, when 38.3% of women reported first experiencing rape.[5] This is also the age when many young women are in college. A study of campus sexual assault funded by the National Institute of Justice, Krebs and colleagues (2007) found that 19% of women experienced an attempted or completed sexual assault while in college, with freshmen and sophomores being at greatest risk. The rate of attempted or completed sexual assault of male college students was 6.1%. The vast majority of sexual assaults were perpetrated by a male known to the woman, and very few survivors (15%) made formal complaints to campus or community law enforcement.[5] In 2009, only 3,284 forcible sexual offenses were reported by college campuses across the country,[18] numbers that are far lower than those found in campus sexual assault surveys. Such findings suggest that sexual assault survivors on college campuses encounter significant barriers to reporting their experiences to law enforcement or to university employees and are inhibited from doing so.

On January 22, 2014, President Obama issued a Presidential Memorandum that established the White House Task Force to Protect Students from Sexual Assault. He stated,

> *"Sexual violence is more than just a crime against individuals. It threatens our families, it threatens our communities; ultimately, it threatens the entire country. It tears apart the fabric of our communities. And that's why we are here today—because we have the power to do something about it as a government, as a nation. We have the capacity to stop sexual assault, support those who have survived it, and bring perpetrators to justice"* (p. ii).[19]

President Obama's statement and establishment of the Task Force signaled a commitment to addressing sexual violence. He charged his appointed representatives with providing schools with resources to more effectively prevent and respond to campus sexual assault, and with enhancing the federal government's enforcement mechanisms. The primary legal mechanisms that the federal government has to address campus sexual assault are Title IX, the Clery Act, and the Campus Sexual Violence Elimination Act.

Title IX prohibits educational institutions that receive federal funding from discriminating against persons based on their sex; the Title IX prohibition applies across the full spectrum of activities that constitute the educational enterprise.[20] Title IX applies to all students, full and part-time, regardless of sex, sexual orientation, gender identity, physical or mental abilities, race, ethnicity, nationality, and citizenship or documentation status.[21, 22] A student's rights are violated under Title IX when a hostile environment is created that interferes with a student being able to partake in and benefit from the educational programs available. Failure on the part of the educational institution to bring an end to the hostile environment, prevent its reoccurrence, and remedy its negative effects constitutes a violation of Title IX.[22]

Violations of Title IX can be reported to the Office for Civil Rights within the Department of Education, which has the authority to launch an investigation and to enforce compliance. Typically, this process is conducted in a collaborative fashion with hopes of voluntary compliance without the need for withdrawal of federal funding. In the absence of voluntary compliance, however, the Office for Civil Rights can refer the matter to the Department of Justice, which has the authority to initiate litigation.[23] The ability of the Office for Civil Rights to enforce Title IX is derived from the educational institution's agreement to comply as a condition of receiving federal funds.[24]

Title IX regulations require educational institutions to (1) widely disseminate their policies on sexual nondiscrimination; (2) designate one or more employees with responsibility for coordinating and implementing Title IX obligations (Title IX Coordinator); and (3) develop and disseminate grievance procedures to facilitate timely and fair resolution of complaints.[21,22] Although these requirements appear rather straightforward, over time there has been an evolving recognition of how sexual harassment and sexual assault are forms of sex discrimination, which has greatly expanded the recommendations for compliance. These recommendations come from the Office for Civil Rights, which periodically develops documents intended to enhance clarity about compliance expectations. These "guiding documents" are informed by outcomes of investigations by the Office for Civil Rights when claims of sex discrimination have been made; through case law, such as relevant rulings issued by the Supreme Court; consultation with key stakeholders (educators, students, administrators, and researchers); and public comments.[25]

A critically important "guiding document" was the *Sexual Harassment Guidance: Harassment of Students by School Employees, Other Students, or Third Parties* (62 FR 12034), published in March 1997 and revised in January of 2001, which made explicit that sexual harassment is a form of sex discrimination. A decade later, on April 11, 2011, a *Dear Colleague Letter* was released by the Office for Civil Rights that made explicitly clear for the first time that sexual violence (sexual coercion, sexual battery, sexual assault or rape) is a form of sexual harassment, thereby making both sexual harassment and sexual violence forms of sex discrimination.[23,26] This sent shockwaves across college campuses, most of which were not adequately responding to campus sexual assault and consequently were ill-prepared to meet the compliance expectations. The *Dear Colleague Letter* recommended that universities move beyond mere compliance by proactively developing and implementing prevention education programs for faculty, staff, and students; providing comprehensive services for survivors; and developing educational materials on sexual violence that describe resources, policies, and procedures for reporting.[23] Compliance suddenly required much more concerted effort from educational institutions.

Most recently (April 29, 2014), the Office for Civil Rights released a new 46-page document entitled *Questions and Answers on Title IX and Sexual Violence: The 2014 Guidance*[23] to further clarify and expand upon the Dear Colleague Letter and the *2001 Revised Guidance*. Despite the White House Task Force and the substantive guidance from the Office for Civil Rights, many universities continue to fail to meet compliance. As of January 2015, 94 colleges and universities had pending Title IX investigations related to sexual assault. Courts have shown considerable deference to the Office for Civil Rights interpretations in their guiding documents.[27] Consequently, universities wishing to avoid Title IX investigations or litigation should follow the recommendations very closely.

Concerns have been expressed by stakeholders about potential conflicts between Title IX and other federal policies. For example, under Title IX, a student who has been sexually harassed or sexually assaulted has a right to know the outcome of a complaint, including any sanctions imposed by the university against the accused student. Provision of this information to the victim demonstrates the responsiveness of the institution, their effort to address concerns about a hostile environment, and to prevent reoccurrence.[21] However, the *Family Educational Rights and Privacy Act*, 20 U.S.C. 1232g prohibits the disclosure of most information contained in a student record without first obtaining consent from the student. The Office for Civil Rights addresses this potential point of conflict, clarifying that when there are any direct conflicts that might interfere with efforts to prevent or end sex-based discrimination Title IX requirements supersede those of the Family Educational Rights and Privacy Act.[21,23] Furthermore, the Family Educational Rights and Privacy Act allows universities to disclose outcomes of complaints to alleged victims when the allegation involves a nonforcible sexual offense or a violent crime regardless of the conclusion reached through the grievance process. It also allows the university to disclose the results to anyone if it determines the perpetrator committed the alleged violence and violated the university's policies or rules.[22,23]

The Clery Act also informs campus sexual assault programming. In 1990, the *Higher Education Act of 1965* was amended to include the Crime Awareness and Campus Security Act, which requires educational institutions that receive federal financial aid to collect and report information about campus security and crime. This was enacted to hold institutions accountable and to provide faculty and staff, as well as current and prospective students and their families with campus safety information. In 1998, the Act was amended and renamed the Jeanne Clery Disclosure of Campus Security Policy and Campus Crime Statistics Act (20 U.S.C. 1092(f)) in honor of a young woman who was murdered in her dormitory in 1986.[29] Postsecondary educational institutions are required to make public and submit an Annual Security Report (ASR) to the Department of Education based on definitions used by the FBI's *Uniform Crime Reporting Handbook* (UCR) and the *Hate Crime Data Collection Guidelines*. Alternatively, an institution can use the UCR *National Incident-Based Reporting System*. The Clery Act crime reporting requirements also do not violate the Family Educational Rights and Privacy Act.[23] The Federal Student Aid office acts as the investigative and enforcement agency for the Department of Education. The office conducts compliance reviews and has the authority to levy fines against universities for failure to comply.[29]

Campus SaVE Act. The Campus Sexual Violence Elimination Act (Campus SaVE Act) was added to the Reauthorization of the Violence Against Women Act (VAWA) in 2013. Campus SaVE mandated changes to the Clery Act that expand the types of sexual violence that have to be reported and requires universities and colleges to document and report incidents of stalking, dating violence, and domestic violence.[27] After the Reauthorization of Violence Against Women Act (VAWA), the Office for Civil Rights issued another Dear Colleague Letter (July 14, 2014) to clarify that "VAWA did not affect in any way Title IX" and that "Nothing in the Clery Act, as amended by VAWA, alters or changes an institution's obligations or duties under Title IX as interpreted by OCR" (p. 1).[30] However, many of the procedures that had been *recommended* by the Office for Civil Rights for Title IX compliance are now *required* by law for Clery compliance. New requirements brought forth by the Campus SaVE Act include ongoing primary prevention education and awareness training for faculty, staff, and students as well as specialized training for those involved in implementing the grievance process.[27]

It is too early to assess the effectiveness of these policy efforts, and the uneven implementation of the various guidelines[31] hampers our understanding of promising approaches. We do know that sexual violence on college campuses continues to be too prevalent and that it requires a significant university response. ASRs submitted to the Department of Education as required by the Clery Act contain substantially lower numbers of campus sexual assaults than are detected through campus-wide and national surveys. A study of rates provided during audit years as compared with non-audit years confirms the tendency to under-report.[32] Fully implementing the OCR recommendations and the Campus SaVE Act would move universities beyond mere compliance to being proactive agents of institutional change, which could create campus climates that lead to substantial reductions in sexual violence.

Violence Prevention and the Criminal Justice System

The literature on criminal justice system responses to violence against women is more developed than that of sexual violence on college campuses. Criminological perspectives on the reduction of violence share much in common with public health perspectives. Both perspectives search for ways to prevent such incidents from occurring, and their respective research literatures have identified a similar set of social, environmental, familial, and individual correlates of violence. The potential role of the criminal justice system in preventing violence is easy to overlook, however, because the system is commonly viewed as primarily reactive to crime and violence. Over the past few decades, innovative crime and violence reduction policies involving various components of the system (such as the police, prosecutors, and probation officers) have been developed and assessed, and several approaches have been found to be promising for the prevention of violence.

Before discussing the potential role of the criminal justice system in preventing violence, it is important to note briefly the general features of the understandings that criminologists have about patterns in violence and, in particular, violence against women. Criminologists study the characteristics of violent incidents, trends in rates of violence, and the etiology of violent offending and victimization among individuals.

This broad body of research (derived from analyses of administrative records from police departments, victim surveys, and many other data sources) has found that the rates for various types of violent crime generally share similar trends. For example, rates of homicide, rape and sexual assault, robbery, and violence against women have declined since the 1970s, with the majority of the decline occurring during the 1990s. Beginning around 2000, the trends generally exhibit slowing declines or stability.[33] The similarities in the trends across crime types suggest that the broader social and historical factors that are associated with violent crime trends (such as macroeconomic conditions) also may be associated with trends in violence against women.[34] Similarly, community-level research finds that rates of violence against women are higher in places where other forms of violence are higher. Here the key correlates of the rates are factors such as the level of neighborhood socioeconomic disadvantage, the percentage of female-headed households, and the level of collective efficacy in the community.[35,36,37]

Prospective individual-level research has found that men who commit violence against women also are more likely to commit violence against others. In addition, these offenders are more likely to have had temperamental problems in childhood, harsh and inconsistent parenting, poor family backgrounds, difficulties in school, and trouble with the law in adolescence, as compared with men who do not commit violence against women.[38] These studies also find that the women who are most likely to be victims of intimate partner violence share important similarities in their life-course profiles They, too, are more likely to have had temperamental problems in childhood, difficult family backgrounds and school experiences, as well as contact with the juvenile justice system as adolescents.[3] The most consistent findings from longitudinal research suggest that the two strongest predictors of violent victimization (regardless of type) are prior experiences with victimization (especially recent victimization) as well as one's own level of involvement in violence perpetration. Conversely, the strongest predictors of violent offending are prior involvement in violence, either as an offender or as a victim.[39]

Obviously, this very brief description of the patterns and predictors of violence against women compared to other forms of violence is not meant to be exhaustive or to suggest that there are no unique causal forces involved in violence against women versus other forms of violence. Rather, it is intended to reveal the context and challenges that policymakers and program developers must confront as they work to develop ways to prevent violence. Development of broad social policies assumes that there is a good understanding of the factors that account for much of the change over time in violence against women, but sound knowledge of these issues is in the early stages of development.[33]

Most of the efforts designed to reduce violence against women have been programs and policies targeted at individual offenders or victims. Programs aimed at changing offender behavior have generally emphasized legislative efforts, such as mandatory arrest, no-drop prosecution, or increasing the availability of orders of protection; or, they have stressed mandatory batterer treatment programs for offenders convicted of domestic assault in an effort to deter future violence perpetration. Criminologists and others have conducted numerous assessments of the effects of these legislative changes and programmatic efforts and most of these evaluations show limited, null, or even counterproductive effects on offenders' future behaviors. For example, contrary to expectations, most batterer treatment programs tend not to be successful at reducing partner violence,[40,41] and studies of the effects of mandatory-arrest policies have often found limited, or even mixed, effects on future domestic violence.[42] Such findings warn against simplistic hopes that mandatory treatment or legislative changes to deter offending can prevent violence from occurring.

Other policies and programs intended to reduce and prevent violence against women (especially intimate partner violence) have been focused on providing services and resources to victims, in the hopes that such services can help to remove women from violent environments and, therefore, reduce their future risk. Some of the most well-designed and evaluated of these efforts are referred to as "second-responder" programs. After an initial police response to a family violence incident, a second visit—typically including a police officer and a victim advocate or family violence specialist—is made with the victim to provide information about her legal rights and the available services in the area that she might need, including shelters, counseling, and other forms of assistance. These second responder programs are targeted at preventing re-victimization under the premise that victims are most receptive to help and assistance in the period immediately following a violent incident. A systematic review of 10 second-responder programs that contained key methodological features (such as having a control group for comparison) found that these program interventions did *not* reduce the likelihood of subsequent violence, though they did appear to increase victims' willingness to *report* incidents to the police, perhaps because victims came to have more confidence in the police as a result of the extra concern and attention they received.[43] A large issue confronting such efforts is that many victims state that they want the violence to stop, but they want the relationship to continue.

Though the results of intensive batterer and victim services programs often have been disappointing, much has been learned about the ineffectiveness of these efforts. An alternative approach to preventing violence against women has been inspired by the success of criminal justice strategies known as "focused deterrence" programs. A long line of criminological evidence suggests that the most serious violent crime is disproportionately committed by relatively few offenders with criminal records; thus, targeting these offenders effectively should have the greatest influence on violence rates. Initially created to reduce gun violence and homicide, focused-deterrence programs involve multipronged strategies, in which "every lever is pulled" when violence occurs.[44,45]

First developed in the 1990s in Boston by David Kennedy and colleagues, these problem-oriented policing projects were designed to halt escalating gang violence. In working-group meetings with the police, probation and parole officers and community-based organizations and practitioners met with the most serious gang members to target them with the message that violence will no longer be tolerated by the community. Backed by a variety of both formal and informal sanctions, gang members were told during the meetings why they were receiving special attention from the criminal justice system and the community, and the consequences of their actions. Sanctions (such as immediate arrest, and strictly enforced revocations of probation and parole, which resulted in returns to prison) were applied swiftly if violence re-emerged among the gangs. Involvement from community groups, along with the coordinated offering of social services and community resources, was found to be critical to maintaining the legitimacy and effectiveness of the criminal justice component of the effort. Without such legitimacy, threats from the criminal justice system often prompted gang members and their communities to feel as though they were under siege by outside forces.

These coordinated focused-deterrence efforts have been shown to reduce gang violence, gun violence, and homicide significantly and at noteworthy levels.[45] Only recently, however, has the success of such efforts for the most serious forms of offending led to the initial development and testing of a focused-deterrence effort to reduce domestic violence. The first effort is currently underway in High Point, North Carolina.[46] As in many jurisdictions and communities, the police department there reports that they receive a large number of domestic violence calls, that the criminal histories of the domestic abusers are extensive and similar to those of other serious offenders, and that repeat calls to the same residence are common despite victim services and resources. The logic of this domestic violence reduction program follows that of the earlier focused-deterrence programs. The targeted offender meets with a team of criminal justice personnel and representatives of the community who inform the offender that any future incident will be met with a coordinated and swift response, using every legal lever available, including revocations of probation and parole, and a return to prison.

The program is in the early stages of evaluation and, thus far, the data on calls for police service, arrests, and harms to victims suggest there have been significant declines in domestic violence.[47] For example, the *recidivism rate* of those offenders targeted by the program is averaging approximately 9%. Other criminal justice treatments, such as anger management, counseling, and incarceration, exhibit recidivism rates that are often about 2 to 5 times higher. Importantly, this focused-deterrence intervention has been associated with decreases in domestic violence homicides rather than increasing harm to victims.

Clearly it is necessary to replicate the program elsewhere before widening its broader adoption, and efforts to do so are underway. This is necessary because, as noted above, there is a long history of mixed and counterproductive outcomes from various types of violence-reduction programs. However, the successes of the earlier focused-deterrence programs in reducing other forms of serious violence, along with the early evidence from the High Point, North Carolina domestic violence program, provide some hope that a targeted response that relies on coordination between the criminal justice system and other community resources can help improve the lives of women by significantly reducing domestic violence.

Healthcare Policy and Violence Against Women

The passage of the Affordable Care Act has led to increased attention to two forms of intervention in cases of intimate partner violence: (1) home visitation and

(2) screening and referral in primary care. These are evolving areas of policy and programming and are more permissive in nature than either college campus responses to sexual assault or criminal justice responses to domestic violence.

Home Visitation

The early years of life are a period of great vulnerability to injury and developmental harm. Home-visiting programs are considered an extremely promising approach to improve these and a broad range of other child and family health outcomes.[48,49,50] Yet, significant gaps remain in our understanding of the effectiveness of such programs to prevent serious threats to healthy development, such as family violence.[51] Many home visiting models name child maltreatment prevention as a goal, but success in this area has been mixed.[52,53,54,55] One of the oft-mentioned barriers to success in maltreatment prevention has been the co-occurrence of domestic violence.[56] Although estimates of the rates of co-occurrence vary, there is significant evidence that domestic violence and child maltreatment frequently co-occur.[10,57]

Home visitation, albeit with adaptations, is thought to hold promise for addressing domestic violence in perinatal populations as well as among mothers with very young children.[59] The Affordable Care Act (PL 111-148) amended Title V of the Social Security Act to create the Maternal Infant and Early Childhood Home Visitation (MIECHV) Program and required grantees to address domestic violence. It also allowed states to use up to 25% of the funding for in-home visitation to test new models that could address issues like mothers and children experiencing domestic violence.[60]

A 2003 review of the published home visitation literature examined the impact on prevention of domestic violence and found insufficient evidence to assess its effectiveness.[61] Subsequently, program development has increased and evaluation research is improving. One program with a home vistation component has been included in the California Evidence-based Clearinghouse, Domestic Violence Home Visitation Intervention.[62] This program, however, is limited to outreach visits combined with law enforcement efforts. A randomized trial of Healthy Families America in Hawaii found that participation in home visitation was associated with maternal perpetration of domestic violence but not victimization.[63] The Nurse–Family Partnership model developed an additional module to address domestic violence.[64] A recently published randomized study from Holland found the Dutch Nurse–Family Partnership model to be effective in reducing self-reported intimate partner violence.[65] This version of Nurse–Family Partnership, however, included a different intimate partner violence module adapted from a study by Langhinrichsen-Rohling and Turner (2012).[66] A training curriculum for home visitation programs was developed in collaboration with Futures Without Violence, but it is unclear whether this has been tested.[67] Certain states have also created protocols and programs such as "Project Connect Texas" and the domestic violence protocol for Baltimore, Maryland (2011).[68] The latter protocol originates from a study of "Domestic Violence Enhanced Home Visitation" that showed promising preliminary results.[68]

Over a decade after the 2003 review, it still appears too early in the evolution of this approach to prevent domestic violence or prevent recurrence to provide compelling evidence for or against this innovation. Despite the need for additional research to support the approach overall, several initiatives now exist to promote addressing domestic violence within home visitation programs.[68] Some states, such as Tennessee, include the reduction in domestic violence as a required reported outcome for their statewide home-visitation program.[69] It may be that the MIECHV program is the necessary catalyst for further development and evaluation. Should the funding to encourage research and development through the MIECHV program continue long enough, in the near future we may be able to assess this as a policy approach to domestic violence among women with young children.

Healthcare Providers

Healthcare policy concerning IPV has focused mostly around the issues of mandatory reporting and the utility of universal screening for violence. The Affordable Care Act included legislation that allowed screening for domestic violence to be reimbursed as a preventive service. More recently, the U.S. Preventive Services Task Force changed their recommendation on screening for domestic violence so that this is now recommended for women of reproductive age.[70]

Family violence, both current and past, has been linked to mental health problems such as post-traumatic stress disorder (PTSD), depression, and an array of anxiety disorders, as well as physical health problems such as heart disease, diabetes, many types of cancer, and chronic pain syndromes leading to disability and early mortality.[71] We also know that victims of IPV use the healthcare system significantly more often than nonvictims, and that this increased use persists long after the violence ceases. This pattern of use provides many opportunities to intervene.[72] There is significant evidence that screening or case finding for IPV does result in disclosure, that women who are victims desire that their healthcare providers ask, and that when asked, they will disclose.

Because of the association of family violence across the lifespan to disease and premature mortality, healthcare providers generally agree that this screening should be included in periodic health exams. Education of healthcare professionals and resources for referral and treatment are often lacking, however, preventing its incorporation into practice. For example, a visit to the doctor's office usually includes only about 15 minutes for the patient to interact with the physician, leaving very little time to discuss relationships. The ability of healthcare providers to connect victims with community and healthcare resources is also variable. Because of this, public health facilities with coordinated care approaches, such as Federally Qualified Health Centers, may be much better equipped to provide appropriate support and resources for those who are in violent relationships than are healthcare providers in private practice.

There is no standard response or established standard of care for healthcare providers' responses to IPV identified in the office, and practices vary across settings.[73] For example, to comply with Joint Commission on Accreditation of Hospital

Organizations (JCAHO) standards, most hospitals have developed a system to screen all patients. In reality, however, this is often implemented by a checklist of questions asked at the time of emergency department intake or admission by a nurse, and in such a way that the patient is urged to simply reply that, "Things at home are fine." The questions are often asked in front of the potential perpetrator, and in a leading manner, as in, "You're safe at home, aren't you?" Furthermore, in a recent meta-analysis of studies of IPV screening, although screening does result in disclosure, there was no evidence that it resulted in decreased IPV long-term.[74] None of the studies included were conducted after the U.S. Preventive Services Task Force released its new guidelines in 2012; thus, we do not yet know the effect of these new guidelines.

Another variable related to screening in healthcare settings is mandatory reporting. All states require healthcare personnel to report suspected child and elder abuse to a state authority. Though this requirement has been in place for decades, many healthcare professionals may lack confidence in their state's ability to handle these incidents well. As a result, they may be reluctant to file a report unless they are fairly sure child neglect or abuse, or elder abuse, has definitely occurred.[75] In some states, domestic violence can be reported as a form of child abuse.[76] In Utah, for instance, an incident of domestic violence that occurs with a child present constitutes child abuse. More recently, reporting female victims of domestic violence has become mandatory in some states, including California. The utility of mandatory reporting of women as potential victims of domestic violence has been controversial. Many healthcare providers worry that universal screening in states with mandatory reporting will cause patients to end up in the legal system and result in poorer outcomes.[77] If large-scale screening and mandated reporting systems are to be implemented and tested, better and more coordinated systems are needed in order to provide services in response to identified need and in order to have a preventive impact.

CONCLUSION

Although federal, state, and agency-based policies related to violence against women exist, much remains unknown about the relative effectiveness of programs and interventions put in place in response to these policies. Three things are clear. There is great variability by region and system in the implementation of policies in criminal justice, higher education, and health care. Rigorous research like that profiled in the criminal justice section is needed across all systems attempting to prevent or intervene in the area of sexual assault and domestic violence. Finally, there is also a need to build effective bridges between prevention programming, reporting, and screening efforts, and services for survivors.

The recent CDC report,[2] *Connecting the Dots*, reminds us that many forms of violence co-occur and may share root causes. Policy remains fragmented and largely focused on responses to violence rather than on prevention. On the other hand, many of the efforts reviewed here are relatively recent, which leaves us with hope that we are headed in the direction of a more coordinated approach to this costly public health problem.

REFERENCES

1. Finkelhor D. *Childhood Victimization: Violence, Crime and Abuse in the Lives of Young People.* New York: Oxford University Press; 2008.
2. Wilkins N, Tsao B, Hertz M, Davis R, Klevens J. *Connecting the Dots: An Overview of the Links Among Multiple Forms of Violence.* Atlanta, GA: National Center for Injury Prevention and Control, Centers for Disease Control and Prevention; Oakland, CA: Prevention Institute; 2014.
3. Centers for Disease Control and Prevention. Understanding sexual violence. 2006; http://www.cdc.gov/violenceprevention/pub/sv_factsheet.html
4. Breiding M, Smith S, Basile K, Walters M, Chen J, Merrick M. Prevalence and characteristics of sexual violence, stalking, and intimate partner violence victimization—National Intimate Partner and Sexual Violence Survey, United States, 2011. *MMWR.* 2014; 63(SS08): 1–18.
5. Krebs C, Lindquist C, Warner T, Fisher B. Martin S. *The Campus Sexual Assault (CSA) Study: Final Report.* 2007. http://www.ncjrs.gov/pdffiles1/nij/grants/221153.pdf
6. Truman J. Criminal Victimization, 2010. Washington, DC: U.S. Department of Justice. 2011; http://aia.berkeley.edu/media/2011_teleconferences/ipv/IPVwebinarslides.pdf
7. Bureau of Justice Statistics. *Violent Crime Rates Declined for Both Males and Females since 1994.* 2006; http://www.ojp.usdoj.gov/bjs/glance/vsx2.htm.
8. Wenzel SL, Hambarsoomian K, D'Amico EJ, Ellison M, Tucker JS. Victimization and health among indigent young women in the transition to adulthood: A portrait of need. *J Adol Health.* 2006;38(5):536–543.
9. Noll JG, Trickett PK, Harris WW, Putnam FW. The cumulative burden borne by offspring whose mothers were sexually abused as children: descriptive results from a multigenerational study. *J Interpers Violence.* 2009 Mar;24(3):424–449.
10. The White House Council on Women and Girls (January 2014). Rape and sexual assault: A renewed call to action. http://www.whitehouse.gov/sites/default/files/docs/sexual_assault_report_1-21-14.pdf
11. Centers for Disease Control and Prevention, National Center for Injury Prevention and Control. *Understanding intimate partner violence: Fact sheet.* 2006; http://www.cdc.gov/ncipc/dvp/ipv_factsheet.pdf.\
12. Buzawa E, Buzawa C, Stark E. *Domestic Violence: The Criminal Justice and Societal Response.* Thousand Oaks, CA: Sage Publications; 2012.
13. Crossland C, Palmer J, Brooks A. NIJ's program of research on violence against American Indian and Alaska Native women. *Violence Against Women.* 2013;19(6):771–790.
14. Rivara F, Anderson M, Fishman P, et al. Intimate partner violence and health care costs and utilization for children living in the home. *Pediatrics.* 2007;120(6):1270–1277.
15. Moore AM, Frohwirth L, Miller E. Male reproductive control of women who have experienced intimate partner violence in the United States. *Soc Sci Med.* 2012;70(11):1737–1744.
16. Saftlas AF, Wallis AB, Shochet T, Harland KK, Dickey P, Peek-Asa C. Prevalence of intimate partner violence among an abortion clinic population. *Am J Pub Health.* 2010;100(8):1412–1415.
17. American Bar Association. Domestic violence arrest policies by state. 2007; http://www.americanbar.org/content/dam/aba/migrated/domviol/docs/Domestic_Violence_Arrest_Policies_by_State_11_07.authcheckdam.pdf

18. de Boinville M. Screening for domestic violence in health care settings. *ASPE Policy Brief.* 2013; http://aspe.hhs.gov/hsp/13/dv/pb_screeningdomestic.cfm.

19. United States Department of Education. Office of Postsecondary Education. Summary Crime Statistics. 2010; http://www2.ed.gov/admins/lead/safety/criminal2007-09.pdf

20. White House Task Force to Protect Students from Sexual Assault. *Not alone: The First Report of the White House Task Force to Protect Students from Sexual Assault.* April 2014.

21. Title IX of the Education Amendment of 1972, 20 U.S.C.XX 1681 et seq. (Title IX).

22. Title IX of the Civil Rights Act of 1964. Statute: 20 U.S.C. 1681. Regulations: 34 C.F.R. Part 106.

23. Office of Civil Rights. *Questions and Answers on Title IX and Sexual Violence.* 2014; http://www2.ed.gov/about/offices/list/ocr/docs/qa-201404-titlt-ix.pdf

24. Office of Civil Rights. Dear Colleague Letter on Sexual Violence. 2011; http://www2.ed.gov/about/list/ocr/letters/colleague-201104.html

25. Cantalupo N. Institution-specific victimization surveys: Addressing legal and practical disincentives to gender-based violence reporting on college campuses. *Trauma, Violence, & Abuse.* 2014. Online version. doi: 10.1177/1524838014521323.

26. Office of Civil Rights. Revised sexual harassment guidance: Harassment of student by school employees, other students, or third parties. 2001; http://www.ed.gov/offices/OCR/archives/pdf/shguide.pdf

27. Johnson L, Walesby A. Beyond the "Dear Colleague" Letter: A summary of several recent OCR enforcement actions. The National Association of College and University Attorneys. 2013.

28. Nolan, J. Title IX, meet CLERY, CLERY, meet Title IX: Implementing campus SaVE. The National Association of College and University Attorneys. 2014; http://counsel.cua.edu/res/docs/NACUA-paper.pdf

29. Keller J, Foerster A. Defending (and winning) a Title IX lawsuit: Student claims arising out of alleged sexual violence. The National Association of College and University Attorneys. 2014.

30. Ward D, Mann J. *The Handbook for Campus Security and Reporting.* 2011; https://www2.ed.gov/admins/lead/safety/handbook.pdf

31. Information for Financial Aid Professionals. Dear Colleague Letter, July 14, 2014; http://ifap.ed.gov/dpcletters/GEN1413.htlm

32. Streng TK, Kamimura A. Sexual assault prevention and reporting on college campuses in the U.S.: a review of policies and recommendations. *J Ed Pract.* 2015;6(3):65–71.

33. Yung, CR. Concealing campus sexual assault: An empirical examination. *Psych Pub Policy Law.* 2015;21(1):1–9.

34. Goldberger A,Rosenfeld R, Eds. *Understanding Crime Trends.* Washington, DC: The National Academies Press; 2009.

35. Lauritsen J, Rezey M, Heimer K. Violence and economic conditions in the U.S., 1973–2011: Gender, race, and ethnicity patterns in the NCVS. *Journal of Contemporary Criminal Justice.* 2014;30:7–28.

36. Benson M, Fox G, DeMaris A, Van Wyk J. Neighborhood disadvantage, individual economic distress and violence against women in intimate relationships. *J Quant Criminology.* 2003;19:207–235.

37. Browning C. The span of collective efficacy: Extending social disorganization theory to partner violence. *J Marriage Family.* 2002;64:833–850.

38. Lauritsen J, Carbone-Lopez K. Gender differences in risk factors for violent victimization: An examination of individual-, family-, and community-level predictors. *J Res Crime Delinq*. 2011;48:538–565.

39. Moffitt T, Caspi A. *Findings About Partner Violence from the Dunedin Multidisciplinary Health and Development Study*. National Institute of Justice Research in Brief. Washington, DC: U.S. Department of Justice; 1999.

40. Lauritsen J, Laub J. Understanding the link between victimization and offending: New reflections on an old idea. *Crime Prev Studies*. 2007;22:55–76.

41. National Institute of Justice. Interventions for domestic violence offenders: Cognitive behavioral therapy. 2015; http://www.crimesolutions.gov/PracticeDetails.aspx?ID=16.

42. MacLeod D, Pi R, Smith D, Rose-Goodwin L. Batterer intervention systems in California: an evaluation. Final report to the National Institute of Justice. 2010; https://www.ncjrs.gov/pdffiles1/nij/grants/230702.pdf

43. Garner J, Fagan J, Maxwell, C. Published findings from the spouse assault replication program: A critical review. *J Quant Criminology*. 1995;11:3–28.

44. Davis R, Weisburd D, Taylor B. 2008. Effects of second responder programs on repeat incidents of family abuse. Campbell Collaborative Systematic Review. 2008; http://www.ncjrs.gov/pdffiles1/nji/grants/224991.pdf.

45. National Institute of Justice. Focused deterrence strategies. 2015; http://www.crimesolutions.gov/PracticeDetails.aspx?ID=11

46. Braga A, Weisburd D. *Pulling Levers: Focused Deterrence Strategies to Prevent Crime*. No. 6 of Crime Prevention Research Review. Washington, DC: Office of Community Oriented Policing Services. U.S. Department of Justice; 2012.

47. High Point, North Carolina Police Department. (nd). Domestic violence initiative. Available at: http://www.highpointnc.gov/police/how_to/domestic_violence_initiative.cfm

48. Sechrist S, Weil JD. The High Point Offender Focused Domestic Violence Initiative: Preliminary evaluation results. In: Kennedy D (Chair), *Using Focused Deterrence to Combat Domestic Violence*. Symposium presented at the John Jay College of Criminal Justice International Conference: The Rule of Law in an Era of Change: Security, Social Justice, and Inclusive Governance. Athens, Greece. 2014.

49. Brown CH, Sturgeon S. Promoting a healthy start in life and reducing early risks. In: Hosman C, Jané-Llopis E, Saxena S (Eds.). *Prevention of Mental Disorders: Effective Interventions and Policy Options: Summary Report*. Geneva, Switzerland: World Health Organization. Department of Mental Health and Substance Abuse in collaboration with the Prevention Research Centre of the Universities of Nijmegen and Maastricht.

50. Stagner MW, Lansing J. Progress toward a prevention perspective. *The Future of Children*. 2009;19(2):19–38.

51. Howard KS, Brooks-Gunn J. The role of home-visiting programs in preventing child abuse and neglect. *The Future of Children*. 2009;19(2):119–146.

52. Astuto J, Allen L. Home visitation and young children: An approach worth investing in? *Social Policy Report*. 2009;23(4):3–21.

53. Reynolds A, Mathieson L, Topitzes J. Do early childhood interventions prevent child maltreatment? A review of research. *Child Maltreatment*. 2009;14(2):182–206.

54. LeCroy C, Whitaker K. Improving the quality of home visitation: An exploratory study of difficult situations. *Child Abuse and Neglect*. 2005;29:1003–1013.

55. Zielinski D, Eckenrode J, Olds D. Nurse home visitation and the prevention of child maltreatment: Impact on the timing of officials reports. *Dev Psych*. 2009; 21:441–453.

56. Eckenrode B, Ganzel CR, Henderson E, et. al. Preventing child abuse and neglect with a program of nurse home visitation: the limiting effects of domestic violence. *JAMA: Journal of the American Medical Association.* 2000;84(11):1385–1391.

57. Kohl PL, Barth RP, Hazen A, Landsverk J. Child welfare as a gateway to domestic violence services. *Child Youth Services Rev.* 2005;27:1203–1221.

58. Family Violence Prevention Fund. *Realizing the Promise of Home Visitation: Addressing Domestic Violence and Child Maltreatment.* 2010; http://www.futureswithoutviolence. org/userfiles/file/Children_and_Families/Realizing%20the%20Promise%20of%20 Home%20Visitation%202-10.pdf

59. Sharps PW, Campbell J, Baty ML, Walker KS, Bair-Merritt MH. Current evidence on perinatal home visiting and intimate partner violence. *J Obstet Gynecol Neonatal Nurs.* 2008;37(4):480–491.

60. Adirim T, Supplee L. Overview of the federal home visiting program. *Pediatrics.* 2013;132(Suppl 2):559–564.

61. Hahn RA, Bilukha OO, Crosby A, et al. First reports evaluating the effectiveness of strategies for preventing violence: early childhood home visitation. Findings from the Task Force on Community Preventive Services. *MMWR.* 2003;52(RR-14):1–9.

62. Stover CS, Berkman M, Desai R, Marans S. The efficacy of a police-advocacy intervention for victims of domestic violence: 12 month follow-up data. *Violence Against Women.* 2010;16(4):410–425.

63. Bair-Merritt MH, Jennings JM, Chen R, Burrell L, McFarlane E, Fuddy L, Duggan AK. Reducing maternal intimate partner violence after the birth of a child: a randomized controlled trial of the Hawaii Healthy Start Home Visitation Program. *Arch Ped Adolesc Med.* 2010;164(1):16–23.

64. Jack S, Ford-Gilboe M, Wathen C, Davidov D, McNaughton D, et.al. Development of a nurse home visitation intervention for intimate partner violence. *BMC Health Services Research.* 2012;12:50.

65. Mejdoubi J, van den Heijkant SC, van Leerdam FJ, Heymans MW, Hirasing RA, Crijnen AA. Effect of nurse home visits vs. usual care on reducing intimate partner violence in young high-risk pregnant women: a randomized controlled trial. *PLoS One.* 2013;8(10):e78185.

66. Langhinrichsen-Rohling J, Turner LA. The efficacy of an intimate partner violence prevention program with high-risk adolescent girls: a preliminary test. *Prev Sci.* 2012;13: 384–394.

67. Chamberlein L, Levenson R. (nd). *Healthy Moms: Happy Babies.* Futures without Violence. Project Connect. http://www.futureswithoutviolence.org/userfiles/file/HealthCare/ HV_Trainer's_Guide_Low_Res_FINAL.pdf

68. Project Connect. http://www.tcfv.org/our-work/project-connect & Domestic Violence Enhanced Visitation. https://clinicaltrials.gov/ct2/show/NCT00465556

69. McCabe BK, Potash D, Omohundro E, Taylor CR. Design and implementation of an integrated, continuous evaluation, and quality improvement system for a State-based home-visiting program. *Maternal Child Health J.* 2012;16(7):1385–1400.

70. Nelson HD, Bougatsos C, Blazina I. Screening women for intimate partner violence: a systematic review to update the U.S. Preventive Services Task Force recommendation. *Ann Int Med.* 2012;156(11):796–809.

71. Filetti VJ, Anda RF, Nordenberg D, et al. Relationship of childhood abuse and household dysfunction to many of the leading causes of death in adults. *Am J Prev Med.* 1998;14(4):245–258.

72. Singh V. Intimate Partner Violence victimization: identification and response in primary care. *Primary Care*. 2014;41(2):261–281.

73. Plichta SB. Interactions between victims of intimate partner violence against women and the health care system. *Trauma Violence Abuse*. 2007;8(2):226–239.

74. O'Doherty LJ, Taft A, Hegarty K, Ramsay J, Davidson LL, Feder G. Screening women for intimate partner violence in healthcare settings: Abridged Cochrane systematic review and meta-analysis. *BMJ*. 2014;348:g2913.

75. Sege RD, Flaherty EG. Forty years later: inconsistencies in reporting of child abuse. *Arch Dis Child*. 2008;93:822–824.

76. United States Department of Health and Human Services. Administration for Children & Families. (nd). State Statutes Search: Child welfare gateway. https://www.childwelfare.gov/topics/systemwide/laws-policies/state/

77. Davi S. U.S. Guidelines for domestic violence screening spark debate. *Lancet*. 2010; 379:506.

13

Public Policy and Sexual Behavior

Bradley Stoner

LEARNING OBJECTIVES

1. Define sexual behavior as it relates to public policy.
2. Explore historical context of sexual behavior policy.
3. Describe current policy strategies related to sexual behavior policy.

IDENTIFYING THE PROBLEM: SEXUAL
BEHAVIOR AND CONSEQUENCES

Sexual behavior policy is an important topic with deep implications for a variety of arenas in public health, including family planning, sexually transmitted infection control, and blood-borne pathogen transmission. Policy issues related to sexual behavior affect public health directly and indirectly. For example, policy can be directly targeted toward the regulation and control of sexual behavior itself, or it can be indirectly targeted, as in policy that is implemented to affect other health concerns (such as blood donation).

Defining Sexual Behavior

For the purposes of this chapter, sexual behavior is defined as the specific behavioral acts through which human beings experience and express their sexuality.[1] Sexual behavior is quite often reductively thought of as heteronormative penile vaginal intercourse, but actually involves a broad range of behaviors, which may include oral intercourse, anal intercourse, and a variety of nonintercourse stimulative activities. In all societies, these specific behavioral acts are imbued with special meaning owing to their close association with procreation and societal continuity.[2,3]

Governments have a strong interest in regulating and controlling sexuality and sexual behavior, and have implemented a variety of policies over the years to ensure "appropriate" sexual behavior among the population. Of course, what is considered normal and appropriate is fluid and dynamic, and subject to changing historical and situational circumstances. One need only look at the trend toward legalization

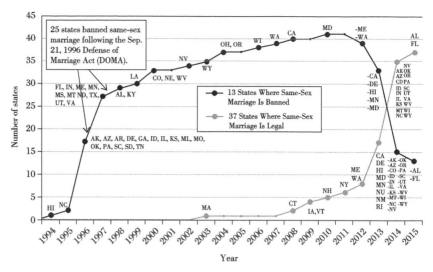

Figure 13.1 Timeline of same-sex marriage bans and legalizations by effective date of laws.
Source: http://gaymarriage.procon.org/ Accessed May 6, 2015.

of same-sex marriage in the United States for an example of how societal norms and expectations around sexuality can change within a very short time period.[4] In the mid-1990s, a total of 25 states quickly moved to ban same-sex marriage after passage of the federal Defense of Marriage Act in 1996, with several other states following suit over the next few years (Figure 13.1). Yet in less than 20 years, public opinion toward same-sex marriage changed dramatically. Numerous court challenges led to judicial rulings in several states overturning same-sex marriage bans as unconstitutional, and several other states have proactively affirmed the legality of same-sex marriage through legislative action or popular vote. By 2015, same-sex marriage was legal in 37 states.

In this context, policy with regard to sexual behavior is implemented with the goal of ensuring the socially defined health and welfare of the populace. This may involve disease prevention strategies such as condom promotion to prevent HIV transmission, or wellness promotion strategies such as positive sexuality messaging for advancing sexual health. In all cases, policy is a reflection of, and a response to, wider societal forces that are prevalent in the community at large.

PUBLIC POLICY STRATEGIES RELATED TO SEXUAL BEHAVIOR

Same-sex Sexual Behavior

Some of the earliest and best-known examples of state regulation of sexual behavior are laws that prohibit specific forms of sexual contact between individuals, primarily contact that is societally deemed deviant, immoral, or otherwise undesirable. Sodomy laws, for example, criminalized certain forms of "unnatural" sexual behavior (such as oral intercourse, anal intercourse, or bestiality), and participants in such acts could be subject to prosecution, imprisonment, or death. Historians date these laws to Roman times or even earlier, and they were widely codified into law in Western countries in the late Middle Ages and early Enlightenment period.[5,6] In England, the Buggery Act of 1533 made sodomy a capital offense punishable by hanging, a punishment that remained on the books until the 1861 Offenses Against the Person Act reduced the sentence to life in prison.[7] These laws did not define sodomy or buggery, but rather left it to the courts to interpret the offense according to judicial precedent. Conviction required that penetration must occur but that actual ejaculation was not necessary. Decriminalization of anal intercourse did not occur in the United Kingdom until 1967.[8]

In the United States, regulation of sexual behavior was largely under control of the individual states, rather than the federal government. These laws date to the founding of the Republic; hence, the criminalization of sodomy was universal and harsh. Until 1962, sodomy was a felony in all 50 states, punishable by prison terms and, in some cases, hard labor.[9] At that point, Illinois became the first state to adopt recommendations put forth by the American Law Institute's Model Penal Code proposal, which sought to decriminalize consensual sodomy (Box 13.1). In time, other states repealed their sodomy laws or reduced the penalty for consensual homosexual contact.[10]

In the mid-20th century, many states enforced sodomy laws that relegated penalties of imprisonment for up to 10 years and fines of up to $2,000. By 2002, a total of 36 states' sodomy laws were repealed or overturned by court rulings. All remaining state laws were rendered unenforceable in 2003 after the U.S. Supreme Court's *Lawrence v. Texas* ruling, in which the court ruled 6–3 that Texas' same-sex sodomy law is unconstitutional because private sexual contact is an implicitly protected liberty guaranteed by the due process clause of the Constitution.[11] An important exception to state regulation of sexual behavior is the proscription against same-sex sexual contact in the U.S. military, enforced by the federal government. Article 125 of the Uniform Code of Military Justice, passed in 1951, forbids sodomy (defined as unnatural carnal copulation with another person of the same or opposite sex or with an animal) among all military personnel.[12] It was essentially rendered moot by *Lawrence v. Texas*, except in circumstances where "factors unique to the military environment" can be demonstrated to override the protected liberty interests of individuals.[13]

Commercial Sexual Behavior

Prostitution has been called "the world's oldest profession," and has been recognized and regulated since biblical times. Examples of prostitution appear in the writings of ancient cultures across the world, from Mesopotamia to the Far East.[14] Regulation of prostitution emerged in the Middle Ages, when sex work by and large was institutionalized in brothels, and sumptuary laws required sex workers to wear distinctive forms of dress. Criminalization soon followed, spurred in part by the perceived link between prostitutes and sexually transmitted diseases such as syphilis, although the legal status of prostitution varied from jurisdiction to jurisdiction.[15,16] In the United States, state laws prohibiting commercial sex work appeared in the early

Box 13.1 American Law Institute—Model Penal Code

The Model Penal Code was developed in 1962 as statutory text to assist state legislatures in their efforts to update and standardize penal law. Section 213.2 defines "deviate sexual intercourse" as "sexual intercourse per os or per anus between human beings who are not husband and wife, and any form of sexual intercourse with an animal." Such behavior would be criminalized if performed by force or imposition. Consensual activity would not be subject to criminal penalties. States were free to adopt the Model Penal Code provisions or to develop their own language.

Model Penal Code—Section 213.2. Deviate Sexual Intercourse by Force or Imposition

(1) **By Force or Its Equivalent.** A person who engages in deviate sexual intercourse with another person, or who causes another to engage in deviate sexual intercourse, commits a felony of the second degree if:

(a) he compels the other person to participate by force or by threat of imminent death, serious bodily injury, extreme pain or kidnapping, to be inflicted on anyone; or

(b) he has substantially impaired the other person's power to appraise or control his conduct, by administering or employing without the knowledge of the other person drugs, intoxicants or other means for the purpose of preventing resistance; or

(c) the other person is unconscious; or

(d) the other person is less than 10 years old.

(2) **By Other Imposition.** A person who engages in deviate sexual intercourse with another person, or who causes another to engage in deviate sexual intercourse, commits a felony of the third degree if:

(a) he compels the other person to participate by any threat that would prevent resistance by a person of ordinary resolution; or

(b) he knows that the other person suffers from a mental disease or defect which renders him incapable of appraising the nature of his conduct; or

(c) he knows that the other person submits because he is unaware that a sexual act is being committed upon him.

Source: http://www.law-lib.utoronto.ca/bclc/crimweb/web1/mpc/mpc.html. Accessed May 8, 2015.

20th century, and to this day the exchange of sex for money remains illegal in all states except Nevada. The policy implications of criminalizing prostitution are twofold: first, for the protection of society by preventing the spread of "licentious" (i.e., immoral) behavior and diseases that may follow, and second for the protection of the individual, because prostitution is inherently exploitative and degrading. Nevertheless, emerging critiques of prostitution have posited that commercial sex work may be empowering in certain circumstances, by allowing individuals to generate an income that permits a standard of living far higher than would normally be accessible to them under prevailing economic conditions.[17] Despite these critiques, commercial sex work remains criminalized in most jurisdictions.

Unwanted Sexual Behavior: Title IX in the United States

A more recent example of policy toward sexual behavior has been the emergence of allegations of the failure of colleges and universities in the United States to protect the sexual rights of women attending their institutions. Specifically, women are asserting their right to freedom from unwanted sexual advances under the federal law known as Title IX. This law, implemented as part of the Education Amendments of 1972, was implemented to ensure women's equal access to educational programs and activities at institutions that receive federal financial assistance.[18] In practice, this applies most specifically to providing women with intercollegiate sports venues, facilities, and opportunities equal to those enjoyed by men on college and university campuses. Because most schools in the United States receive federal funds to support at least some of their operations, the law has far-reaching implications.

Title IX also ensures that women will enjoy a safe environment free from harassment and unwanted sexual pressures. (See Chapter 12 on Title IX and violence against women.) A number of court cases have been brought under Title IX, alleging that colleges and universities have not done enough to prevent on-campus rape and sexual assault, and have endangered women's well-being by failing to provide appropriate oversight of sexual misconduct occurring on their campuses. These cases follow from a 2011 complaint against Yale University, in which a sexual assault victim and several other students alleged that the university failed to eliminate a "hostile sexual environment" and did not adequately respond to concerns about sexual harassment on campus.[19] This triggered the Office for Civil Rights of the Department of Education to issue an open letter to U.S. colleges and universities stating, in part, that "the sexual harassment of students, including sexual violence, interferes with students' right to receive an education free from discrimination and, in the case of sexual violence, is a crime." [20] A number of institutions have been implicated in Title IX violations related to on-campus sexual assault, including Amherst College, University of North Carolina, and several other elite institutions. By January 2015, 94 colleges and universities were under investigation by the Department of Education for allegedly not having properly handled cases of sexual assault.[21]

Title IX complaints are an important example of the way in which nonhealth policies can have important health ramifications. The initial purpose of Title IX was to create parity of opportunity in education and sports. However, the law is now being applied to ensure parity of safety—specifically, safety with regard to unwanted sexual behavior, and to ensure freedom from sexual assault on college and university campuses. Title IX compliance is now a major focus of higher education administrators across the country and includes efforts to train faculty and staff on mandates for reporting suspected sexual harassment and sexual assault.

Condom Policy for STI/HIV Prevention

A good example of sexual behavior policies designed to reduce the spread of infectious diseases are those related to promotion and funding of the long-standing public health recommendation for consistent and correct condom use to prevent sexually transmitted infections (STIs), including HIV. Policies promoting condom use have been implemented for decades, and even predate the HIV epidemic, to the extent that syphilis and gonorrhea were prioritized as public health problems for much of the 20th century.[22,23] Originally developed as a means of contraception, the condom was a cloth or sheath, fashioned from linen, animal intestine, or other materials, and placed on the penis to prevent insemination during intercourse. Historians suggest several instances in which condoms were reportedly used in Renaissance Europe for the prevention of venereal diseases such as syphilis.[24] Rubber condoms appeared in the 19th century, and governments began to recognize the value of condoms for preventing disease in the military and maintaining fighting force readiness. By the 1930s, condoms were widely promoted within the U.S. military for venereal disease prevention.[23] Health departments in the United States included condom promotion as part of their sexually transmitted disease prevention strategies, including efforts to deal with surging rates of gonorrhea and syphilis in the 1960s and 1970s.

The AIDS era brought a renewed emphasis on condom promotion, as the newly identified human immunodeficiency virus (HIV) became recognized as transmissible through sexual contact and blood exposure. An early advocate of this strategy was C. Everett Koop, U.S. Surgeon General, whose landmark 1986 Report on AIDS strongly recommended the use of condoms as an effective means of preventing or reducing the transmission of HIV infection in sexually active individuals.[25] In a 1987 statement to a skeptical committee of the U.S. House of Representatives, Koop acknowledged that although "scientific evidence indicates that abstinence is the only completely safe way to avoid acquiring AIDS sexually," nevertheless "the use of a condom is the best method of reducing or preventing HIV infection" for persons who are not abstinent or monogamous.[26]

Despite opposition from some who objected on religious or philosophical grounds, condom promotion remains an important cornerstone of STI/HIV prevention policy in the United States and worldwide. Currently, correct and consistent condom use at the individual level, as well as condom distribution and accessibility at the structural level, are foundational components of national policies such as the U.S. National HIV/AIDS Strategy,[27] the Centers for Disease Control and Prevention (CDC) Division of HIV/AIDS Prevention Strategic Plan,[28] and the CDC Division of Sexually Transmitted Disease (STD) Prevention recommendations.[29] The scientific basis of common efficacy was examined by a National Institutes of Health (NIH) workshop in 2000, which concluded that condoms, when used consistently and correctly, significantly reduce the likelihood of transmission of HIV and other sexually transmitted infections.[30] Moreover, a recent meta-analysis of U.S. and international-based structural-level condom distribution interventions showed that increasing condom availability and accessibility significantly increases appropriate condom-use behaviors.[31]

Sexual education policy is another highly politicized arena in the United States, in which many states have exerted their right to mandate the content and messaging of classroom instruction around sex and sexuality. Often, sexual education instruction is coupled with information about HIV prevention. Table 13.1 provides a state-by-state listing of mandated sexual education and HIV instruction in the classroom. Currently, 22 states require sex education as a part of the formal school curriculum, and 33 states require some form of HIV-prevention instruction.[32] While specific educational content is left up to individual school districts, only 13 states require instruction to be "medically accurate," and 25 states require abstinence to be "stressed" within the curriculum when sex education is taught.

Interestingly, states' political leanings often are reflected in specific aspects of the mandated sexual education policies. More conservative Southern states, for example, often require the curriculum to emphasize the importance of sex only within marriage, and may include modules on negative outcomes of teen sex. More liberal states, such as those on the West coast, mandate that discussion of sexual orientation be inclusive rather than negative. Most states allow parents to "opt out" of mandated sex and HIV instruction if they find it objectionable for their children. In the absence of a unified national curriculum, states are left to develop and implement their own policies for sexual behavior instruction in the classroom. Tellingly, 15 states do not require any form of instruction in sexual behavior or HIV-prevention education.

CASE STUDY

Blood Donation Policy: Regulating the Consequences of Sexual Behavior

The AIDS era brought with it new concerns regarding the safety of the blood supply in the United States and abroad. In the early 1980s, AIDS was increasingly recognized among persons who had received transfusions of blood or blood products, and the U.S. Food and Drug Administration (FDA), the regulatory agency overseeing the collection and distribution of blood donation in the United States, quickly moved to protect the blood supply. In 1983, the FDA imposed a ban on blood donations from members of certain high-risk groups, including injection drug users as well as men who have sex with men (MSM).[33] Although not a policy that addresses sexual behavior per se, this policy does address the consequences of sexual behavior by stipulating a lifetime ban on blood donations from any man who has ever had sex with another man since 1977.

The policy dates to a time when tests for HIV were just emerging, and epidemiologic concerns about "window period" transmission were developing. The FDA argued that MSM, as a group, were at increased risk not only for HIV, but also for hepatitis B and other blood-borne infectious conditions. Moreover, blood donations taken from a newly infected individual could still be contagious even in the face of a negative HIV test, because of the protracted time period between acquisition of infection

Table 13.1 Sex Education and HIV Mandates in the United States

State	Sex Education* Mandated	HIV Education Mandated	When Provided, Sex Education or HIV Education Must:				Parental Role		
			Be Medically Accurate	Be Age Appropriate	Be Culturally Appropriate and Unbiased	Cannot Promote Religion	Notice	Consent	Opt-Out
Alabama		X		X					X
Arizona				X			HIV	SEX	HIV
Arkansas									
California		X	X	X	X	X	X		X
Colorado			X	X	X		X		X
Connecticut		X							X
Delaware	X	X							
District of Columbia	X	X		X			X		X
Florida				X					X
Georgia	X	X					X		X
Hawaii			X	X					
Idaho				X					X
Illinois†		X	X	X					X
Indiana		X							
Iowa	X	X	X	X	X		X		X
Kentucky	X	X							
Louisiana				X		X	X		X
Maine	X	X	X	X					X
Maryland	X	X							X
Massachusetts							X		X
Michigan		X	X‡	X			X		X
Minnesota	X	X							X
Mississippi^Ω	X			X			X		X

State									
Missouri		X		X			X		X
Montana	X	X							
Nevada	X	X		X			X	X	X
New Hampshire		X							X
New Jersey	X	X	X	X	X		X		X
New Mexico	X	X							X
New York		X		HIV					HIV
North Carolina	X	X	X	X					
North Dakota	X								
Ohio	X	X							X
Oklahoma		X					X		X
Oregon	X	X	X	X	X		X		X
Pennsylvania		X		HIV			X		X
Rhode Island	X	X	X	X					X
South Carolina	X	X		X			X		X
Tennessee	X[ψ]	X		HIV					X
Texas									
Utah[ζ]	X	X	X		X		X	X	
Vermont	X	X		X	X		X		X
Virginia							X		X
Washington				X			X		X
West Virginia	X	X		X			X		X
Wisconsin		X					X		X
TOTAL	22+DC	33+DC	13	26+DC	8	2	22+DC	3	35+DC

*Sex education typically includes discussion of STIs.

†Sex education is not mandatory, but health education is required and it includes medically accurate information on abstinence.

‡Sex education "shall not be medically inaccurate."

Ω Localities may include topics such as contraception or STIs only with permission from the State Department of Education.

ψ Sex education is required if the pregnancy rate for 15- to 17-year-old women is at least 19.5 or higher.

ζ State also prohibits teachers from responding to students' spontaneous questions in ways that conflict with the law's requirements.

and seroconversion. This overarching policy excludes not only those MSM who are currently sexually active, but also those persons who are no longer sexually active, as well as those whose last sexual encounter may have been months, years, or even decades prior. The policy was reframed and restated in 1992, and a lifetime donation ban remains the current position of the U.S. Food and Drug Administration.

However well-intended this may have been at the time, the policy has been roundly criticized in recent years by scientists, gay-rights activists, and others who argue that the policy as stated is ill-conceived, discriminatory, and regressive now that better tests for HIV are available and scientific understanding of HIV epidemiology and transmission has improved.[34] Additionally, critics suggest that the policy is inconsistent and unfairly reduces the potential pool of blood donors without significantly reducing the likelihood of blood-borne HIV transmission. Some of the criticisms include:

(1) Rather than focus on recent or ongoing high-risk sexual behavior, the policy applies to any man who has ever had sex with a man since 1977. This means that a person who had one sexual encounter with another man more than 30 years ago would still be excluded as a potential blood donor for life, even if he has repeatedly tested negative for HIV, hepatitis B, hepatitis C, and other infectious pathogens.

(2) Although the policy excludes any man who has ever had sex with a man, the same is not true for female sex partners of MSM. A woman who was the sexual partner of an MSM may freely donate blood if the last sexual exposure was more than one year ago. Many advocates have suggested this policy is flawed, given that it denies the same logic to MSM who have had remote exposures more than one year prior.

(3) The policy excludes MSM in stable monogamous relationships, where transmission risk is nonexistent if both partners have tested negative for HIV.

Over the past decade, an ever-growing number of voices have been speaking out against the MSM lifetime blood donation ban. Protests on college campuses across the United States have brought attention to the fact that many MSM would gladly donate if given the opportunity. Moreover, professional organizations such as the American Medical Association have challenged the scientific justification for continuing such a ban.[35] In December 2014, the FDA announced a revision of the policy, to be implemented sometime in 2015. Under the revised policy, any MSM whose last sexual exposure was greater than one year ago will be allowed to donate blood. Some have argued that this policy does not go far enough, for it still disallows sexually active MSM in stable monogamous relationships who have tested negative for HIV. Advocates suggest that many of these individuals would be willing and able blood donors, and the risk of HIV transmission is nonexistent. This experience has shown that health policy focusing on the consequences of sexual behavior (in this case the ability of MSM to donate blood) is responsive to advances in scientific understanding, as well as advocacy and awareness in the political arena.

THE FUTURE OF SEXUAL BEHAVIOR POLICY:
THE SEXUAL HEALTH PARADIGM

A new movement is slowly but surely gaining ground in the United States—the movement toward sexual health as a public health goal (Box 13.2). Proponents of a sexual health framework argue that for too long U.S. policy has been focused on sexual disease, and its attendant messages about prevention, protection, avoidance, and fear. These negative consequences of sexual behavior engender a policy approach that is essentially negative in its outlook: markers of success include such things as how quickly disease rates fall, how many cases of infection are prevented, how many risky sexual liaisons are interrupted? Instead, the focus on sexual health allows us to emphasize the benefits of sexual behavior as part of a healthy normal human existence, something that occurs normally and regularly across the lifespan.[36,37,38]

The roots of the sexual health movement in the United States date to 2001 when the U.S. Surgeon General, David Satcher, issued a call to action to promote sexual health and responsible sexual behavior.[39] This model advances and builds upon the World Health Organization definition of health and applies a sexual dimension: that is, sexual health is a state of physical, emotional, mental, and social well-being in relation to sexuality, and not merely the absence of disease, dysfunction, or infirmity. Unfortunately, progress has been intermittent with regard to operationalizing sexual health within bureaucratic structures and organizations in the United States. For example, the

---

Box 13.2 Sexual Health Paradigm

The sexual health paradigm recognizes that multiple domains affect personal and interpersonal well-being with regard to sex and sexuality. Experts are working to develop up-to-date, inclusive definitions of the term, which recognize the importance of socio-ecological influences on individual wellness.

Sexual health is a state of well-being in relation to sexuality across the lifespan that involves physical, emotional, mental, social, and spiritual dimensions. Sexual health is an inextricable element of human health and is based on a positive, equitable, and respectful approach to sexuality, relationships, and reproduction; an approach that is free of coercion, fear, discrimination, stigma, shame, and violence. It includes the ability to understand the benefits, risks, and responsibilities of sexual behavior; the prevention and care of disease and other adverse outcomes; and the possibility of fulfilling sexual relationships. Sexual health is impacted by socioeconomic and cultural contexts—including policies, practices, and services—that support healthy outcomes for individuals, families, and their communities.

Source: CDC/HRSA [Health Resources and Services Administration] Advisory Committee on HIV, Viral Hepatitis and STD Prevention and Treatment. Record of the proceedings, May 8–9, 2012. Atlanta, Georgia. http://www.cdc.gov/maso/facm/pdfs/CHACHSPT/20120508_CHAC.pdf. Accessed on May 8, 2015.

Centers for Disease Control and Prevention (CDC), as well as state and local health departments across the country, still maintain a disease-centered approach to STI and HIV prevention and have yet to embrace sexual health as an organizing concept. The lack of uptake for using a sexual health model instead of a disease model may be related to funding policies. Monies for public health activities are often appropriated for specific targeted disease-control efforts.

Still, the potential for a sexual health approach in policy development is profound, and there are great opportunities for collaboration across multiple agendas. For example, adolescent sexual growth and development are closely related to psychosocial adaptation and integration, particularly with regard to issues of gender identity and maturation. Similarly, reproductive health is closely linked to aging, menopause, and postmenopausal sexuality as more elders remain sexually active later in life. One important instance of collaborative success has been the extent to which public health officials in sexually transmitted infection prevention have been able to include experts in reproductive health in important projects that address both areas. Reproductive health specialists now routinely are included in developing and vetting the CDC's quadrennial STD Treatment Guidelines,[40] and the World Health Organization has embraced sexual and reproductive health as an organizing construct for prevention work in global contexts.[41] At this time, tremendous opportunity remains to engage advocates and experts from other arenas in promoting sexual health and wellness across the lifespan, including men's health, adolescent health, and elder health, to name but a few. Indeed, as people live longer and remain sexually active later in life, policies based on a sexual health approach undoubtedly will have a deeper and more positive impact on people's lives than would a negative, disease-focused approach.

CONCLUSION

Sexual behavior policy is a complex and contested arena in which normal human expressions of sexuality are controlled, regulated, and surveilled by governments acting, ostensibly, in the best interests of the wider population. What is considered normal and acceptable sexual behavior changes across time and space, and responds to advances in science as well as pressures imposed within the political arena. Sexual health may be a promising new framework for developing sexual behavior policy that respects the rights of individuals and emphasizes the normalcy and ubiquity of sexual behavior across human communities and across the lifespan.

REFERENCES

1. Bancroft, J (Ed.). *Researching Sexual Behavior.* Bloomington, IN: Indiana University Press; 1997.
2. Malinowski B. *Sex and Repression in Savage Society.* London, UK: Routledge Classics; 1927.
3. Mead M. *Coming of Age in Samoa.* New York, NY: William Morrow Paperbacks; 1928.
4. Same-sex marriage laws. National Conference of State Legislatures. http://www.ncsl.org/research/human-services/same-sex-marriage-laws.aspx. Accessed March 31, 2015.

5. McGinn TAJ. *Prostitution, Sexuality and the Law in Ancient Rome.* New York, NY: Oxford University Press; 1988.

6. Boswell J. *Christianity, Social Tolerance, and Homosexuality.* Chicago, IL: University of Chicago Press; 1980.

7. Hyde HM. *The Love that Dared Not Speak Its Name: A Candid History of Homosexuality in Britain.* Boston, MA: Little Brown; 1970.

8. United Kingdom Sexual Offences Act 1967. http://www.legislation.gov.uk/ukpga/1967/60/pdfs/ukpga_19670060_en.pdf. Accessed March 31, 2015.

9. Eskridge WN. *Dishonorable Passions: Sodomy Laws in America, 1861–2003.* New York, NY: Viking; 2008.

10. Canaday M. We colonials: sodomy laws in America. *The Nation* Sept. 22, 2008. http://www.thenation.com/article/we-colonials-sodomy-laws-america. Accessed March 30, 2015.

11. *Lawrence v. Texas,* 539 US 558 (2003). https://supreme.justia.com/cases/federal/us/539/558/. Accessed March 31, 2015.

12. Uniform Code of Military Justice, 925, Article 125. Sodomy. http://www.ucmj.us/subchapter-10-punitive-articles/925-article-125-sodomy. Accessed March 31, 2015.

13. U.S. Court of Appeals for the Armed Forces, U.S. v. Marcum (No. 02-0944, Crim. App. No. 34216), 2004. http://www.armfor.uscourts.gov/newcaaf/opinions/2004Term/02-0944.htm. Accessed March 31, 2015.

14. Ringdal NJ. *Love for Sale: A World History of Prostitution.* New York, NY: Grove Press; 2005.

15. Sanger WW. *The History of Prostitution: Its Extent, Causes and Effects Throughout the World.* New York, NY: American Medical Press, 1895 (orig. 1858).

16. Grant MG. *Playing the Whore: The Work of Sex Work.* London, UK: Verso; 2014

17. Nagle J (Ed.), *Whores and Other Feminists.* London, UK: Routledge, 1997.

18. U.S. Dept. of Justice, Title IX of the Education Amendments of 1972. http://www.justice.gov/crt/about/cor/coord/titleix.php. Accessed March 31, 2015.

19. Gasso J. Yale under federal investigation for possible Title IX violation. *Yale Daily News.* April 1, 2011. http://yaledailynews.com/blog/2011/04/01/yale-under-federal-investigation-for-possible-title-ix-violations/. Accessed March 30, 2015.

20. Ali R. Dear Colleague Letter: Sexual Violence. April 4, 2011. http://www2.ed.gov/about/offices/list/ocr/letters/colleague-201104.pdf. Accessed March 30, 2015.

21. Kingkade T. Barnard College joins list of 94 colleges under Title IX investigation. *Huffington Post.* January 7, 2015. http://www.huffingtonpost.com/2015/01/07/barnard-college-title-ix-investigations_n_6432596.html. Accessed March 31, 2015.

22. Brandt AM. *No Magic Bullet: A Social History of Venereal Disease in the United States Since 1880.* New York, NY: Oxford University Press; 1987.

23. Lord AM. *Condom Nation: The U.S. Government's Sex Education Campaign from World War I to the Internet.* Baltimore, MD: Johns Hopkins University Press; 2009.

24. Collier A. *The Humble Little Condom: A History.* Amherst, NY: Prometheus Books; 2007.

25. U.S. Public Health Service. Surgeon General's Report. Acquired Immune Deficiency Syndrome. 1986; http://profiles.nlm.nih.gov/ps/access/NNBBVN.pdf. Accessed March 31, 2015.

26. Koop CE. Statement before the Committee on Energy and Commerce, U.S. House of Representatives, February 10, 1987. http://profiles.nlm.nih.gov/ps/access/QQBDPH.pdf. Accessed March 31, 2015.

27. White House Office of National AIDS Policy. National HIV/AIDS Strategy for the United States, July 2010. https://www.whitehouse.gov/sites/default/files/uploads/NHAS.pdf. Accessed May 8, 2015.

28. Centers for Disease Control and Prevention. Division of HIV/AIDS Prevention. Strategic Plan 2011 through 2015. August 2011; http://www.cdc.gov/hiv/pdf/policies_DHAP-strategic-plan.pdf. Accessed May 8, 2015.

29. Centers for Disease Control and Prevention. Division of STD Prevention. Sexually Transmitted Disease Surveillance 2013. December 2014; http://www.cdc.gov/std/stats13/surv2013-print.pdf. Accessed May 8, 2015.

30. National Institute of Allergy and Infectious Disease. National Institutes of Health. Workshop Summary: Scientific Evidence on Condom Effectiveness for Sexually Transmitted Disease Effectiveness. July 2001; http://www.niaid.nih.gov/about/organization/dmid/documents/condomreport. Accessed April 1, 2015.

31. Charania MR, Crepaz N, Guenther-Gray C, et al. Efficacy of structural-level condom distribution interventions: a meta-analysis of U.S. and international studies. *AIDS and Behavior.* 2011;15(7):1283–1297.

32. Sex and HIV education. State policies in brief. Guttmacher Institute, May 2015; http://www.guttmacher.org/statecenter/spibs/spib_SE.pdf. Accessed May 8, 2015.

33. Food and Drug Administration. Blood donations from men who have sex with men—questions and answers. http://www.fda.gov/BiologicsBloodVaccines/BloodBloodProducts/QuestionsaboutBlood/ucm108186.htm. Accessed on April 1, 2015.

34. Gay Men's Health Crisis. A Drive for Change: Reforming U.S. Blood Donation Policies. 2010; http://www.gmhc.org/files/editor/file/a_blood_ban_report2010.pdf. Accessed on April 2, 2015.

35. American Medical Association. Opposition to the Lifetime Ban on Blood Donations for Gay Men. 2013; http://www.ama-assn.org/ama/pub/news/news/2013/2013-06-18-new-ama-policies-annual-meeting.page. Accessed on April 5, 2015.

36. Edwards MA, Coleman E. Defining sexual health: a descriptive overview. *Archives of Sexual Behavior.* 2004;33(3):189–195.

37. Swartzendruber A, Zenilman JM. A national strategy to improve sexual health. *JAMA: Journal of the American Medical Association.* 2010;304:1005–1006.

38. Satcher D, Hook EW III, Coleman E. Sexual health in America: improving patient care and public health. *JAMA: Journal of the American Medical Association.* 2015;314:765–766.

39. Satcher D. The Surgeon General's Call to Action to Promote Sexual Health and Responsible Sexual Behavior. 2001; http://www.ncbi.nlm.nih.gov/books/NBK44223/. Accessed on April 5, 2015.

40. Centers for Disease Control and Prevention. Sexually Transmitted Diseases: Treatment Guidelines, 2010. *MMWR.* 2010;59(RR-12).

41. World Health Organization. Sexual and reproductive health. Department of Reproductive Health and Research. http://www.who.int/reproductivehealth. Accessed April 5, 2015.

14

Public Policy and Illicit Drugs

Duane C. McBride, Yvonne M. Terry-McElrath,
and Curtis J. VanderWaal

LEARNING OBJECTIVES

1. Describe illicit drug use as a public health problem.
2. Explain illicit drug use policy strategies in terms of the ecological systems approach.
3. Describe the continuum of U.S. illicit drug policy.
4. Explore the application of an ecological systems approach to policies related to marijuana and methamphetamine.

IDENTIFYING THE PROBLEM: ILLICIT DRUG USE

This chapter focuses on substances that are—by *policy* definition—illegal. They have been defined as such because of the perceived public health risks associated with their use. Users are at risk from immediate physiological consequences (e.g., accidents, overdose). Longer-term risks may include permanently impaired cognition, tolerance (needing an increasingly larger dose of a substance to achieve the same effect), dependence (wherein the brain physically adapts to repeated use and cannot function normally without the substance), and/or addiction (a chronic, relapsing brain disease characterized by compulsive drug seeking and use despite harmful consequences).[1] Significant health risks can be associated with modes of administration, such as transmission of hepatitis and HIV infection via shared injection equipment.[2] Illicit drug use consequences are particularly significant for adolescents. Compared with individuals who initiate illicit drug use as adults, adolescent initiators are more likely to develop dependence,[3,4] have lower educational and earnings achievement as adults,[5] and become involved in other deviant/criminal behaviors and poly-drug use.[6,7]

The public health risks of illicit drug use reach beyond individual physiological and psychopharmacological effects to significant social costs. Nonusers are at risk from crimes committed by illicit drug users to obtain money or drugs for continued use, or committed while intoxicated, such as impaired driving. Nonusers are also at risk from crimes committed by illicit drug manufacturers and/or distributors (e.g., the threat of toxic fumes and explosions inherent in small-scale methamphetamine production).

Children are often at highest risk, whether from exposure in utero, accidental ingestion of drugs used by others in the household, or abuse and neglect suffered while under the care of illicit drug users, manufacturers, or distributors.[8] All members of society are affected by increased public safety and healthcare costs associated with illicit drug use, as well as lost productivity. To be specific, estimates place the total cost of illicit drug use in the United States at more than $193 billion in 2007: approximately $52 billion for incarceration and premature mortality from homicide and more than $61 billion for other crime-related costs, $68 billion for lost productivity excluding homicide, and $11 billion for health-related costs.[9] Indeed, the economic impact of illicit drug use on American society is on par with other serious chronic health problems in the United States, including diabetes, obesity, and smoking.[9]

The costs and nature of illicit drugs result in complicated connections across sectors, particularly the health and criminal justice systems. A primary complication arises from the shifting understanding of which substances should be classified as illegal. Because the definition is based on *perceived* harm, substances move in or out of the illicit classification based on new scientific research, political and ideological shifts of opinion, and/or changes in perceived risk of use. For example, alcohol is not illicit now—but was illegal from 1920 to 1933 during Prohibition. Designer drugs known as bath salts emerged in the early 2000s, but federal legislation classifying many of the active chemical ingredients as illicit was not enacted until 2012.

Illicit drugs comprise a wide range of substances. Some are naturally derived from plants (e.g., marijuana, opium), others are semisynthetic substances (e.g., heroin, which is a chemical manipulation of opium), and still others are entirely synthetic (e.g., methamphetamine; LSD). Illicit drugs include narcotics, stimulants, depressants or sedatives, hallucinogens, and substances with combined effects. The United States is the world's largest consumer of cocaine, Colombian heroin, Mexican heroin and marijuana; a major consumer of Ecstasy and Mexican methamphetamine; and a minor consumer of Southeast Asian heroin.[10] The United States is also an illicit producer of marijuana, depressants, stimulants, hallucinogens, and methamphetamine.[10] Illicit drug use incidence and prevalence have varied significantly throughout U.S. history and undoubtedly will continue to change. (See Figure 14.1.) Illicit drug use prevalence is highest among individuals in their late teens and early twenties.[11] As of 2014, past 12-month use of any illicit drug was reported by 15%, 30%, and 39% of 8th, 10th, and 12th graders, respectively.[12] In 2013, 36% of all young adults aged 19 to 28 years reported similar use.[13] Marijuana was the illicit drug most commonly used among these age groups; other frequently reported illicit drugs included inhalants (for 8th graders), synthetic marijuana, amphetamines, and narcotics other than heroin.

U.S. POLICY STRATEGIES FOR ADDRESSING ILLICIT DRUG USE

The Structure of U.S. Illicit Drug Policy

The United States is a democratic federal constitutional republic: the power to govern is shared among national, state, and local governments. Although states cede

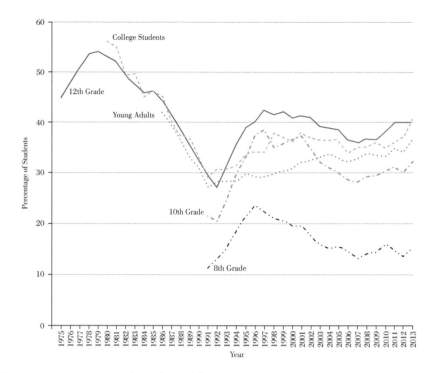

Figure 14.1 Trends in annual prevalence of illicit drug use, 1976–2013.

Adapted and reproduced with permission.[14] For 12th graders, college students, and young adults: any use of marijuana, LSD, other hallucinogens, crack, other cocaine, or heroin; or any use of narcotics other than heroin, amphetamines, sedatives (barbiturates), or tranquilizers not under a doctor's orders. For 8th and 10th graders: use of narcotics other than heroin and sedatives (barbiturates) has been excluded (younger respondents appear to over-report use).

responsibility for some matters to the federal government (e.g., foreign policy, national defense), they retain considerable autonomy in other matters. States and governmental subdivisions within states (counties/parishes, townships, municipalities) hold powers of taxation, education, and infrastructure.[15] There are frequent tensions among federal, state, and local authorities in many areas of policy and practice, including education, public health, and law enforcement.[16]

U.S. illicit drug policy is a combination of federal, state, and local policy. One way to conceptualize this involves an ecological systems approach composed of macro, mezzo, and micro levels.[17] The *macro level* refers to federal and state government policy. The *mezzo level* involves municipal policies and institutional practices (e.g., city ordinances, public health, drug treatment, and criminal justice systems). The *micro level* includes individual actions and collective advocacy leading to macro- and mezzo-level policies/practices. Each level—macro, mezzo, and micro—exerts a direct or indirect influence across other levels (see Figure 14.2).

Macro Level 1: Federal Policy

The primary legislation guiding current federal illicit drug policy is the 1970 Controlled Substances Act (CSA) (21 U.S.C. 811 et seq.). The CSA identifies which

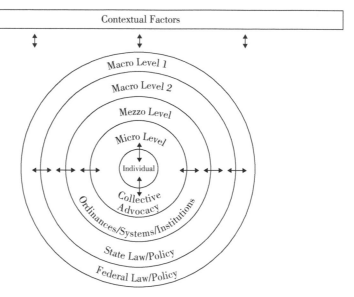

Figure 14.2 Ecological systems map of U.S. illicit drug policy.
Adapted and reproduced with permission.[17] Arrows indicate cross-level reciprocal influences. Contextual factors include sociodemographic characteristics, funding resources, political priorities, etc.

substances are illicit at the federal level using controlled substance schedules, a classification system based on a complex combination of scientific knowledge (abuse potential, medical utility, health consequences of misuse) and political considerations (public perceptions). Federal controlled substance schedules range from Schedule I to Schedule V. Each schedule identifies types of use and distribution allowed under law (if any), and specifies penalties for illicit use (based on quantity; possession vs. sales; first or subsequent offense, etc.). Substances are added, removed, or transferred from one schedule to another via legislation or—more recently—through the judicial system.[18] Updated federal schedules are published annually (Title 21 Code of Federal Regulations [C.F.R.] §§ 1308.11 through 1308.15). When illicit drugs are discussed, Schedule I and II drugs are the primary focus.

- Schedule I—the most restrictive classification—includes substances defined as having high abuse potential leading to severe psychological or physical dependence. Schedule I drugs either have no accepted medical use or lack accepted safety for use in treatment under medical supervision. Examples include heroin and LSD as well as marijuana. Prescriptions cannot be written for Schedule I substances.
- Schedule II substances also have high abuse potential, but do have currently accepted medical use. Examples include opiates used for pain management, many medications used to treat attention deficit hyperactivity disorder, and cocaine (which is very rarely prescribed). Schedule II substances are closely monitored and have considerable restrictions on prescriptions, refills, and distribution.

- Schedules III, IV and V contain substances that have decreasing abuse potential with each successive schedule level. These substances have accepted medical use, but are monitored closely.

Federal schedules attempt to reduce demand for illicit drugs by labeling identified substances as illegal and specifying increasingly severe penalties for use and distribution. Federal policy via the CSA also addresses demand reduction by funding research on drug use, treatment (reducing demand among users), and prevention education (reducing demand among the general population). Federal policy (again via the CSA) addresses illicit drug supply reduction by specifying which entities are allowed to manufacture/distribute/dispense and import/export controlled substances, as well as which are designated to enforce CSA provisions. The U.S. Coast Guard seizes billions of dollars worth of drugs each year and accounts for the majority of drug seizures in international waters. The U.S. Customs Department is responsible for drug law enforcement along the U.S. borders. Inside the United States, the primary federal agency of interdiction is the Drug Enforcement Administration (DEA), responsible for CSA enforcement and for preventing, disrupting, and seizing illicit drug trade crossing state lines.

Macro Level 2: State Law and Policy

Under the 10th amendment to the U.S. constitution, states have responsibility for developing rapid and innovative policies to address health, social, and economic issues, except in cases where the issue has been preempted by federal legislation.[19] States have been—and continue to be—the innovative actors in developing illicit drug policy. For example, the club drug GHB (Gamma-Hydroxybutyrate) was made a Schedule I substance at the federal level in 2000. However, 24 states had already scheduled GHB by that time.[20] Each state has its own controlled substance scheduling framework assigning penalties for illicit use and distribution. Not all states base their schedules on abuse potential and medical utility. In addition, variation from federal schedules and between states exists in the number of schedules and classification of substances within schedules.[20] For example, the federal government listed GHB as a Schedule I substance. Eleven states also classified it as a Schedule I substance, but five states listed GHB in Schedule II, two states in Schedule III, and six states in Schedule IV.[20] Even when a substance is classified in the same schedule, between-state penalties can differ widely.

The importance of the variance in state illicit drug policy stems from the differential impact state policy has compared with federal policy on a person's daily life. If federal schedules address a substance, federal law generally supersedes state law.[21] However, in 2006, only 6% of all U.S. adult felony convictions occurred in federal court, while 94% occurred in state courts, and drug offenders made up the largest percentage (33%) of state court felony convictions.[22] The majority of arrests for illicit drug possession, sales, and manufacturing are made by local or state police.[23] In order for local and/or state police to make an arrest for a specific act, that act must be illegal under state—not federal—law. State illicit drug arrests are usually for small quantity offenses; violations prosecuted at the federal level are predominately related to trafficking and conspiracy.[24] The importance of differences between federal and state policies (and variation among state policies) is nowhere better illustrated than by the current marijuana policy landscape, as will be discussed in the case study presented later in this chapter.

Mezzo Level: Municipal Ordinances and Institutions Implementing Policy—Public Health, Treatment, and Criminal Justice Systems

Consider a state where policy prohibits a particular substance's use, specifying high fines and long incarceration. In one community, the criminal justice system may have developed policies and practices facilitating diversion to treatment for the noted offense. Municipal ordinances frequently govern the establishment of substance abuse treatment programs (via authorizing permitted use through zoning and land use ordinances). Unless a group of concerned individuals advocates for quality treatment, however, it is unlikely that treatment services will be available to individuals most in need of those services, whether privately desired or court-referred. In another community, a municipal ordinance may make the use of the same state-prohibited substance within city limits subject merely to a small fine. Alternatively, the local prosecutor in yet another community may decide not to prosecute offenders arrested for low-level possession, and police may cease to arrest offenders. The mezzo level is especially relevant for juvenile illicit drug offenders. No separate body of law focuses on penalties specific to juvenile illicit drug offenders; case outcomes are almost entirely at the discretion of prosecutors and vary considerably.[25] Two juveniles arrested for possession of one ounce of marijuana (who are the same age and have the same sociodemographic backgrounds and drug use histories) could have markedly different case outcomes depending on the particular jurisdiction of their arrest, ranging from being diverted to treatment and having their record expunged, to transfer to adult criminal court for a lengthy prison sentence.[17]

Micro Level: Individual and Collective Actions that Impact Mezzo and Macro Policymaking and Implementation

The individual actions and treatment/other needs of drug users form the basis for social concerns about drug use, and drive calls for policy changes at all levels. Individual actions and financial contributions also start and/or support collective advocacy via informal or formal organizations and coalitions (e.g., Community Anti-Drug Coalitions of America [CADCA]; National Organization for the Reform of Marijuana Laws [NORML]) addressing issues such as substance abuse treatment, diversion programming, or drug policy reform. Individual citizens in the United States also vote—for elected officials who support specific drug policies (prosecutors, judges, and legislators), as well as in direct democracy efforts to change policies. Direct democracy refers to individual citizens collectively, actively, and directly making law and policy via initiatives, referenda, or recalls, thereby complementing the process of representative democracy. Two forms of direct democracy especially relevant for drug policy are ballot initiatives and referenda.

Ballot initiatives involve citizens collecting signatures for petitions to place statutes or constitutional amendments on the ballot for public vote.[26] In contrast, a referendum is when citizens have the power to reject specific legislation enacted by their legislature.[26] Significant initiative and referendum (I&R) activity exists at state, county, and city/town levels. Twenty-four states in the United States allow initiatives (18 allow constitutional initiatives; 21 allow statutory initiatives), and public referenda are available in 23 states.[26] The I&R aspects of direct democracy allow micro-level efforts to directly affect drug policy at the state level, which may then affect the federal level. The I&R process in the United States has been used successfully in five main illicit drug policy related areas: medical marijuana, diversion to treatment, reform of civil asset forfeiture laws (the majority of such cases are drug related), marijuana decriminalization, and marijuana legalization.[27] In a democratic society that emphasizes and allows for individual and collective initiatives to change law and policy, and even change state constitutions through ballot initiatives, the micro level of policy development and action is a crucial part of understanding U.S. illicit drug policy.

The Continuum of U.S. Illicit Drug Policy

Illicit drug policies across and within macro, mezzo, and micro levels can move in similar directions. In some cases, however, policy moves in different—even oppositional—directions based on conceptual positions about various substances. These positions can be viewed as existing along a continuum from mercantilism at one extreme through legalization/regulation, decriminalization, to prohibition at the other extreme (see Figure 14.3). Public health/harm reduction and medicalization positions frequently overlap with a variety of legalization/regulation and decriminalization positions.

Mercantilism

Drug policy in the Thirteen Colonies and early years of U.S. history can be characterized as mercantilism: unregulated commercial sales and use. Many later prohibited substances initially were a significant part of U.S. agriculture, manufacturing, and trade. An extensive and well-organized patent medicine industry emerged. By the end of the 19th century, the Sears catalog sold opium, barbiturates, and cocaine (and

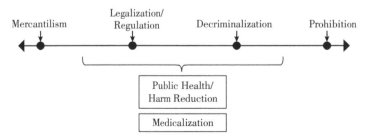

Figure 14.3 Conceptual positions in the drug policy debate.

syringes needed for injection), marketing these substances as useful for both children and adults.[28] Early American society successfully integrated powerful narcotics, stimulants, and sedatives into daily work and leisure life.[29]

Prohibition

At the other end of the drug policy spectrum is prohibition, and the first prohibition policies emerged in response to mercantilism. Prohibitionist policies prohibit the use, possession, sale, or manufacture of a specified substance for any reason (medical or recreational). Prohibition supporters argue that the individual and social harms associated with drug use and abuse (crime, violence, economic costs) require strong deterrence to prevent drug availability, use, and harmful consequences. Severe, mandated punishment for drug offenses is often part of prohibitionist policies. Prohibition is currently used at both federal and state levels for some substances (e.g., heroin), and at the federal level and only some states for other substances (e.g., marijuana). Critics note that prohibition policies lead to swelling state prison populations from those convicted of drug offences, primary marijuana possession.[30,31] The remaining policy positions have emerged in response to prohibition.

Decriminalization

Decriminalization supporters maintain that punishing illicit drug users is destructive to individuals and society, and results in prisons filled with those who have violated only drug possession laws. Although a policy of prohibition likely remains in place for selling or manufacturing specified drugs under decriminalization, individual use and/or possession of small amounts of specific substances is either overlooked or subject only to civil penalties such as fines.[32] Decriminalization may occur without formal policy change via local law enforcement practices (i.e., police not arresting offenders for individual use/possession), prosecutorial discretion (i.e., prosecutors deciding not to prosecute individual use/possession violations), or by local ordinance. For example, in the state of Michigan, possession of marijuana for recreational use is a criminal misdemeanor, with a penalty of up to one year in prison. In the city of Ann Arbor, however, local ordinances have decriminalized marijuana since 1972. Possession infractions result in only a civil penalty of $25 for a first offense and $50 for a second offense.[33]

Legalization/Regulation

This position argues for legalizing substances via regulations for use, possession, growing/manufacturing, and distribution; this policy approach currently governs tobacco and alcohol. Legalization/regulation generally includes restrictions by age, amounts that can be sold/possessed, and licensing for manufacturing/distribution.[34] Virtually all legalization proponents reject providing adolescents unrestricted drug access. Supporters argue legalization/regulation (a) enables regulations to ensure substance quality, potency, and legal access, thus promoting public health and safety; (b) removes violence associated with illegal distribution because of access to legal drug markets; and (c) generates state tax revenue. Much of the current legalization policy debate focuses on marijuana, with ballot initiatives being the policy mechanism employed. In 2012, ballot initiatives legalized recreational marijuana use in Colorado and Washington. In 2014, similar initiatives passed in Alaska, Oregon, and Washington DC.

Public Health/Harm Reduction

This approach views illicit drug use as a public health issue and attempts to reduce drug use initiation and continued use through prevention education, treatment instead of incarceration, and teaching methods designed to reduce the harms associated with drug use (e.g., needle cleaning or exchange programs for heroin injectors). The Institute of Medicine has called for a public health approach to U.S. drug policy.[35] It has been argued that public health agencies should assume major responsibility for drug abuse prevention as well as be policy advocates for diversion to treatment from the criminal justice system and engage in harm reduction programs.[36] Local public health agencies do frequently provide community- and school-based drug prevention education, are involved with providing treatment alternatives to incarceration, and advocate for diversion to treatment and harm reduction programs including needle exchange.[37]

Medicalization

Medicalization views drug addiction as a medical issue that cannot be addressed effectively through prohibition, decriminalization, or regulations. Medicalization argues that physicians should be allowed to use currently prohibited illicit drugs with legitimate medical utility, and that physicians—not politicians—should determine medical utility (e.g., medical use of marijuana, as discussed later). Medicalization further argues that addiction is a disease that should be treated by approaches such as prescription drugs that block the intoxicating effects of the illegal drug or through substitute drug maintenance. For example, opiate addiction is seen as a chronic medical condition that is best managed by using long-acting opiates such as methadone.[38] From this perspective, heroin addiction is seen as a "metabolic disease" requiring a synthetic long-acting opiate (heroin is relatively rapidly metabolized) in the form of methadone in order for those with this condition to function in a job or a relationship and not be involved in crime to support their heroin use. Methadone is available in many areas at clinics and is prescribed by physicians.

CASE STUDIES OF U.S. ILLICIT DRUG POLICY: MARIJUANA AND METHAMPHETAMINE

To illustrate the complex U.S. illicit drug policy process, we examine policies for two substances: marijuana (a "classic" non-synthetic drug with a long policy history) (see Box 14.1) and methamphetamine (a more recently appearing, fully synthetic drug) (see Box 14.2). Although the specific policies in place for both substances will have evolved further than described here by the time you read this chapter, the policy levers and processes available to affect change will have remained the same. It is particularly important to note the interplay among macro, mezzo, and micro policy levels and changes in conceptual positions.

Case Study Conclusions

These case studies illustrate the complexity and asynchronous development of U.S. illegal drug policies at macro, mezzo, and micro levels. Understanding of the public health consequences of using either marjiuana or methamphetamine has changed dramatically over time, and resulting policy responses are sometimes at odds across federal, state, and local levels. What was once illegal becomes legal, while what was once legal becomes illegal. The federal government may choose to loosen restrictions on a substance during one presidential administration, crack down on that same substance during several succeeding administrations, only to have the next administration turn a blind eye to enforcing state and local laws that directly conflict with federal laws, thereby essentially decriminalizing the substance (i.e., marijuana). One state—such as Oregon—may adopt a strict prohibitionist policy with strong access limits and penalties for one substance (methamphetamine) while simultaneously adopting a legalization policy toward another substance (marijuana). Counties and cities sometimes enact ordinances in defiance of federal and state policies, while at other times they support and cooperate with those same governmental agencies to combat a new drug threat to the community. Local prosecutors have a great deal of discretion in deciding which drug offenses to prosecute and what outcomes to seek. In one jurisdiction, the prosecutor may recommend diversion to treatment for a low-level marijuana offender, while in the neighboring jurisdiction, the prosecutor may aggressively enforce prohibitionist state laws and have a similar defendant incarcerated.[17] In addition, drug policy advocates such as NORML actively work to create support for local, state, and national policy changes by forming coalitions and developing ballot initiatives for actions such as marijuana decriminalization or diversion to drug treatment for drug offenders.[52] Once a ballot reaches state voters, individual citizens may vote in favor or against a particular initiative, or may vote a policymaker out of office because they do not approve of the policy approach used. Given the variance at macro, mezzo, and micro levels, it is little wonder that illegal drug policies are confusing and often contradictory.

Box 14.1 Case Study: Marijuana (*Cannabis sativa* L.)

This section describes the overall flow of U.S. marijuana policy as of the date of this writing and identifies the main macro, mezzo, and micro policy levers used: federal and state legislature-initiated bills, regulations, court decisions, municipal ordinances, and voter-initiated ballot initiatives and constitutional amendments.

Mercantilism and Early Regulation. Cannabis—known commonly as hemp—played a key role in the early American economy. Stem fibers were essential for rope, canvas, and other goods, and the plant had long been recognized for its medicinal qualities (hemp was listed as a recognized medication in the 1851 U.S. Pharmacopeia).[39] Major social reform movements of the early 20th century included an attack on the pharmaceutical industry for widespread marketing of dangerous, addictive drugs.[40] Resulting regulatory actions included the federal Pure Food and Drugs Act of 1906, which required labeling of all medicines, including cannabis. Occurring simultaneously with major social reform efforts (but unrelated to them) was growing societal fear of immigrants and minority groups. African Americans, Mexicans, and Chinese were portrayed as marijuana- and opium-using offenders who were corrupting youth and attacking young women.[41] Fears of addiction and violence, along with anti-immigrant sentiment, moved the public to demand policies addressing drug use, including marijuana use.

Early Prohibition: State Legislatures, Federal Policy, and Public Standards. States first legislated prohibitionist marijuana policy beginning with Massachusetts in 1911. In 1914, the federal Harrison Narcotics Tax Act was signed targeting opium and coca; as legal access to narcotics decreased, concerns rose over recreational marijuana use.[42] The National Conference of Commissioners on Uniform State Laws added marijuana to opium and coca under the 1934 Uniform Narcotic Drug Act. Four years later—by 1937—the Act had been adopted by 35 states (although every state had enacted some form of prohibitionist marijuana legislation by then).[42] The federal government joined the marijuana prohibition movement through the Marihuana Tax Act of 1937, wherein a tax was levied on anyone commercially dealing, prescribing, or possessing marijuana. Although the tax itself was minimal (approximately $1), punitive penalties (five years imprisonment and/or $2,000 fine) and complex reporting/inspection requirements effectively prohibited medical and recreational marijuana use.[43] In 1942, marijuana was removed from the U.S. Pharmacopeia due to concerns regarding its addiction potential and beliefs that it caused "psychoses, mental deterioration, and violent behavior."[44] In the 1950s, two additional federal laws established mandatory minimum sentences for marijuana offenses: The Boggs Act of 1951 and the even stricter Narcotic Control Act of 1956, which moved a first offense marijuana possession charge to a felony carrying a minimum 5- to 10-year prison sentence.[45,46] The Federal Bureau of Narcotics urged states to increase their penalty structures to be in line with the new federal laws. By 1956, 28 states had strengthened their existing laws to meet or exceed federal mandatory guidelines.[46]

1960s and 1970s: Cultural Revolution, Prohibition, Decriminalization, and Medicalization. Prohibitionist drug policy was generally accepted until the cultural revolution of the 1960s questioned many established social norms, including drug use. Public concerns about increasing drug use led to calls for new federal legislation preventing the use of dangerous substances. In 1971, President Nixon stated, "Public enemy number one in the United States is drug abuse. In order to fight and defeat this enemy, it is necessary to wage a new, all-out offensive."[47] Under the 1970 Controlled Substances Act (CSA) (21 U.S.C. 811 et seq.), all components and derivatives of *Cannabis sativa* L. became federal Schedule I substances identified as having high abuse potential and no accepted medical use. The CSA made it illegal to manufacture, distribute, dispense, or possess marijuana. CSA-specified penalties largely eliminated prior mandatory minimum sentences set in the 1950s; new penalties included up to five years imprisonment and/or $15,000 fine for a first manufacturing/distribution/dispensing offense, and up to one year imprisonment and/or $5,000 fine for simple possession.

There was debate as to how to schedule marijuana: should it be listed as a Schedule I substance (with no recognized medical utility) or as a Schedule II substance (with potential medical use)? Under the CSA, the National Commission on Marihuana and Drug Abuse (NCMDA) was ordered to review the issue; it was recommended that marijuana be temporarily classified as a Schedule I drug pending the NCMDA report. In 1972, the NCMDA concluded marijuana use should be discouraged, but advocated for penalty reductions and studies on marijuana's medical efficacy.[48] The year also saw a petition submitted to what was to become the Drug Enforcement Agency (DEA) to reschedule marijuana as a Schedule II substance, thereby allowing physician prescription. In 1976, Robert Randall won a landmark DC Superior Court case using a medical necessity defense for use of marijuana to deal with glaucoma. It appeared the United States might move away from strict prohibition of marijuana use. Several states took note of the NCMDA recommendations and the Randall case. Eleven state legislatures in some way decriminalized marijuana possession during the 1970s,[20] and 31 states and the District of Columbia passed some sort of medical marijuana legislation by 1982.[49]

Marijuana use rates by the end of the 1970s were high: 50% of high school seniors in 1978 and 1979 reported using marijuana in the past 12 months.[14]

1980s: Renewed Prohibition. President Ronald Reagan's inauguration in 1981 brought unprecedented expansion of the federal war on drugs begun under President Nixon. Many states increased drug-related offense penalties. By the mid-1980s, most state-level medical marijuana laws had been allowed to expire or were repealed, largely due to continued federal rejection of the appeal to reschedule marijuana and to the 1985 approval of the brand-name drug Marinol, which contained the active ingredient delta-9-tetrahydrocannabinol (THC), found in marijuana. The U.S. Congress passed the Anti-Drug Abuse Acts of 1986 and 1988, bringing back mandatory minimum sentences for marijuana trafficking and establishing federal civil penalties for personal marijuana use. Dramatic increases in arrest and incarceration rates for illicit drug offenses occurred at state and federal levels.

Marijuana use rates dropped steadily during the 1980s; by 1989, 30% of high school seniors reported using marijuana in the past 12 months.[14]

1990s: Diversion, Medicalization, and Continued Prohibition. The 1990s brought nonlegislated marijuana policy approaches. Scientists discovered cannabinoid receptors in the brain in

1990,[50] and a state court upheld the application of a medical necessity defense for personal marijuana use in 1991 (Jenks v. State 582 SO.2D 676). Micro-level voter-driven ballot initiatives began to take center stage as ways to change the existing marijuana policy landscape. The first "modern" medical marijuana initiative appeared as Proposition P on the City of San Francisco's 1991 ballot (and passed with 80% of the vote). In 1996, California became the first state to legalize medical marijuana through ballot Proposition 215. Using ballot initiatives, four other states successfully legalized medical marijuana by 1999 (Alaska, Oregon, Washington, Maine); voters in the District of Columbia also voted in a medical marijuana ballot initiative, but implementation was blocked by the U.S. Congress. The enacted policies varied significantly as to illnesses and symptoms covered and source of supply (a problematic issue in an environment where possessing or prescribing marijuana was illegal under federal law). In 1997, the Office of National Drug Control Policy asked the Institute of Medicine to conduct a review of scientific evidence related to medical marijuana use. The final report was released in 1999, and called for continued research into the effects of both synthetic and plant-derived cannabinoids.[44]

The other dramatic policy movement of the 1990s focused on diversion to treatment. Significant increases in drug-related arrests and incarcerations had strained state budgets and resulted in overcrowded prisons and sentencing disparities. Further, simply incarcerating offenders did nothing to address dependence/addiction or drug-related crime. In the late 1980s and 1990s, diversion to treatment for nonviolent drug offenders was made possible in seven states through both macro-level state legislation and micro-level ballot initiatives.[51] In 1996, Arizona voters passed the first successful state diversion-to-treatment ballot measure. California passed the second successful state ballot initiative in 2000 (Proposition 36). Large-scale studies indicated that even coerced treatment proved beneficial, resulting in lower re-arrest and re-incarceration rates, and significant cost savings over incarceration.[52,53] Although diversion policies were not specific to marijuana, they significantly impacted case processing for nonviolent marijuana offenders.

Past 12-month high school senior marijuana use prevalence continued to decrease in the early 1990s, reaching a low of 22% in 1992. Rates then rose steadily, plateauing between 1997 and 1999 at 38%–39%.[14]

2000s: Location, Location, Location. By 2000, the federal government remained steadfastly prohibitionist regarding marijuana. Meanwhile, states were involved in a tremendous natural marijuana policy experiment. State-level marijuana policy was completely dependent on geographic location as to drug scheduling, severity of use and sales penalties, use of diversion to treatment as an alternative to incarceration, and medical marijuana use. Although most state legislatures followed the federal CSA marijuana scheduling framework, a significant number diverged from federal precedent in developing state-specific schedules; seven states avoided scheduling marijuana altogether.[20] For a standard retail amount of marijuana, maximum imprisonment times ranged from one day to five years for possession, and from six months to life for sales; maximum fines ranged from $100 to $150,000 for possession and from $100 to $500,000 for sales.[20] Diversion-to-treatment legislation continued to expand; by mid-2004, 14 states had passed ballot initiatives or enacted diversion laws.[51]

Medical marijuana moved beyond ballot initiatives. In 2000, Hawaii's state legislature legalized medical marijuana; Colorado and Nevada legalized medical marijuana via constitutional amendments. The tension between federal prohibition and state medicalization was considerable. In 2001, the U.S. Supreme Court ruled there was no medical exception to the federal CSA, thus clarifying the illegality of selling or dispensing marijuana for medical purposes even when state law allowed (USA v. Oakland Cannabis Buyers' Cooperative and Jeffrey Jones, 2001). Federal agents conducted raids on medical marijuana dispensaries.[54] Likewise, the U.S. Supreme Court ruled in 2005 that Congress had authority to prohibit an individual's medical marijuana use despite existing state medical marijuana laws (Gonzalez v. Raich 545 U.S. 1, 2005). Supreme Court support for federal prohibition notwithstanding, the U.S. Attorney General announced that DEA raids on medical marijuana dispensaries would end,[55] and the Department of Justice (DOJ) announced that it would no longer prioritize prosecution of state-authorized medical marijuana patients.[56] Thirteen states legalized medical marijuana use by 2009.

Past 12-month high school senior marijuana use prevalence dropped somewhat over the decade, ending at 33% in 2009.[14]

2010 to 2014: Re-emergence of Decriminalization and Emerging Legalization/Regulation. As noted earlier, 11 state legislatures in some way decriminalized marijuana possession during the 1970s.[20] In 2008, Massachusetts became the first state in decades to enact policy defining the possession of a small amount of marijuana for nonmedical personal use as a civil—not criminal—offense. From 2010 through December 2014, five additional states enacted similar laws. Penalties for infractions in these states range from a $25 fine (and parental notification for minors) to a $200 fine for adults (and diversion to treatment for minors).[57]

The medical marijuana movement has expanded to 23 states, and—for the first time in more than 30 years—the U.S. Congress enacted policy that supports state decision-making power in regards to marijuana. On December 17, 2014, President Obama signed a fiscal appropriations bill including a provision blocking the DOJ from spending money to enforce federal bans on growing or selling marijuana in states that have legalized medical use.[58]

In 2012, a voter-approved Washington state ballot initiative legalized adult personal use and possession of cannabis, and in Colorado a voter-approved constitutional amendment legalized adult personal use and possession of cannabis, as well as required state lawmakers to enact regulations for licensing marijuana commercial production and sales. In 2013, the Respect State Marijuana Laws Act of 2013 (H.R. 1523) was introduced in the U.S. House. The Act would amend the CSA so that individuals acting in compliance with their state marijuana laws would not be subject to CSA penalties. The Act was referred to committee; no further action was taken. In the 2014 November elections, however, voters approved marijuana legalization ballot measures in Alaska and Oregon for adult personal use and commercial production/sales, and in Washington, DC for adult personal use and cultivation (commercial production/sales was not addressed). New policy issues related to regulating legal marijuana use now arise for these states: taxation, advertising, licensing, distribution, regulation of purity and potency, etc.

	Supporters	**Opponents**
Individuals:	• Former US Attorney • Former Oregon Supreme Court Justice • Travel entrepreneur	• Judges (2) • State Representatives (2) • State Senator • Former US Attorney for Oregon • District Attorneys (3) • County Sheriffs (4)
Organizations: 	• Drug Policy Action of Oregon • New Approach Oregon • Cascade Policy Institute • American Federation of State County and Municipal Employees Local 88 and 328 • United Food & Commercial Workers Local 555 • Northwest Oregon Labor Council • Moms for Yes on 91	• Oregon Pediatric Society • American Academy of Pediatrics • American Academy of Child & Adolescent Psychiatry • American Medical Association • American Society of Addiction Medicine • Oregon Republican Party • Restore America • Parents Opposed to Pot • Oregon State District Attorney's Association • Oregon State Sheriff's Association • Oregon Narcotics Enforcement Association • Oregon Catholic Conference
$ Total campaign cash:	$9,246,174	$179,673
Final vote: Passed	**847,865 (56.11%)**	**663,346 (43.89%)**

Figure 14.4 Oregon Legalized Marijuana Initiative, Ballot Measure 91 (2014).[59]

In all of these cases, it is important to remember how complex successful passage of the initiative was (for example, see Figure 14.4). Many individual and organizational policy-change advocates worked for years, through numerous failed attempts, to get legislators to change laws or—failing that—to get initiatives on the ballot. Advocates included not only groups one would expect, such as NORML and the Drug Policy Alliance,[60] but also less-expected actors including parental groups and, in some cases, even law enforcement.[61] The mainstream media often played a crucial role in giving voice to advocacy groups; and the use of social media allowed widespread distribution of advocacy positions.

Past 12-month high school senior marijuana use prevalence has risen somewhat since the start of the decade; by 2013, the rate was 36%.[14]

Research is conclusive that marijuana impairs short-term memory and judgment, distorts perception, and has addictive properties; effects on long-term cognitive development among adolescent users are especially concerning.[62] What will the results of recent policy change be on use rates and health/social outcomes? Research indicates that early state decriminalization policies in the 1970s were not associated with changes in adolescent marijuana use or attitudes,[63] and that more recent medicalization policies are not associated with increased violent/property crime.[64] Yet, other research indicates that higher severity of local marijuana offense processing is associated with less marijuana use, higher disapproval rates, and increased perceptions of great risk of using marijuana among adolescents.[65] Research examining effects of state legalization/regulation on use rates, treatment demand, health care utilization, crime rates, and other public health concerns is not available. The marijuana policy experiment continues at all levels from micro-level voter initiatives to macro-level executive orders.

Box 14.2 Case Study: Methamphetamine (N-methyl-alpha-methylphenethylamine)

Methamphetamine—a highly addictive synthetic stimulant—has a relatively recent history of use and abuse. In low doses, it can improve mood and increase energy, concentration, and alertness. At higher doses, it can produce psychosis, damage muscle tissue, and produce permanent brain damage.[66] We briefly describe policy efforts to control conventional large-scale methamphetamine production/distribution; however, we primarily focus on policy efforts to control crystal methamphetamine produced in small toxic laboratories because this allows us to illustrate simultaneous macro, mezzo, and micro policy actions.

Legalization/Regulation to Prohibition. Although methamphetamine was first synthesized in 1919, it was not used extensively until it was given to German, Japanese, and Allied armed forces in the 1930s to promote extended wakefulness and aggressive performance.[67] The American public discovered the drug in the 1950s and 1960s when the brand-name medication Obetrol was marketed for obesity treatment.[67] Methamphetamine's popularity increased rapidly; "pep pills" and "bennies" were used by truckers, homemakers, college students, and athletes to stay awake or enhance energy. Methamphetamine's addictive properties soon became widely recognized, and strict regulations on production and distribution accompanied the drug's listing as a Schedule II substance under the Controlled Substances Act of 1970 and in almost all state schedules. Use decreased, although methamphetamine continued to be used illegally by subcultures such as outlaw biker gangs and men who have sex with men at "raves" or extended dance parties.

1980s and 1990s: Emerging Use and Large-scale Supply Reduction Policy. In the 1980s, Mexican drug cartels began producing methamphetamine in large batches and bringing it to the United States. Illegal methamphetamine "super labs" began large-scale production in California, with gangs expanding distribution throughout the West and Southwest. The federal government attempted to reduce large-scale methamphetamine production via supply reduction: regulating the bulk sales of precursor chemicals needed to synthesize methamphetamine and setting strong manufacturing/trafficking penalties. These federal efforts started with the Chemical Diversion and Trafficking Act of 1988, and continued with the Crime Control Act of 1991, the Domestic Chemical Diversion and Control Act of 1993, the Comprehensive Methamphetamine Control Act of 1996, the Methamphetamine Trafficking Penalty Enhancement Act of 1998, and the Methamphetamine Anti-Proliferation Act of 2000.[68]

Creative drug users and small-time dealers soon discovered ways to cook small batches of crystal methamphetamine in small toxic labs (STLs) located in homes and remote locations. The process required common household chemicals, anhydrous ammonia (farm fertilizer), and—the key ingredient—ephedrine or pseudoephedrine, found in cold medicines such as Sudafed and Tylenol Cold.[69] STL crystal methamphetamine production resulted in direct exposure to toxic chemical fumes and burns, and other health-related consequences including dental disease and addiction.[70,71] STLs frequently exploded, causing fires, chemical burns, property damage, environmental pollution, and health and safety consequences for first responders (police, firefighters) and cleanup crews.[72] Resulting increases in methamphetamine use led to increased, sustained, and violent criminal behavior,[73] increased risk of child abuse and neglect,[74] homelessness, and removal of children from homes by the child welfare system.[75] STLs rapidly became a serious public health threat.

2000–2007: Small Toxic Lab Precursor Policies and Community Coalitions. Small toxic labs (STLs) spread quickly through the Northwest and Midwest.[76] The Drug Enforcement Agency (DEA) documented 2,122 methamphetamine STL seizures in 1999 (labs, dumpsites, and chemicals/glass/equipment); seizure rates rapidly escalated to 23,829 in 2004.[77,78] The health and safety costs associated with STLs in 2005 were almost 23.5 million dollars.[79] By 2006, STLs were estimated to provide approximately 20% of the U.S. methamphetamine supply.[19]

Policymakers in states most affected by STLs responded by passing methamphetamine precursor laws targeting small-scale precursor access. Although these laws addressed a wide range of precursor chemicals, they especially focused on ephedrine and pseudoephedrine, and addressed some or all of the following: (1) state scheduling, (2) retail sales quantity limits, (3) personal possession limits, and (4) retail sales environment restrictions (such as requiring buyer identification).[68] Other state policy provisions included regulatory agency specification for monitoring compliance and tracking precursor purchases using centralized electronic databases. Existing state policies differed widely. Oregon passed the most restrictive law, classifying pseudoephedrine as a Schedule III substance and requiring physician prescription to obtain products containing pseudoephedrine. Most state policy action occurred from 2001 onwards; by late 2005, 35 states had scheduled ephedrine and/or pseudoephedrine, or set retail sales quantity or environment restrictions.[68]

The federal government began regulating methamphetamine STL precursors by passing the 2005 Combat Methamphetamine Epidemic Act (CMEA). Among other things, the CMEA regulated retail ephedrine and pseudoephedrine sales by setting daily sales limits and 30-day purchase limits, product placement out of direct customer access, sales logbooks, customer ID verification, employee training, and self-certification of regulated sellers. The CMEA provided a national approach to controlling access to precursor chemicals but did not preempt more stringent state laws.[68]

A variety of mezzo-level demand reduction strategies were developed. Many communities established collaborative partnerships among pharmacists, child welfare agencies, media organizations, law enforcement agencies, and other community groups, often creating local, regional, or state methamphetamine task forces or coalitions. For example, the Montana Meth Project,[80] whose programs are implemented in eight other states, attempts to reduce methamphetamine use through often graphic public service messaging, public policy advocacy, and community outreach. With the understanding that it was impossible to incarcerate their way out of the problem, law enforcement personnel and legislators agreed that treatment and education were the primary avenues of reducing methamphetamine use and its consequences.[81] They worked to educate the media, local business, schools, and other groups about the dangers of methamphetamine.[82] Many officials advocated for diverting arrested methamphetamine addicts to treatment instead of incarceration, an approach that has shown strong evidence of success in helping drug-addicted individuals receive needed treatment without serving long prison sentences.[83,84] Legislators and judges called for drug courts as a viable incarceration alternative for methamphetamine offenders in order to provide drug treatment and monitoring with lower costs, more support, strong sanctions, and clear treatment expectations.[85]

Significant decreases in methamphetamine STL seizures followed the enactment of these initial precursor policies.[8,86] Nationwide, STL seizure rates dropped approximately 71% between 2004 and 2007;[78] some states almost completely eliminated STL seizures, while other states reduced rates by less than one-fourth.[78]

2008–2013: State Policy, Corporate Response, and Municipal Ordinances. Small-time methamphetamine producers soon found ways around the precursor laws. To bypass pseudoephedrine purchasing limits and elude poor and/or inconsistent retail purchase monitoring, STL operators began "smurfing," or having multiple shoppers travel from store to store, sometimes even crossing state lines, purchasing the maximum allowable number of cold medicine packages.[87] A simpler process for making STL methamphetamine also evolved. Called "one-pot" or "shake and bake," it made production simpler and detection more difficult.[88]

Precursor laws had only limited, short-term impacts, leading to temporarily reduced methamphetamine use rates, hospital admissions, and arrests.[89] STL seizure rates quickly rebounded, more than doubling from 6,858 in 2007 to 15,196 in 2010.[78] As STL seizure rates rose again, state legislators responded in several ways. Some strengthened pseudoephedrine tracking mechanisms to better share real-time purchase information between pharmacies; others passed additional laws designed to further restrict pseudoephedrine access.

Numerous other states noticed Oregon's successful prescription-only law and, between 2010 and 2013, 85 bills in 24 other states attempted to pass laws requiring physician prescription for pseudoephedrine-containing cold medicines.[90] Massive lobbying efforts designed to anger voters over "the violation of their civil rights" to purchase legal products resulted. Pseudoephedrine products bring in an estimated $605 million to the pharmaceutical industry; some legislators who had relationships with large pharmaceutical corporations blocked bills from moving forward.[91,92] To date, the only state other than Oregon to pass a prescription-only law has been Mississippi, which observed a 66% STL seizure rate reduction the first year the law was in effect.[87]

Where macro state-level prescription-only laws have been unsuccessful, counties and cities have begun to pass mezzo-level local ordinances requiring prescriptions for purchasing pseudoephedrine-containing products. Since 2009, 63 Missouri cities or counties have passed laws or ordinances requiring prescriptions.[87,90] Although STL seizures across Missouri increased almost 7% between 2010 and 2011, seizures dropped by nearly 50% in southeastern Missouri where the majority of prescription-only ordinances were adopted.[87] In 2013, 18 cities in Tennessee voted for prescription-only ordinances. Illustrating the complexity of drug policies and the conflicts that can occur between state and local governments, Tennessee's Attorney General ruled that the ordinances violated state law.[93] Recently, however, "meth-resistant" pseudoephedrine products have been developed using technology that makes it more difficult to convert pseudoephedrine into methamphetamine. Nearly 30,000 pharmacies across the nation, including West Virginia and parts of Tennessee, have banned traditional single-ingredient pseudoephedrine products and carry only meth-resistant formulations.[94]

Despite extensive U.S. and Mexican interdiction efforts and tough Mexican laws banning pseudoephedrine importation,[95] seizures of powder and crystal methamphetamine at the U.S./Mexico border increased 200% between 2009 and 2013 as drug trafficking organizations found new ways to acquire precursor chemicals and discovered non-ephedrine-based production methods.[78] The DEA is also working to restrict manufacture and import of ephedrine and pseudoephedrine by countries such as China, India, and South Korea.[95] Law enforcement officials and U.S. drug enforcement authorities continue to search for policy levers that will reduce both methamphetamine supply and demand.

CONCLUSION

U.S. governmental structure allows illicit drug policymaking to be shared among federal, state, and local governments. In addition, it permits citizen-based policy initiatives. The conceptual positions guiding U.S. illicit drug policies have ranged from mercantilism to legalization/regulation to decriminalization to prohibition, along with public health/harm reduction and medicalization. Frequently, each of these conceptual positions can be found operating at the same time for different substances at various levels of government. States act as natural laboratories for federal drug policy. This has been the case as far back as the first prohibition policies of the early 20th century when existing state-level prohibition policies were adopted at the national level, and continues today with current experiments with marijuana legalization at the state level at the beginning of the 21st century. The case studies demonstrate how policy emerges at the macro national/state level, the mezzo municipal/systems/institutional level, and at the micro citizen and collective advocacy level. The case studies also illustrate how various substances can simultaneously move in opposite policy directions at all of these levels. U.S. illicit drug policy is complex, dynamic, and ever-changing. At its best, it strives to use both demand and supply reduction policies at macro, mezzo, and micro levels to lower the individual and public health harms resulting from substance use.

REFERENCES

1. National Institute on Drug Abuse. *Drugs, Brains and Behavior: The Science of Addiction.* NIH Pub. No. 14-5605. Bethesda, MD: National Institute on Drug Abuse. Published 2007. Updated July 2014.
2. Wood E, Kerr T, Spittal PM, et al. The potential public health community impacts of safer injecting facilities: Evidence from a cohort of injection drug users. *J Acquir Immune Defic Syndr.* 2003;32:2–8.
3. Lopez-Quintero C, Pérez de los Cobos J, Hasin DS, et al. Probability and predictors of transition from first use to dependence on nicotine, alcohol, cannabis, and cocaine: results of

the National Epidemiologic Survey on Alcohol and Related Conditions (NESARC). *Drug Alcohol Depend.* 2011;115(1–2):120–130.

4. Chen C-Y, Storr CL, Anthony JC. Early-onset drug use and risk for drug dependence problems. *Addict Behav.* 2009;34(3):319–322.

5. Ellickson PL, Martino SC, Collins RL. Marijuana use from adolescence to young adulthood: Multiple developmental trajectories and their associated outcomes. *Health Psychol.* 2004;23(3):299–307.

6. Lynskey M, Hall W. Age of initiation to heroin use: cohort trends and consequences of early initiation for subsequent adjustment. NDARC Technical Report No.61. Sydney, Australia: National Drug and Alcohol Research Centre, Sydney; 1998. https://ndarc.med. unsw.edu.au/sites/default/files/ndarc/resources/T.R%20061.pdf. Accessed February 5, 2015.

7. VanderWaal CJ, McBride DC, Terry YM, VanBuren H. *Breaking the Juvenile Drug Crime Cycle: A Guide for Practitioners and Policymakers.* NCJ 186156. Washington, DC: U.S. Department of Justice, Office of Justice Programs; 2001.

8. McBride DC, Terry-McElrath YM, Chriqui JF, O'Connor JC, VanderWaal CJ, Mattson KL. State methamphetamine precursor policies and changes in small toxic lab methamphetamine production. *J Drug Issues.* 2011;41(2):253–282.

9. National Drug Intelligence Center. *The Economic Impact of Illicit Drug Use on American Society.* Washington, DC: United States Department of Justice; 2011.

10. Central Intelligence Agency. *The World Factbook 2013–14.* Washington, DC: Central Intelligence Agency; 2013.

11. National Institute on Drug Abuse. *DrugFacts: Nationwide Trends.* Bethesda, MD: Author; 2014. http://www.drugabuse.gov/publications/drugfacts/nationwide-trends. Accessed February 5, 2015.

12. Johnston LD, Miech RA, O'Malley PM, Bachman JG, Schulenberg JE. Use of alcohol, cigarettes, and a number of illicit drugs declines among U.S. teens [news release]. Ann Arbor, MI: University of Michigan News Service; December 16, 2014. http://ns.umich.edu/new/ multimedia/videos/22574-use-of-alcohol-cigarettes-number-of-illicit-drugs-declines-among-u-s-teens. Accessed February 5, 2015.

13. Johnston LD, O'Malley PM, Bachman JG, Schulenberg JE, Miech RA. *Monitoring the Future. National Survey Results on Drug Use, 1975–2013: Volume 2, College Students and Adults Ages 19–55.* Ann Arbor: Institute for Social Research, The University of Michigan; 2014.

14. Johnston LD, O'Malley PM, Bachman JG, Schulenberg JE, Miech RA. *Monitoring the Future National Survey Results on Drug Use, 1975–2013: Volume I, Secondary School Students.* Ann Arbor: Institute for Social Research, The University of Michigan; 2014.

15. Onuf PS. *The Origins of the Federal Republic: Jurisdictional Controversies in the United States, 1775–1787.* Philadelphia: University of Pennsylvania Press; 2001.

16. Bardhan P. Decentralization of governance and development. *J Econ Perspect.* 2002;16(4): 185–205.

17. McBride DC, Terry-McElrath YM. Drug policy in the U.S.: a dynamic multi-level experimental environment. In: Brownstein H, Ed. *Wiley Handbook on Drugs and Society.* Hoboken, NJ: John Wiley & Sons, Inc; in press.

18. Federal judge weighs marijuana's classification. ABC News; January 12, 2015. http://abc-news.go.com/US/wireStory/federal-judge-weighs-marijuanas-classification-28169478. Accessed January 23, 2015.

19. O'Connor JC, Chriqui JF, McBride DC. Developing lasting legal solutions to the dual epidemics of methamphetamine production and use. *N D Law Rev.* 2006;82:1165–1194.

20. ImpacTeen Illicit Drug Team. *Illicit Drug Policies: Selected Laws from the 50 States.* Berrien Springs, MI: Andrews University; 2002. http://www.impacteen.org/generalarea_PDFs/IDTchartbook032103.pdf

21. Gray H. Commentary: Federal preemption of state laws regarding medical marijuana. Partnership for Drug-Free Kids. January 21, 2015. http://www.drugfree.org/join-together/commentary-federal-preemption-state-laws-regarding-medical-marijuana/?utm_source=Stay+Informed+-+latest+tips%2C+resources+and+news&utm_campaign=58b3e37e64-JTWN_FedJdgRuleMarijuanaSchedule_I_Drug1_22_2015&utm_medium=email&utm_term=0_34168a2307-58b3e37e64-223220225. Accessed January 23, 2015.

22. Rosenmerkel S, Durose M, Farole D Jr. *Felony Sentences in State Courts, 2006—Statistical Tables.* NCJ 226846. Washington, DC: U.S. Department of Justice, Office of Justice Programs, Bureau of Justice Statistics; 2009.

23. Bureau of Justice Statistics. Drugs and crime facts. http://www.bjs.gov/content/dcf/enforce.cfm. Accessed February 4, 2015.

24. Glaeser EL, Kessler DP, Piehl AM. What do prosecutors maximize? An analysis of drug offenders and concurrent jurisdiction. National Bureau of Economic Research. Working Paper W6602. June 1998. http://www.nber.org/papers/w6602. Accessed February 5, 2015.

25. Terry-McElrath YM, McBride DC, Ruel E, Harwood EM, VanderWaal CJ, Chaloupka FJ. Which substances and what community? Differences in juvenile disposition severity. *Crime Delinq.* 2005;51:548–572.

26. Initiative and Referendum Institute. *State-by-State List of Initiative and Referendum Provisions.* Los Angeles: University of Southern California School of Law, Initiative and Referendum Institute; 2014.

27. Ehlers S. Drug policy reform initiatives and referenda. In: Waters MD, Ed. *Initiative and Referendum Almanac.* Durham, NC: Carolina Academic Press; 2003:484–487.

28. Sears, Roebuck and Co. *Consumers Guide* (Catalogue No. 104). Chicago, IL: Sears, Roebuck and Co. New York: Chelsea House Publishers; Published 1897. Reprinted 1968.

29. Musto DF. *The American Disease.* New York: Oxford University Press; 1999.

30. Federal Bureau of Investigation. Crime in the United States 2013. Uniform Crime Reports. http://www.fbi.gov/about-us/cjis/ucr/crime-in-the-u.s/2013/crime-in-the-u.s.-2013. Accessed February 5, 2015.

31. People sentenced for drug offenses in the US correctional system. http://www.drugwarfacts.org/cms/Prisons_and_Drugs#Drugs. Accessed February 5, 2015.

32. Inciardi JA (Ed.). *The Drug Legalization Debate.* 2nd ed. Thousand Oaks, CA: Sage Publications, Inc; 2002.

33. Michigan laws and penalties. NORML. http://norml.org/laws/item/michigan-penalties-2. Accessed May 2, 2015.

34. MacCoun RJ, Reuter P. *Drug War Heresies: Learning from Other Vices, Times, and Places.* New York: University of Cambridge; 2001.

35. Institute of Medicine. *The Future of Public Health.* Washington, DC: The National Academies Press; 1998.

36. Des Jarlais D. Prospects for a public health perspective on psychoactive drug use. *Am J Public Health.* 2000;90(3):335–337.

37. McBride DC, Terry-McElrath YM, VanderWaal CJ, Chriqui JF, Myllyluoma, J. United States public health agency involvement in illicit drug policy, planning, and prevention, 1999–2003. *Am J Public Health*. 2008;98(2):270–277.

38. Centers for Disease Control and Prevention. Methadone maintenance treatment. IDU HIV Prevention. February 2002. http://www.cdc.gov/idu/facts/MethadoneFin.pdf. Accessed May 4, 2015.

39. National Medical Convention. *The Pharmacopeia of the United States of America*. Philadelphia, PA: Lippincott, Grambo, & Co; 1851.

40. Adams SH. The great American fraud. *Collier's*. 1905;36(2):14–15, 29. http://college.cengage.com/history/ayers_primary_sources/americanfraud_adams_1905.htm. Accessed February 4, 2015.

41. Inciardi JA. *The War on Drugs IV: The Continuing Saga of the Mysteries and Miseries of Intoxication, Addiction, Crime and Public Policy*. 4th ed. Upper Saddle River, NJ: Prentice Hall; 2007.

42. Bonnie RJ, Whitebread CH. Forbidden fruit and the tree of knowledge: an inquiry into the legal history of American marijuana prohibition. *Va Law Rev*. 1970;56:971–1203.

43. Solomon D. The Marihuana Tax Act of 1937: Introduction. Schaffer Library of Drug Policy. http://www.druglibrary.org/schaffer/hemp/taxact/mjtaxact.htm. Accessed February 5, 2015.

44. Joy JE, Watson SJ, Benson JA Jr. (Eds.). *Marijuana and Medicine: Assessing the Science Base*. Washington, DC: The National Academies Press; 1999.

45. Cameron JM, Dillinger RJ. Narcotic Control Act. In: Kleiman MAR, Hawdon JE, Eds. *Encyclopedia of Drug Policy*. Thousand Oaks, CA: SAGE Publications, Inc; 2011:543–545.

46. Rothwell VL. Boggs Act. In: Kleiman MAR, Hawdon JE, Eds. *Encyclopedia of Drug Policy*. Vol 2. Thousand Oaks, CA: SAGE Publications, Inc; 2011:96–98.

47. Nixon R. Remarks about an intensified program for drug abuse prevention and control. June 17, 1971; http://www.presidency.ucsb.edu/ws/?pid=3047. Accessed February 5, 2015.

48. National Commission on Marihuana and Drug Abuse. *Marihuana: A Signal of Misunderstanding*. Washington, DC: Government Printing Press; 1972.

49. Pacula RL, Chriqui JF, Reichmann DA, Terry-McElrath YM. State medical marijuana laws: Understanding the laws and their limitations. *J Public Health Policy*. 2002;23(4):413–439.

50. Herkenham M, Lynn AB, Little MD, et al. Cannabinoid receptor localization in brain. *Proc Natl Acad Sci USA*. 1990;87:1932–1936.

51. VanderWaal CJ, Chriqui JF, Bishop RM, McBride DC, Longshore DY. State drug policy reform movement: the use of ballot initiatives and legislation to promote diversion to drug treatment. *J Drug Issues*. 2006;36(3):619–648.

52. General Accounting Office. *Drug Abuse: Research Shows Treatment is Effective, But Benefits May Be Overstated*. GAO/HEHS_98_7. Washington, DC: United States General Accounting Office; 1998.

53. Rydell CP, Caulkins JP, Everingham SS. Enforcement or treatment? Modeling the relative efficacy of alternatives for controlling cocaine. *Oper Res*. 1996;44(5):687–695.

54. Authorities raid 11 medical pot suppliers. *Los Angeles Times*. December 13, 2005. http://articles.latimes.com/2005/dec/13/local/me-sbriefs13.3. Accessed February 5, 2015.

55. Johnson MA. DEA to halt medical marijuana raids. NBCNEWS.com. February 27, 2009; http://www.nbcnews.com/id/29433708/ns/health-health_care/t/dea-halt-medical-marijuana-raids/#.VNOENWjF98E. Accessed February 5, 2015.

56. U.S. Department of Justice. Memorandum for selected United States attorneys on investigations and prosecutions in states authorizing the medical use of marijuana. October 19, 2009; http://www.justice.gov/opa/blog/memorandum-selected-united-state-attorneys-investigations-and-prosecutions-states. Accessed January 15, 2015.

57. Marijuana Policy Project. State laws with alternatives to incarceration for marijuana possession. http://www.mpp.org/assets/pdfs/library/State-Decrim-Chart.pdf. Accessed February 5, 2015.

58. Berman R. Why Congress gave in to medical marijuana. *The Atlantic* December 17, 2014; http://www.theatlantic.com/politics/archive/2014/12/a-congressional-surrender-in-the-medical-marijuana-fight/383856/. Accessed February 4, 2015.

59. Oregon Legalized Marijuana Initiative, Measure 91 (2014). http://ballotpedia.org/Oregon_Legalized_Marijuana_Initiative,_Measure_91_%282014%29. Accessed May 4, 2015.

60. Ten most influential legalization groups. https://www.dinafem.org/en/blog/cannabis-marijuana-legalization-groups/. Accessed May 4, 2015.

61. Colorado Marijuana Legalization Initiative, Amendment 64 (2012). http://ballotpedia.org/Colorado_Marijuana_Legalization_Initiative,_Amendment_64_%282012%29#Supporters. Accessed May 4, 2015.

62. National Institute on Drug Abuse. *Research Report Series: Marijuana.* NIH Pub. No. 12-3859. Bethesda, MD: National Institute on Drug Abuse. Published 2012. Updated December 2014.

63. Johnston LD, O'Malley PM, Bachman JG. Marijuana decriminalization: the impact on youth, 1975–1980. Monitoring the Future Occasional Paper 13. Ann Arbor, MI: Institute for Social Research, The University of Michigan; 1981. http://www.monitoringthefuture.org/pubs/occpapers/occ13.pdf. Accessed February 5, 2015.

64. Morris RG, TenEyck M, Kovandzic TV. The effect of medical marijuana laws on crime: evidence from state panel data, 1990–2006. *PLoS One.* 2014;9(3):e92816. doi: 10.137/journal.pone.0092816.

65. Terry-McElrath YM, McBride DC, Chriqui JF, et al. Evidence for connections between prosecutor-reported marijuana case dispositions and community youth marijuana-related attitudes and behaviors. *Crime Delinq.* 2009;55(4):600–626.

66. National Institute on Drug Abuse. *Research Report Series: Methamphetamine.* NIH Pub No. 13-4210. Bethesda, MD: National Institute on Drug Abuse. Published 1998. Updated September 2013.

67. Rasmussen N. *On Speed: The Many Lives of Amphetamine.* 1st ed. New York: New York University Press; 2008.

68. O'Connor J, Chriqui J, McBride D, et al. *From Policy to Practice: State Methamphetamine Precursor Control Policies.* NCJ 228133. Washington, DC: U.S. Department of Justice, Office of Justice Programs, National Institute of Justice; 2007.

69. Hunt DE. Methamphetamine abuse: challenges for law enforcement and communities. *Nat Inst Justice J.* 2006;254:24–27.

70. Shetty V, Mooney LJ, Zigler CM, Belin TR, Murphy D, Rawson R. The relationship between methamphetamine use and increased dental disease. *J Am Dent Assoc.* 2010;14:307–318.

71. Barr AM, Panenka WJ, MacEwan GW, et al. The need for speed: an update on methamphetamine addiction. *J Psychiatry Neurosci.* 2006;31(5):301–313.
72. McFadden D, Kub J, Fitzgerald F. Occupational health hazards to first responders from clandestine methamphetamine labs. *J Addict Nurs.* 2006;17:169–173.
73. Sommers I, Baskin D. Methamphetamine use and violence. *J Drug Issues.* 2006;Winter:77–96.
74. Dube SR, Felitti VJ, Dong M, Chapman DP, Giles WH, Anda RF. Childhood abuse, neglect, and household dysfunction and the risk of illicit drug use: the adverse childhood experiences study. *Pediatrics.* 2003;111:564–572.
75. Connell-Carrick K. Methamphetamine and the changing face of child welfare: practice principles for child welfare workers. *Child Welf.* 2007;86(3):125–143.
76. Lineberry TW, Bostwick JM. Methamphetamine abuse: a perfect storm of complications. *Mayo Clin Proc.* 2006;81:77–84.
77. Office of National Drug Control Policy. The national drug control strategy: 2001 annual report. https://www.ncjrs.gov/ondcppubs/publications/policy/ndcs01/chap2.html#5. Accessed February 6, 2015.
78. Methamphetamine lab incidents, 2004–2012. Drug Enforcement Administration. http://www.justice.gov/dea/resource-center/meth-lab-maps.shtml. Accessed January 9, 2015.
79. Dobkin C, Nicosia N. The war on drugs: methamphetamine, public health, and crime. *Am Econ Rev.* 2009;99(1):324–349.
80. Montana Meth Project. http://www.montanameth.org/. Accessed May 4, 2015.
81. Rawson RA, Anglin MD, Ling W. Will the methamphetamine problem go away? *J Addict Dis.* 2002;21(1):5–19.
82. VanderWaal CJ, Bishop RM, McBride DC, et al. *Controlling Methamphetamine Precursors: The View from the Trenches.* NCJ 223480. Washington, DC: U.S. Department of Justice, Office of Justice Programs, National Institute of Justice; 2008.
83. VanderWaal CJ, Taxman F, Gurka M. Reforming drug treatment services to offenders: cross-system collaboration, integrated policies, and a seamless continuum of care model. *J Soc Work Pract Addict.* 2008;8(1):127–153.
84. Gottfredson DC, Najaka SS, Kearley B. Effectiveness of drug treatment courts: evidence from a randomized trial. *Criminol Public Policy.* 2003;2(2):171–196.
85. Listwan SJ, Shaffer DK, Hartman JL. Combating methamphetamine use in the community: the efficacy of the drug court model. *Crime Delinq.* 2009;55(4):627–644.
86. VanderWaal CJ, Young RM, McBride DC, Chriqui JF, Terry-McElrath YM. Smurfing in small toxic meth labs: impact of state methamphetamine precursor policies. *J Policy Pract.* 2013;12(3):231–255.
87. Government Accountability Office. *State Approaches Taken to Control Access to Key Methamphetamine Ingredient Show Varied Impact on Domestic Drug Labs.* GAO-13-204. Washington, DC: United States Government Accountability Office; 2013.
88. Saulny S. With cars as meth labs, evidence litters the roads. *The New York Times.* April 14, 2010.
89. Cunningham JK, Liu L, Callaghan R. Impact of US and Canadian precursor regulation on methamphetamine purity in the United States. *Addiction.* 2009;104:441–453.
90. Pseudoephedrine: legal efforts to make it a prescription-only drug. Public Health Law Issue Brief. Centers for Disease Control and Prevention; Office for State, Tribal, Local and Territorial Support. 2013; http://www.cdc.gov/phlp/docs/pseudo-brief112013.pdf. Accessed February 4, 2015.

91. Engle J. Merchants of meth: How big pharma keeps the cooks in business. *Mother Jones*. July/August, 2013. http://www.motherjones.com/politics/2013/08/meth-pseudoephedrine-big-pharma-lobby. Accessed February 5, 2015.

92. Sisk C. Drug firms spend millions to lobby state. *The Tennessean*. March 3, 2014.

93. Tamburin A. Tennessee cities go it alone in the anti-meth crusade. *The Tennessean*. March 3, 2014.

94. Join Together. Pharmacies stock "meth-resistant" cold medications—and see drop in community meth labs. Partnership for Drug-Free Kids. http://www.drugfree.org/join-together/pharmacies-stock-meth-resistant-cold-medications-see-drop-community-meth-labs/ Accessed January 19, 2015.

95. National Drug Intelligence Center. *National Drug Threat Assessment 2010*. Product No. 2010-Q0317-001. Johnstown, PA: U.S. Department of Justice, National Drug Intelligence Center; 2010.

Part 3
Next Steps in Public Health through Policy

15

Public Policy Tracking and Surveillance
Assessing Policy Adoption and Content for Advocacy and Evaluation Purposes

Jamie F. Chriqui and Amy A. Eyler

LEARNING OBJECTIVES

1. Explain why on-the-books policies are assessed for use in public health advocacy and evaluation.
2. Describe what is meant by policy tracking and surveillance.
3. Identify policy tracking and surveillance system resources.
4. Provide examples of tools developed for evaluating on-the-books policies in public health policy evaluation and impact studies.
5. Describe how to assess the incorporation of evidence-based elements in on-the-books policies.

WHY ASSESS POLICY ADOPTION AND CONTENT FOR USE IN PUBLIC HEALTH?

Most of the leading public health achievements of the 20th and 21st centuries can be attributed to public policy solutions or "interventions."[1,2] As a result, in recent years, governmental agencies and quasigovernmental bodies such as the Institute of Medicine have recommended policy and environmental change approaches for addressing large-scale public health problems given their population-wide impact.[3-10] Throughout this book, the authors have identified a wide range of public policy solutions that have been utilized for prevention and public health purposes, including but not limited to, tobacco control, illicit drug control and use, obesity prevention and food access, alcohol use and misuse, physical activity and inactivity, and motor vehicle accidents. When a problem is deemed worthy of governmental attention, advocates and policymakers often search for "evidence" that a given policy solution will work, what it will cost, and how it would be implemented. In such instances, they typically rely on lessons learned from other states or localities or from scientific evidence documenting the prevalence and impact of a given policy solution on the problem at hand. This chapter provides an introduction to key tools that are often used for (1) identifying what policies exist (policy tracking) and how they have changed over time (policy surveillance); (2) determining whether policy solutions incorporate the best available scientific evidence; and (3) evaluating policy impact.

POLICY TRACKING AND POLICY SURVEILLANCE SYSTEMS: KEY TOOLS IN THE PUBLIC HEALTH ARSENAL

The public health community often has a need to track and evaluate public policy actions across jurisdictions (e.g., across states, across counties, across localities) for advocacy, reporting, and research purposes. Advocates working to encourage new policy action or policy change within and across jurisdictions utilize and rely on *policy tracking systems* (e.g., the National Conference of State Legislatures, LexisNexis StateNet, the Centers for Disease Control and Prevention [CDC] Chronic Disease Policy Tracking Database, and the Rudd Center on Obesity and Food Policy Legislative Tracking Database) to monitor and report on policy actions. Many topical policy tracking systems (e.g., the CDC Chronic Disease Policy Tracking Database and the Rudd Center database) incorporate policy tracking data catalogued in commercial legal research service databases such as the LexisNexis StateNet database. In other cases, advocacy organizations may develop their own policy tracking system to inform their stakeholders of policy actions on a given topic.

In policy tracking systems, the goal is to monitor the policy status (e.g., introduced, amended, repealed, referred to committee, vetoed, or passed) of a given piece of legislation, regulation, or topic of interest. Policy tracking systems contain "data" on individual policy measures but the policies are not linked to any outcomes (e.g., individual health, system changes). Most policy tracking systems are qualitative systems relying on keywords and basic search schemes to enable end-users to search for policy actions within the jurisdictions of interest and on the topics of interest. Typically, policy tracking systems are updated on a regular basis to enable users to monitor changes in policy status and/or actions.[11] Policy tracking systems are particularly useful for advocates seeking to promote policy actions in their specific jurisdictions (e.g., adopting policies requiring healthy food procurement, requiring a certain amount of time per week for physical education, mandating insurance coverage for certain cancer screening services, and taxes on alcohol or tobacco products). The tracking systems can provide useful information on policies already being introduced or implemented in other places and the content of those policies. In another example, *Healthy People 2020* includes specific objectives for state legislatures and the District of Columbia (DC) city council to enact laws that prohibit smoking in public places and worksites (Objective TU-13), as well as baseline and target data on the number of states with such laws and the target goal of all states and Washington, DC[4] The data for the objectives were obtained from the CDC's State Tobacco Activities Tracking and Evaluation System (STATE System). Examples of policy tracking systems relevant for public health are presented in Table 15.1. With one exception, the table examples focus on systems that monitor and report on state laws and policies nationwide (the exception is the American Nonsmokers' Rights Foundation U.S. Tobacco Control Laws Database[12]). Similar systems may exist on a wide range of federal and local policy topics and readers are encouraged to identify such systems for their specific needs.

Policy surveillance systems, on the other hand, are typically designed for evaluating longitudinal changes in the adoption and scope of policies on a given topic, across jurisdictions and over time, for use in larger-scale policy impact and evaluation studies. Policy surveillance systems, like epidemiologic and public health surveillance systems, typically measure the current status of laws and policies as of a specific point in time for each measurement period (e.g., as of January 1, July 1, or December 31 of each year of data in the system) and typically will include a unique geographic identifier (e.g., state abbreviation or federal information processing standards code) to enable the policy data to be linked to other data, such as epidemiologic data on disease prevalence.[11] In contrast to public health policy tracking systems, public health policy surveillance

Table 15.1 Examples of Health Policy Tracking Systems

Database Name	Source
Chronic Disease State Policy Tracking System	Centers for Disease Control and Prevention (CDC) http://nccd.cdc.gov/CDPHPPolicySearch/Default.aspx
State Food Policy and Obesity-related Legislative Database	UConn Rudd Center for Food Policy and Obesity http://www.uconnruddcenter.org/legislation-database
State HPV vaccination laws	National Conference of State Legislatures (NCSL) http://www.ncsl.org/research/health/hpv-vaccine-stat e-legislation-and-statutes.aspx
State laws regarding alternative nicotine products: electronic cigarettes	NCSL http://www.ncsl.org/research/health/alternativ e-nicotine-products-e-cigarettes.aspx
State laws regarding prevention of prescription drug overdose and abuse	NCSL http://www.ncsl.org/research/health/prevention-o f-prescription-drug-overdose-and-abuse.aspx
State laws related to dietary sodium	NCSL http://www.ncsl.org/research/health/analysis-of-state-l aws-related-to-dietary-sodium.aspx
State School Health Policy Database	National Association of State Boards of Education http://www.nasbe.org/healthy_schools/hs/index.php`
State Tobacco Activities Tracking and Evaluation System (STATE)	CDC http://apps.nccd.cdc.gov/statesystem/Default/Default.aspx
U.S. Tobacco Control Laws Database	American Nonsmokers' Rights Foundation http://www.no-smoke.org/pdf/ USTobaccoControlLawsDatabase.pdf

systems typically include quantitative measures or data related to policy existence, ordinal measures of policy strength, and other quantitative markers that can be used in analyses linked to public health outcomes. Typical measures of policy strength are often based on scientific evidence as to what strategies will have the broadest reach, impact, and effect on the outcome of interest (e.g., reducing smoking rates).[11] The Robert Wood Johnson Foundation (RWJF)-supported Public Health Law Research Program at Temple University was established to enhance surveillance of public health law. In other examples, policy surveillance data from the National Institute on Alcohol Abuse and Alcoholism's Alcohol Policy Information System have been used to study the implementation and impact of state alcohol policies on the alcohol environment and alcohol consumption.[13-16] Policy surveillance data from the National Cancer Institute's Classification of Laws Associated with School Students (C.L.A.S.S.) system have been used to examine the association between state school-based nutrition and physical education-related laws and effects on student body mass index (BMI), school food practices, student diet, and student activity levels.[17-20] Similarly, policy surveillance data from the RWJF-supported Bridging the Gap research program have been used to study the impact of state beverage taxes and state laws governing school food, physical activity, and school wellness on school environments and practices as well as on student diet, physical activity, and BMI.[21-40] Examples of public health policy surveillance systems are provided in Table 15.2.

Using Policy Tracking Versus Policy Surveillance Data for Prevention and Public Health Policy Evaluation and Advocacy

The decision whether to use policy tracking or policy surveillance typically will depend on the purpose for which the data are being used. Advocates and policy-makers looking to see which states, for example, have enacted a law on a given topic often will rely on policy tracking or dichotomous (yes/no) data. Public health researchers, on the other hand, often want to be able to examine the breadth and depth of a given law on a specific topic. This information will help differentiate among correlates of policy impact such as levels of policy comprehensiveness (i.e., topics addressed) and strength (i.e., extensiveness of required provisions in a given policy or law). Systems for evaluating public health policy comprehensiveness and strength have been developed in recent years related to a wide range of policy topics including but not limited to tobacco control, school nutrition, physical education, school wellness, and alcohol policy.[41-47] Table 15.3 provides two examples (one related to obesity prevention and the other to tobacco control) to illustrate the variability in the data that may be produced with policy tracking or dichotomous (yes/no) measures as compared with more in-depth policy evaluation or surveillance measures that assess the comprehensiveness and strength of a policy on a given topic across jurisdictions.

Table 15.2 Examples of Public Health Policy Surveillance Systems

Database Name	Source
Classification of Laws Associated with School Students (C.L.A.S.S.)	National Cancer Institute http://class.cancer.gov
LawAtlas: Distracted Driving	Public Health Law Research (PHLR) Program http://lawatlas.org/query?dataset=distracted-driving
LawAtlas: Child Car Safety Seat Laws	PHLR http://lawatlas.org/query?dataset=child-restraint
LawAtlas: Communicable Disease Intervention Protocol	PHLR http://lawatlas.org/query?dataset=communicable-dise ase-intervention-protocol
LawAtlas: Good Samaritan Overdose Prevention Laws	PHLR http://lawatlas.org/query?dataset=good-samarita n-overdose-laws
LawAtlas: HIV Criminalization Statutes	PHLR http://lawatlas.org/query?dataset=hiv-criminalizatio n-statutes
LawAtlas: Syringe Distribution Laws	PHLR http://lawatlas.org/query?dataset=syring e-policies-laws-regulating-non-retail-distribu tion-of-drug-paraphernalia
State Obesity-related Laws	Bridging the Gap Research Program http://www.bridgingthegapresearch.org/research/ state_obesity-related_policies/
State Sales Taxes on Soda, Bottled Water, and Snack Foods	Bridging the Gap Research Program http://www.bridgingthegapresearch.org/research/ sodasnack_taxes/

EVALUATING POLICIES FOR EVIDENCE-BASED CONTENT

Policies based on the best available evidence are essential for the most effective improvements in population health.[48] As indicated in Chapter 1, getting the policies to be based on this evidence can be challenging for several reasons. Although rigorous research syntheses such as the United States Guide to Clinical Preventive Services[49] and The Guide to Community Preventive Services[50] have resulted in evidence-based recommendations, the amount and quality of evidence varies tremendously among health topics. According to the Community Guide,[50] for example, there is enough evidence to recommend maintaining limits on hours of sale to prevent excessive alcohol consumption, but insufficient evidence related to over-service law enforcement (i.e., enforcing laws that prohibit the service of alcoholic beverages to intoxicated customers). The Community Guide also reports that improving the quality and quantity

Table 15.3 Difference between Evaluating Policies Using a Dichotomous Versus an In-depth Policy Evaluation Approach

Question	Approach 1: Dichotomous Coding (Policy Tracking)	Approach 2: Policy Evaluation/ Surveillance Coding	Difference in Understanding of Policy Status
Is there a state law governing availability of sugar-sweetened beverages (SSBs) in schools?	1=Yes, law exists 0=No law	3=SSBs are banned in schools 2=SSBs are prohibited at certain times/locations 1=SSB restrictions are encouraged 0=No law	Approach 1 simply tells whether a law exists but does not provide the nuances. Approach 2 tells both whether a law exists and how detailed the law is.
Is there a law restricting smoking in public places?	1=Yes, law exists 0=No law	4=Ban in all locations 3=Ban with exceptions for employee break rooms 2=Smoking restricted to separately ventilated, separately enclosed areas 1=Smoking restricted to designated smoking areas 0=No law	

of physical education in schools increases physical activity among children and adolescents; therefore, a policy that specifies the required amount and type of physical education is evidence-based. Yet, there is insufficient evidence on school-based obesity prevention programs for these latter programs to be recommended.[50] For some topics, evidence emerges over time or the need for evidence changes. Electronic Nicotine Delivery Systems (ENDS), on the U.S. market since 2007, have gained considerable popularity and public health attention. The benefits and consequences of their use compared with traditional cigarettes are being debated, but as the debate unfolds so does related policy development and implementation to reduce access and public use.[51,52] Because public health harms associated with ENDS are unclear, research is needed to provide evidence for the most effective public policies.[53]

Lack of evidence-based policies may be related to the inherent differences between the process of research to gain evidence and the process of policymaking. The culture of policymaking is not methodological or systematic like research, but instead reactive and related to the demands of constituents.[54,55] Timing can be a challenge, too. Research tends to progress at a deliberate pace, often taking several years from project initiation to thorough dissemination of results. Policymaking moves much more quickly and within short legislative and election cycles. By the time research findings arise to support policy changes, the topic may no longer be relevant or be a policymaker priority. Additionally, research information can be complex. The evidence may be presented, but not communicated appropriately to policy stakeholders. (See Chapter 16 for more information on communication and policy.)

In spite of these challenges, assessing the quality and quantity of evidence within policies is important for identifying trends, comparative analysis, and measuring outcomes. This information can help inform both future research and advocacy efforts. Looking at the trends of evidence-based policy over time can show progress (or lack of) on specific public health initiatives. Results from a study of state-level evidence-based physical education policies from 2006 to 2012 showed that although the number of bills relating to physical education doubled during this time, the number of *evidence-based* bills increased only slightly.[56] Comparing specific policies based on the inclusion of evidence-based content also may provide insight for model policy development. This type of analysis also can identify evidence-based correlates of enactment, which can be helpful for prioritizing advocacy efforts.[56] For example, what aspect of an evidence-based food policy is present in the policies that are more likely to be enacted in schools? Perhaps one of the most important, yet difficult, types of evidence to gather related to policies is evidence of an intended (or unintended) health outcome. How can we say with certainty that an evidence-based policy was the reason for the decrease in disease prevalence or improvements in population health? Due to practical and ethical reasons, traditional methodologically rigorous randomized controlled trails are not appropriate for most policy interventions; yet, there is a definite need for well-designed evaluations to identify whether evidence-based policies result in the desired outcome. (See Chapter 4 for more information on types of studies that can provide evidence on policy-related health outcomes.) Assessing evidence-base in policies can be conducted through a series of steps:

1. Identify components of evidence for the topic of interest from reports such as CDC Guide to Community Preventive Services,[50] research syntheses, systematic reviews, or other published research. (For example, enforcing 0.08% blood alcohol content is an evidence-based component of policies to reduce alcohol related crashes.)
2. Develop a way to quantify or categorize these components. (For example, does the policy contain a provision for 0.08% blood alcohol content? Yes/No)
3. Create an abstraction tool or checklist that includes the information to be assessed from each policy. In addition to the evidence-based components, other policy characteristics may be of interest, too (e.g., year introduced, year enacted or policy progress, or sponsors of the policy).
4. Collect policies of interest through appropriate tracking systems (e.g., all state-level bills introduced in all 50 states in 2015 related to blood alcohol content and driving).
5. Assess the content of each policy using the abstraction tool or checklist, taking measures that ensure reliability (e.g., have more than one person assess each policy and compare results).
6. Compile and disseminate results.

CONCLUSION

This chapter provided examples of tools that can be used by prevention and public health advocates, decision-makers, and researchers interested in identifying and/or studying the impact of on-the-books prevention and public health policies. Although policy tracking and surveillance systems are useful tools for prevention and public health practitioners to use in daily practice, they also are critical tools for use in prevention and public health policy research and evaluation studies seeking to identify which policy strategies may work best under specific situations and for specific populations. As this chapter has briefly discussed, it is important to consider the type of data or system that might be used for the given situation (e.g., tracking or surveillance). And, in order to determine the extent to which on-the-books policies are incorporating the best available scientific evidence, it is also important to consider whether the chosen system captures already identified evidence-based elements. As discussed earlier in Section 1 of this book, being able to identify and study the impact of evidence-based public health policies will be particularly useful for authoritative decision-makers.

REFERENCES

1. Ten great public health achievements—United States, 1900–1999. *MMWR.* 1999;48: 241–243.
2. Brownson RC, Chriqui JF, Stamatakis KA. Understanding evidence-based public health policy. *Am J Public Health.* 2009;99:1576–1583.
3. Khan LK, Sobush K, Keener D, et al. Recommended community strategies and measurements to prevent obesity in the United States. *MMWR Recomm Rep.* 2009;58:1–26.
4. United States Department of Health and Human Services. *Healthy People 2020.* http://www.healthypeople.gov/2020/default.aspx. Updated 2012. Accessed August 28, 2014.
5. Centers for Disease Control and Prevention. *Best Practices for Comprehensive Tobacco Control Programs—2014.* http://www.cdc.gov/tobacco/stateandcommunity/best_practices/index.htm. Updated 2014. Accessed May 1, 2015.
6. Institute of Medicine. *Local Government Actions to Prevent Childhood Obesity.* Washington, DC: The National Academies Press; 2009.
7. Institute of Medicine. Committee on Strategies to Reduce Sodium Intake. *Strategies to Reduce Sodium Intake in the United States.* Washington, DC: The National Academies Press; 2010.
8. Institute of Medicine. Committee to Accelerate Progress in Obesity Prevention. *Accelerating Progress in Obesity Prevention: Solving the Weight of the Nation.* Washington, DC: The National Academies Press; 2012.
9. Institute of Medicine. Committee on Physical Activity and Physical Education in the School Environment. *Educating the Student Body: Taking Physical Activity and Physical Education to School.* Washington, DC: The National Academies Press; 2013.
10. National Prevention Council. *National Prevention Strategy.* http://www.surgeongeneral.gov/initiatives/prevention/strategy/index.html. Updated 2011. Accessed July 1, 2011.
11. Chriqui JF, O'Connor JC, Chaloupka FJ. What gets measured, gets changed: evaluating law and policy for maximum impact. *J Law Med Ethics.* 2011;39 (Suppl 1):21–26.

12. American Nonsmokers' Rights Foundation. *U.S. Tobacco Control Laws Database: Research Applications.* http://www.no-smoke.org/pdf/USTobaccoControlLawsDatabase.pdf. Updated 2015. Accessed May 27, 2015.

13. Naimi TS, Blanchette J, Nelson TF, et al. A new scale of the U.S. alcohol policy environment and its relationship to binge drinking. *Am J Prev Med.* 2014;46:10–16.

14. Xuan Z, Chaloupka FJ, Blanchette JG, et al. The relationship between alcohol taxes and binge drinking: evaluating new tax measures incorporating multiple tax and beverage types. *Addiction.* 2015;110:441–450.

15. Nelson TF, Xuan Z, Blanchette JG, et al. Patterns of change in implementation of state alcohol control policies in the United States, 1999–2011. *Addiction.* 2015;110:59–68.

16. Xuan Z, Blanchette J, Nelson TF, et al. The alcohol policy environment and policy subgroups as predictors of binge drinking measures among U.S. adults. *Am J Public Health.* 2015;105:816–822.

17. Perna FM, Oh A, Chriqui JF, et al. The association of state law to physical education time allocation in U.S. public schools. *Am J Public Health.* 2012;102:1594–1599.

18. Taber DR, Chriqui JF, Perna FM, et al. Weight status among adolescents in states that govern competitive food nutrition content. *Pediatrics.* 2012;130:437–444.

19. Taber DR, Chriqui JF, Perna FM, et al. Association between state physical education (PE) requirements and PE participation, physical activity, and body mass index change. *Prev Med.* 2013;57:629–633.

20. Hennessy E, Oh A, Agurs-Collins T, et al. State-level school competitive food and beverage laws are associated with children's weight status. *J Sch Health.* 2014;84:609–616.

21. Powell LM, Chriqui JF, Chaloupka FJ. Associations between state-level soda taxes and adolescent body mass index. *J Adolesc Health.* 2009;45:S57–S63.

22. Sturm R, Powell LM, Chriqui JF, et al. Soda taxes, soft drink consumption, and children's body mass index. *Health Aff.* 2010;29:1052–1058.

23. Chriqui JF, Taber DR, Slater SJ, et al. The impact of state safe routes to school-related laws on active travel to school policies and practices in U.S. elementary schools. *Health Place.* 2012;18:8–15.

24. Sandoval A, Turner L, Nicholson L, et al. The relationship among state laws, district policies, and elementary school-based measurement of children's body mass index. *J Sch Health.* 2012;82:239–245.

25. Schneider L, Chriqui J, Nicholson L, et al. Are farm-to-school programs more common in states with farm-to-school-related laws? *J Sch Health.* 2012;82:210–216.

26. Slater SJ, Nicholson L, Chriqui J, et al. The impact of state laws and district policies on physical education and recess practices in a nationally representative sample of U.S. public elementary schools. *Arch Pediatr Adolesc Med.* 2012;166:311–316.

27. Taber DR, Chriqui JF, Powell LM, et al. Banning all sugar-sweetened beverages in middle schools: reduction of in-school access and purchasing but not overall consumption. *Arch Pediatr Adolesc Med.* 2012;166:256–262.

28. Taber DR, Chriqui JF, Chaloupka FJ. Differences in nutrient intake associated with state laws regarding fat, sugar, and caloric content of competitive foods. *Arch Pediatr Adolesc Med.* 2012;166:452–458.

29. Taber DR, Chriqui JF, Perna FM, et al. Weight status among adolescents in states that govern competitive food nutrition content. *Pediatrics.* 2012;130:437–444.

30. Turner L, Chriqui JF, Chaloupka FJ. Food as a reward in the classroom: school district policies are associated with practices in U.S. public elementary schools. *J Acad Nutr Diet.* 2012;112:1436–1442.

31. Turner L, Chriqui JF, Chaloupka FJ. Healthier fundraising in U. S. elementary schools: associations between policies at the state, district, and school levels. *PLoS One.* 2012;7:e49890.

32. Chriqui JF, Eyler A, Carnoske C, et al. State and district policy influences on district-wide elementary and middle school physical education practices. *J Public Health Manag Pract.* 2013;19:S41–S48.

33. Taber DR, Chriqui JF, Powell L, et al. Association between state laws governing school meal nutrition content and student weight status: implications for new USDA school meal standards. *JAMA Pediatr.* 2013;167:513–519.

34. Taber DR, Chriqui JF, Chaloupka FJ. State laws governing school meals and disparities in fruit/vegetable intake. *Am J Prev Med.* 2013;44:365–372.

35. Turner L, Chriqui JF, Chaloupka FJ. Classroom parties in U.S. elementary schools: the potential for policies to reduce student exposure to sugary foods and beverages. *J Nutr Educ Behav.* 2013;45:611–619.

36. Turner L, Sandoval A, Chriqui JF, Chaloupka FJ. Competitive foods and beverages in elementary school classrooms: school policies and practices allow access to unhealthy snacks and drinks—a BTG research brief. Chicago, IL: Bridging the Gap Program, Health Policy Center, Institute for Health Research and Policy, University of Illinois at Chicago; 2013.

37. Turner L, Chriqui JF, Chaloupka FJ. Walking school bus programs in U.S. public elementary schools. *J Phys Act Health.* 2013;10:641–645.

38. Turner L, Chriqui JF, Chaloupka FJ. Withholding recess from elementary school students: policies matter. *J Sch Health.* 2013;83:533–541.

39. Taber DR, Chriqui JF, Vuillaume R, et al. How state taxes and policies targeting soda consumption modify the association between school vending machines and student dietary behaviors: a cross-sectional analysis. *PLoS One.* 2014;9:e98249.

40. Terry-McElrath YM, Chriqui JF, O'Malley PM, et al. Regular soda policies, school availability, and high school student consumption. *Am J Prev Med.* 2015;48(4):436–444.

41. LaFond C, Toomey TL, Rothstein C, et al. Policy evaluation research. Measuring the independent variables. *Eval Rev.* 2000;24:92–101.

42. Schwartz MB, Lund AE, Grow HM, et al. A comprehensive coding system to measure the quality of school wellness policies. *J Am Diet Assoc.* 2009;109:1256–1262.

43. Chriqui JF, Frosh M, Brownson RC, et al. Application of a rating system to state clean indoor air laws (USA). *Tob Control.* 2002;11:26–34.

44. Chriqui JF, Frosh MM, Fues LA, et al. State laws on youth access to tobacco: an update, 1993–1999. *Tob Control.* 2002;11:163–164.

45. Mâsse LC, Chriqui JF, Igoe JF, et al. Development of a physical education-related state policy classification system (PERSPCS). *Am J Prev Med.* 2007;33:S264–S276.

46. Mâsse LC, Frosh MM, Chriqui JF, et al. Development of a school nutrition-environment state policy classification system (SNESPCS). *Am J Prev Med.* 2007;33:S277–S291.

47. Alciati MH, Frosh M, Green SB, et al. State laws on youth access to tobacco in the United States: measuring their extensiveness with a new rating system. *Tob Control.* 1998;7:345–352.

48. Brownson RC, Haire-Joshu D, Luke DA. Shaping the context of health: a review of environmental and policy approaches in the prevention of chronic diseases. *Annu Rev Public Health.* 2006;27:341–370.

49. U.S. Preventive Services Task Force. *Guide to Clinical Preventive Services, 2014*. http://www.ahrq.gov/professionals/clinicians-providers/guidelines-recommendations/guide/index.html. Updated 2014. Accessed May 25, 2015.

50. Community Preventive Services Task Force. *The Guide to Community Preventive Services: The Community Guide*. http://www.thecommunityguide.org/index.html. Updated 2015. Accessed May 1, 2015.

51. Marynak K, Holmes CB, King BA, et al. State laws prohibiting sales to minors and indoor use of electronic nicotine delivery systems—United States, November 2014. *MMWR*. 2014;63:1145–1150.

52. Gourdet CK, Chriqui JF, Chaloupka FJ. A baseline understanding of state laws governing e-cigarettes. *Tob Control*. 2014;23(Suppl 3):iii37–iii40.

53. Schmitt CL, Lee YO, Curry LE, et al. Research support for effective state and community tobacco control programme response to electronic nicotine delivery systems. *Tob Control*. 2014;23(Suppl 3):iii54–iii57.

54. Choi BC, Pang T, Lin V, et al. Can scientists and policy makers work together? *J Epidemiol Community Health*. 2005;59:632–637.

55. Brownson RC, Royer C, Ewing R, et al. Researchers and policymakers: travelers in parallel universes. *Am J Prev Med*. 2006;30:164–172.

56. Eyler AA, Brownson RC, Aytur SA, et al. Examination of trends and evidence-based elements in state physical education legislation: a content analysis. *J Sch Health*. 2010;80:326 332.

16

Communicating Research to Help Influence Policy and Practice

Harry T. Kwon and David E. Nelson

LEARNING OBJECTIVES

1. Describe aspects of the policymaking environment as it relates to communicating with policymakers.
2. Explore ways to build relationships with policymakers to enhance communication.
3. Describe the concept of communication planning.
4. Describe challenges and barriers to effectively communicating scientific information to policymakers.

WHY IS COMMUNICATION IMPORTANT?

Public policies, whether in the form of laws or regulations, have a major role, both directly and indirectly, in improving population health across a wide range of issues and topics.[1] Because of knowledge and understanding gained through research, high-quality scientific evidence in the United States and other countries has played, and can continue to play, an important role in decisions to adopt and implement effective policies, and to oppose ineffective or counterproductive policies.[1-7] But for evidence-based scientific information to have an impact on policy decisions, it must be communicated effectively to policymakers.

This chapter provides an overview of communicating with policymakers. It is important to stress that the study of communication is difficult, in general, because communication is influenced by many factors, and because it is both an art and a science. A further challenge is the relatively few quantitative or qualitative research studies about communicating science to policymakers working with health issues.[8-9] That said, research in psychology, communication, health promotion, health education, and other disciplines, along with case studies about health policy efforts across many countries, have been illuminating. Whenever possible, we emphasize practical recommendations regarding more effective communication of evidence-based public health science to policymakers.

COMMUNICATING WITH POLICYMAKERS

Communicating science to policymakers with the goal of persuading them to approve and implement a public policy is difficult. Few policymakers are trained in or familiar with scientific approaches and ways of thinking. Along with a multitude of other powerful factors that influence policymakers, there are inherent differences in how policy systems operate and in how decisions are reached.[3,10–16] Scientific decision-making is based on hypothesis development, study design, data analysis, and synthesis of findings across studies in a fairly systematic way. In contrast, political decision-making is more reactive and usually short-term in nature, based as it is upon past policy experiences, demands of stakeholders, and the perceived available resources and level of support.[11] Fortunately, scientists, public health and healthcare practitioners, advocates, and others can learn how to communicate better with policymakers. Recommendations can broadly be categorized into (1) the policymaking environment and (2) communication planning (Box 16.1).

Policymaking Environment

Begin by understanding the environment in which policymakers operate. This includes learning about formal and informal processes, key individuals, influential factors, and the potential ways science communicators can influence policymakers.

Box 16.1 Recommendations for Communicating with Policymakers

Policymaking Environment

Learn about the formal policymaking process in your jurisdiction
Understand policymaker characteristics and interests
Build relationships with policymakers and gatekeepers
Provide an information subsidy
Know your role
Seek media attention

Communication Planning

Develop the storyline (meta-message)
Consider timing
Select the messenger (source)
Develop and deliver messages
Anticipate potential opposition arguments
Follow up

Adapted from References 3, 11–12.

Learn about the Formal Policymaking Process in the Jurisdiction of Interest

Elected policymakers operate as part of a system with formal rules for legislative or regulatory policymaking, funding decisions, and implementation.[3,12–16] It is essential to learn as much as possible about these formal rules within the specific jurisdiction where one is seeking to encourage the adoption of a new public health policy. There is likely to be a certain time period allowed and a procedure to follow (e.g., when a new bill or regulation may be introduced, or how committee hearings with witnesses are held) for a particular state legislature or city council. In many jurisdictions, the window of opportunity when elected officials can consider new policies is narrow, such as when a state legislature convenes every two years or when legislative sessions are legally restricted to a maximum number of days. This means policy proponents must be well-prepared long before legislative sessions begin. In addition, policymakers are extremely busy[12] and may receive a significant number of legislative bills and other written materials on various issues, so the available time they have to spend on a particular health topic can be very limited.

When it comes to directly communicating with a policymaker in writing or in person about a specific piece of legislation or regulation, it is most important to select someone who actually resides within the policymaker's jurisdiction, especially if the presenter is operating in an unofficial capacity (e.g., not as a representative of a government agency).[3] The "Anywhereville" city council may be unlikely to consider, or accept, testimony at a hearing about a new ordinance from someone who does not live within the city.

Understand Policymaker Characteristics and Interests

As with any communication effort, it is critical to know the audience. The definition of a policymaker has been provided in earlier chapters, but the common underlying characteristic is that policymakers have the authority to make decisions that impact policies or support for programs and efforts. For the purposes of this chapter, the term policymaker refers to an elected official. Most policymakers can be characterized as ambitious, hardworking, savvy, attuned to financial implications, and likely to engage in intuitive decision-making.[12] They also tend to be busy people who are subject to multiple communication efforts and requests from others. Their regular sources of information are primarily interpersonal sources and the news media.[17]

There are also notable demographic characteristics of policymakers, which can vary depending on the level of the policymaking body and the geographic region of the country. Although many policymakers are likely to be middle-aged or older white men, in 2014, women made up 24.2% of all state legislators nationwide.[18] In terms of racial and ethnic diversity, African Americans comprised 9% and Latino elected officials accounted for 3% of total state legislator seats in 2009.[18] Furthermore, only 16% of state legislators work in their positions on a full-time basis,[18] which indicates that the vast majority have concurrent occupations or professions.

When receiving information from experts, policymakers have a strong desire for certainty[12] and for credible, unbiased information.[19] Policymakers are generally familiar with numbers, especially those related to financial costs.[20] Dodson[21] found that state-level policymakers reported that the amount of scientific evidence, and addressing the needs and opinions of their constituents, were important considerations when considering health policy issues.

Every effort needs to be made to learn about the characteristics and preferences of a specific policymaker(s) of interest, for example, someone who could become a champion or a supporter for the policy.[3] The power and potential influence of an individual legislator or council member may depend, for example, on whether he or she is a member of the majority party; holds a prominent committee position (e.g., chairperson); has strong working or personal relationships with influential people; or has expertise with the specific topic or policy issue at hand.

Political party affiliation (where applicable) can provide some idea about ideology and worldviews,[12] but Internet searches will likely be the best way to find detailed information about individual policymakers. After all, most elected officials want to let others know their opinions and beliefs (especially about current issues of great interest to their constituents), voting records, and sponsored or proposed legislative bills. Most national and state elected policymakers are likely to have dedicated websites, and some may have Facebook pages, blogs, or Twitter accounts from which they regularly send or post messages. Information about local policymakers often can be gleaned from news media stories retrieved through Internet searches.

Assessing personal involvement, that is, the personal relevance or level of interest a policymaker has for a specific topic or issue, is another aspect of understanding policymakers, and one definitely worth learning.[3,12] Some of the best champions for specific public health issues are policymakers themselves, or their close family members (e.g., spouses), who have been personally affected by a disease or health issue of concern.[11]

Build Relationships with Policymakers and Gatekeepers (Aides)

In marked contrast to the formal policymaking processes are the "unwritten rules," or informal processes, which also can influence the chances of success in efforts to influence policymakers.[14-16] Most policymakers are busy individuals, which means they are not likely to spend much time reviewing, in detail, written materials on health or other types of policies.[3,11-12,22-23] They also are regularly solicited by many other people and organizations and asked to support policies or funding requests.[3,11,14-16] Not surprisingly, policymakers often rely heavily on gatekeepers, that is, aides or assistants. Gatekeepers have an important role in deciding who has direct access to policymakers, and the information to which they are exposed, especially at the state, national, and international level.[3,9,11-12,14-16] Research and experience have consistently shown the importance of building strong interpersonal relationships with policymakers and their staff members through in-person meetings and other contacts.[3,6,23-29] This also involves regularly communicating with them at times other than when key policy votes or important decisions are pending.[23] To maximize the effect of these efforts, it is important to identify and use the communication channels (e.g., e-mail, text messages, or phone calls) preferred by gatekeepers or policymakers.

Relationships are founded on trust and appreciation. Following through on promises, such as providing requested information or other materials in a timely manner, and remembering to thank policymakers and their staff members, both go a long way in this regard.[3] Diligence in such matters can help build and strengthen a reputation as being trustworthy and reliable, and increase the chances that policymakers will collaborate in the future.

Provide an Information Subsidy

In the fields of mass communication and public relations, an *information subsidy* refers to providing news reporters with information that they can readily use or adapt.[30–31] The same basic concept applies when communicating with policymakers and their aides about a policy issue: the goal is to make their jobs as simple and easy as possible.[3] Because they may be inexperienced or have limited knowledgeable about the science or public health issue of interest, it is important to provide information orally, visually, or in writing, which is clear and concise and offers compelling and actionable reasons (arguments) for supporting the policy.[32] If a strong professional relationship already exists with an aide, for example, one could provide him or her in advance with a written document and ask for suggestions for improvement before sending it on to the policymaker.

Knowing One's Role

Whether in formal or informal settings, it is important to remember the role one plays when communicating with policymakers.[3,33] Individuals acting on their own behalf as private citizens, as well as advocacy organizations, have great leeway in how they express their opinions or beliefs to policymakers. But most communication efforts designed to encourage adoption of public health policies based on evidence-based scientific research will involve people speaking or writing based on their professional qualifications, with individuals often serving as representatives of their organizations, institutions, or agencies.

Scientists are likely to be perceived as credible sources of information in their areas of expertise.[12] (This does not mean, of course, that the science or scientist will not be challenged.) When testifying at a legislative committee hearing, for example, a scientist or healthcare provider should only make comments, or answer questions, directly related to science or healthcare issues.[33] Providing comments outside of one's area of expertise, or speculating without acknowledging it as such, is likely to lead to problems and be counterproductive. Similarly, one needs to be especially careful to portray the "party line" accurately if speaking on behalf of one's agency or organization.

Seek Media Attention

The news media have an agenda-setting function,[34] which means the topics featured in media outlets, and how they are covered, are considered by policymakers and the public as being the most important issues of the day. As a rule, elected policymakers pay close attention to news media stories, especially those they consider relevant to, or on the minds of, their constituents.[12,14–16,35] This means gaining supportive media coverage for a public health policy issue is an important way to get the attention of, and potentially influence, policymakers.[36] National or state-based "report cards" with letter grades are one method used by some organizations and professional societies to try and raise awareness among the news media and policymakers about public health issues (Box 16.2).[3] More information on media advocacy is covered in Chapter 17.

Communication Planning

Communication planning consists of devising the strategy, and creating messages, for policymakers. The three assumptions here are that: (1) The underlying purpose is to persuade policymakers to approve a new public health policy that is evidence-based and highly likely to be effective;[1] (2) An active strategy will be used to engage policymakers and gain their attention (e.g., a fact sheet or report will not simply be placed on a website with the hope that interested people will find it of their own accord); and (3) Communication efforts with policymakers will be coordinated among major supporting organizations, professional societies, and other allies.[39–43] Building partnerships and coalitions provides a united front among supporters and allows the opportunity to share resources for communication and advocacy efforts.

Develop the Storyline (Meta-Message)

Creating a storyline, or meta-message, is the beginning of communication planning.[3,12] The storyline represents the major conclusion one is trying to convey to policymakers. Scientific and other messages (the *premises* or *grounds*, in debate terminology) are then developed to support the storyline. Public health policy storylines are usually straightforward because they are the policies themselves. ("All children must be vaccinated against Disease A before entering elementary school." or "Manufacturers must install Safety Device B in motor vehicles beginning in Year 20XX.")

Nevertheless, it is still important to put the storyline in writing to make sure individuals and organizations supporting the policy, and involved in communicating with policymakers, agree on it. An important corollary is to assess whether alternatives to the desired policy, such as excluding certain population groups or businesses from

---

[1] A similar approach, although with different messages, would be used for communication efforts designed to dissuade policymakers from discontinuing, or reducing funding for, an existing evidence-based public health policy.

Box 16.2 Summary of U.S. Child and Adolescent Physical Activity Report Card

United States Overall Receives a D–

In 2014, the National Physical Activity Plan Alliance, a national coalition of organizations promoting physical activity, released the 2014 United States Report Card on Physical Activity for Children and Youth. The Report Card assesses the level of physical activity and sedentary behaviors among children and youth, facilitators and barriers for physical activity, and related health outcomes.[37] The Report Card reviewed and graded 10 key indicators related to physical activity levels and influencers. Overall physical activity received a D–, indicating that the majority of U.S. children and youth did not meet the physical activity recommendations set forth by the 2008 Physical Activity Guidelines for Americans. These guidelines recommend that children and adolescents should engage in 60 minutes or more of physical activity daily.[38] Additional grades were assigned for the following indicators: Sedentary Behavior (D), Active Transportation (F), Organized Sport Participation (C-), School (C-), and the Community & Built Environment (B-). The four remaining indicators (Active Play, Health Related Fitness, Family & Peers, and Government Strategies and Investments) received a grade of "Incomplete" due to insufficient data.

According to the National Physical Activity Plan Alliance, the Report Card serves as "an advocacy tool which provides a level of accountability and call-to-action for adult decision makers regarding how we, as parents, teachers, health professionals, community leaders, and policy makers can help implement new initiatives, programs, and policies in support of healthy environments to improve the physical activity levels and health of our children and youth." Additional information about the alliance, metrics, methodology, and references can be found in the report.

Source: National Physical Activity Plan Alliance. 2014 United States Report Card on Physical Activity for Children and Youth.[37]

the policy, are acceptable to supporters. These alternatives should also be in writing and circulated in some form to supporters to make sure everyone is on the same page.

Consider Timing

When to communicate with policymakers is another major consideration.[3,12,33] As mentioned earlier in the chapter, timing issues come into play for formal policymaking processes within specific jurisdictions. But timing for communicating with policymakers about a new public health policy also is affected by other current issues, as well as by the likelihood of strong support or opposition for the policy. On the positive side, an excellent time to communicate with policymakers is when a focusing event occurs that is directly germane to the policy.[12,14–16] Focusing events include such things as an infectious disease outbreak, a prominent media celebrity with an injury or illness, or a workplace safety problem (e.g., explosion or hazardous materials release).

Policymakers are often primed to take action because of news media attention and public concern.[36]

On the other hand, a poor time to communicate with policymakers is when they are distracted by more pressing immediate events, such as when they are considering another major health policy issue or facing a budget crisis.[12,26,44] It is also important to consider that despite consensus among scientists about the policy effectiveness, policymakers and the public may require sufficient time to be prepared to accept it. Motor vehicle safety advocates, for example, were surprised by the level of public opposition in the United States to a federal ignition interlock regulation in the 1970s that prevented automobiles from starting unless seatbelts were fastened, which led to a subsequent rapid rollback of this policy by the U.S. Congress.[45]

Select the Messenger (Source)

Figure 16.1 provides a broad overview of the basic model of communication, which consists of the communication source, channel(s) (e.g., written documents, in-person presentations, mass media, Internet websites, and social media), message, audience, and contextual factors. Although most communication planning involves understanding audiences, and message development and delivery (see next section), the selection of the source or messenger(s), that is, who will deliver the messages to policymakers, and the organization or group that the messenger represents, is crucial.[3,12,19,23] Believability of messages by audiences is strongly influenced by the perceived credibility (trustworthiness and expertise) of the messenger.[46] Effective messengers need to have a reputation for fairness and honesty and need to provide accurate, unbiased, and relevant information regarding the issue and questions at hand.

Asking, "To whom will they listen?" is an excellent first step when deciding who should speak to policymakers during interpersonal meetings (including formal testimony), who should send e-mails, or whose name(s) or which organization(s) should appear on written documents such as one-page handouts or correspondence.[3] If a relationship with a specific policymaker and his or her aide(s) has been established, ask who they think would be good choices as messengers.

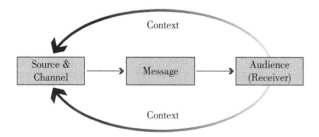

Figure 16.1 Basic communication model.
Source: Nelson DE, Hesse B, Croyle R. *Making Data Talk: Communicating Public Health Findings to the Public, Policy Makers, and the Press.* New York: Oxford University Press; 2009.

Many types of messengers may be used to communicate various aspects of a proposed public policy, depending on the individual situation. As a general rule, the most effective messengers for policymakers are those who reside within the policymakers' jurisdiction, that is, individuals who are more likely to be considered "one of us" because they are from the local area.[3,23]

When communicating about scientific matters, a scientist with strong expertise in the issue and policy is essential, and, in such a case, it is not as important that she or he be from the local area. The scientist may be, for example, a representative from the state or local health agency, or a university professor. A pediatrician might be an excellent choice for a child health issue, especially because he or she may be able to call upon professional experiences with real people (e.g., narratives). Some of the most effective messengers are persons without professional science or health backgrounds, such as a teenager, parent, business owner, community leader, or celebrity figure who can speak from personal experience.[3,26]

Develop and Deliver Messages

General Considerations

Messages provide the rationale (arguments) used to support the storyline (i.e., the public policy). They are created with the goal of convincing policymakers that (1) there is a public health problem, and (2) the new public health policy will solve or alleviate the problem. Messages themselves consist of words, numbers, visual images, or some combination of the three, and they are presented to audiences orally, visually, or in written form.

Message development for communicating with policymakers begins with considering the questions they most often want answered. Questions are likely to be one or more of the following[3,12]:

- Is there a problem?
- If so, is there a solution for the problem? (What do we do?)
- How much will it cost to solve the problem?
- How does this help my constituents?
- Will this make me look good (to the media, to my constituents, and to the powerful interests that shape my region)?

Unlike research studies published in scientific journals, messages should be presented to policymakers using the inverse pyramid approach. This means stating the major conclusion (likely to be the storyline or meta-message) first, followed by the key messages supporting this conclusion. Messages need to contain timely information, be relevant to policymakers, and be easily understood.[3,8–9,11–12,22–23,25–27,35,47–50] They must be scientifically defensible and direct, clearly demonstrating the need for action by policymakers (e.g., enact the policy) that is realistic from a cost and practical perspective.

An especially important point to remember is that messages, including those based on scientific research findings, need to be created and integrated in such a way that they tell a clear, compelling, and simple story about why policymakers should support the new policy. If trying to convince city council members, for example, about the expected benefit of installing red light cameras at major intersections, a message could be used highlighting a 50% reduction in the number of traffic accidents over the past 10 years from another city in the state after the implementation of a red light camera policy.

Information overload is a major problem for policymakers.[11] Data and scientific concepts can be difficult for many policymakers, therefore, presenting and describing one or two major scientific findings simply and clearly will be far more effective than providing lengthy details about scientific studies, using data tables, etc. Phrases such as "logistic regression models" or "statistical significance" will be seen as professional jargon and should be avoided, as should hedging language. ("We are reasonably assured the policy has a high likelihood of having a positive impact.")

Communicating Data

Because science is based on data, a major consideration is whether, and how, to communicate data to policymakers. Although there may be instances when an individual policymaker, for whatever reason, is not interested in scientific data at all, these are likely to be rare. Scientific data can raise awareness, especially if the issue or problem is relatively new. Brownson and colleagues, for example, in a randomized study of policy briefs that presented scientific information in various ways to state legislators, found that the legislators believed data-containing briefs were more useful than narrative-only briefs.[9]

Incorporating data into policy briefs or testimony can help define a particular public health problem, as well as demonstrate the magnitude of the problem (i.e., the number of people impacted and the expected [positive] impact of the new policy). A common and effective strategy is to use public health surveillance data (the more local the data, the better)[8] to highlight the magnitude of a specific health problem (raise awareness), followed by findings from in-depth research studies to demonstrate the cause(s) of the problem or the projected impact of the policy (the solution).[12] Figure 16.2 presents a sample policy brief used to support education efforts on hepatitis B, a liver disease that affects a significant number of Asian American, Native Hawaiian, and other Pacific Islander populations.[51] Note how it uses data to raise awareness about the significance of the disease, bolds text to highlight key messages and actions, and provides a set of clear recommendations. It also does a good job highlighting the magnitude of the disease and provides an overview of the issues that are contributing to the problem.

Whether written in an e-mail or delivered during oral testimony in support or opposition of a proposed policy, communicating research findings primarily with words can help reduce complex scientific research findings into simple messages. Metaphors and narratives are two ways to communicate data and research findings to policymakers using words. Metaphor refers to using words to provide an analogy such that "X is similar to Y."[52] Metaphors can help improve understanding of data when data

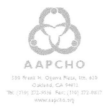

Policy Brief 2009

Hepatitis B

AAPCHO

330 Frank H. Ogawa Plaza, Ste. 620
Oakland, CA 94612
Tel: (510) 272-9536 Fax: (510) 272-0817
www.aapcho.org

Association of Asian Pacific Community Health Organizations

Background

Approximately 350 million people worldwide are infected with hepatitis B, a deadly disease that often goes undetected despite the fact that it causes about 80% of all primary liver cancers.

Hepatitis B, a liver disease caused by the hepatitis B virus (HBV), can lead to lifelong infection, scarring of the liver, liver cancer, and death. In the U.S., it is estimated that 1 in 20 people will become infected with HBV, and 1 in 4 chronic hepatitis B carriers will die of liver cancer or liver failure.

Within Asian American, Native Hawaiian, and other Pacific Islander (AA & NHOPI) populations, this "silent disease" has had an especially devastating health impact. AA & NHOPIs comprise more than half of the 2 million estimated hepatitis B carriers in the United States and, consequently, have the highest rate of liver cancer among all ethnic groups.

Issues

Although infection is preventable with a safe and effective hepatitis B vaccine, many people live with (and often unknowingly pass on) this chronic disease. Compounding this problem, hepatitis B screening and vaccination rates among AA & NHOPIs are alarmingly low, given the disease's disproportionate affect on this population. For example, a 2005 study done in New York City found that more than half (56.6%) of AA & NHOPIs had not been previously screened for HBV and 15% of those unscreened individuals were indeed chronically infected with HBV.

Because many chronic hepatitis B carriers show no symptoms and are generally healthy, the disease progresses, is transmitted unknowingly, and often leaves individuals in the late stages of liver cancer or liver disease without warning, too late for medical intervention.

It is critical that AA & NHOPIs get screened and vaccinated for HBV and those individuals who have been exposed to HBV receive appropriate, ongoing medical care. Increasing the availability of culturally and linguistically appropriate HBV programs will help lower existing barriers that prevent this population from accessing services, from screening and vaccination to disease management and treatment. We must also educate health care providers on the prevalence of HBV among AA & NHOPIs, and replicate successful community-based programs that prevent and manage HBV in these populations.

Recommendations

- Support and promote community and faith-based efforts to educate and mobilize AA & NHOPI communities at risk for and living with hepatitis B
- Support programs that educate health care providers on hepatitis B's high prevalence among AA & NHOPIs
- Support the *Viral Hepatitis and Liver Cancer Control Act of 2009 (H.R. 3974)*, which calls for the prevention, control, and appropriate treatment for hepatitis B through vaccination programs, preventive education, early detection and research. This act also supports expanded outreach and preventative HBV programs specific to AA & NHOPIs and other groups disproportionately affected by hepatitis B.

Figure 16.2 Sample policy brief.

Source: Association of Asian Pacific Community Health Organizations. Hepatitis B Policy Brief 2009. http://www.aapcho.org/wp/wp-content/uploads/2012/12/hep_policy_brief_2009_final_2.pdf. Accessed April 30, 2015.

are related to something with which the audience is familiar,[12] such as traffic, number of certain stores, or schools in one's community. For example, "In Anywhereville, there are more tanning salons than schools, supermarkets, and gas stations combined."

Narratives, such as a personal story about one's experience, have the ability to engage audiences[53] and can serve as a support to report or supplement research findings.[9,54] For example, in a study examining affective and cognitive reactions to organ donation messages using narratives or statistics, Kopfman and colleagues[55] found that narratives had a greater influence on emotions compared with statistical evidence alone. A narrative may improve translation of research evidence into policy by increasing knowledge and awareness of the specific issue, presenting the problem in a real-life example, packaging scientific evidence in a way that is familiar to policymakers, and further augmenting advocacy efforts (Box 16.3).[56]

Visuals

Visual modalities are used to present data and demonstrate magnitude, highlight changes, or make comparisons to enhance understanding and interpretation by an audience. Although various visual modalities exist, pie charts, bar graphs, and line charts are likely to be used most often to present data to policymakers, and these are highlighted here.

Pie charts can be used to show proportions and magnitude by showing how small or large something is in relation to the total. When developing a pie chart, slices should be clearly labeled and no more than six should be used.[12] In a policy brief developed by the CDC to control prescription drug overdose, data were summarized in a pie chart to indicate the main sources of access to prescription painkillers (Figure 16.3). The pie chart clearly shows friends or relatives are the largest source of prescription painkillers, thus highlighting the need for better control of diverting pills to those who were not prescribed them.

Bar charts are great for displaying magnitude, and they can show relative differences or patterns between or across groups.[17] When developing a bar chart, use color or shading to show contrast and include a short and easy to understand title or label that summarizes the key message. For example, in a policy brief to highlight the importance of teen driver safety (Figure 16.4), the bar chart nicely demonstrates that younger drivers are much more likely to be involved in motor vehicle crashes

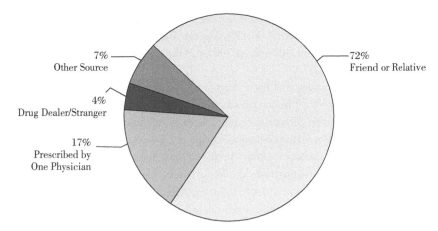

Figure 16.3 People who abuse prescription painkillers get them from various sources.
Source: Adapted from Centers for Disease Control and Prevention. Policy Impact: Prescription Painkiller Overdoses. http://www.cdc.gov/HomeandRecreationalSafety/pdf/PolicyImpact-PrescriptionPainkillerOD. pdf. Accessed March 14, 2015.

compared with older drivers. In addition, a clear and succinct title summarizes the main data finding.

Line graphs are especially helpful for showing trends over time, and to highlight before and after differences such as increases, decreases, or stability (e.g., as a result of a policy). When developing a line graph, use arrows or text to highlight key events or data, place labels close to the lines, and do not use more than four trend lines. For example, the Health Information Technology for Economic and Clinical Health

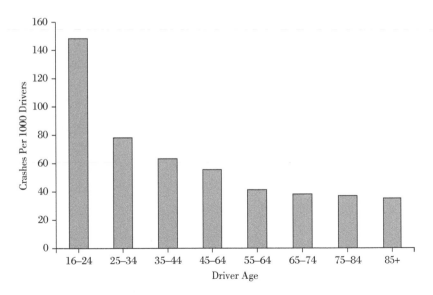

Figure 16.4 Young drivers have more motor vehicle crashes.
Source: Adapted from Centers for Disease Control and Prevention. Policy Impact: Teen Driver Safety. http:// www.cdc.gov/motorvehiclesafety/pdf/policyimpact-teendriversafety-a.pdf. Accessed March 14, 2015.

(HITECH) Act of 2009 authorized incentive payments to increase physician adoption of electronic health record (EHR) systems. Figure 16.5 depicts the adoption trends of EHR system utilizations since 2001 and the trends following the implementation of the policy.

It is helpful to recognize that there is no one "best way" to communicate scientific data to policymakers.[9,12,22,26] In certain situations, one or two key numbers may be all that is needed to convey certain scientific messages adequately.[12] Some people prefer narrative-based information because it helps put a human face to a public health problem or a solution, whereas others prefer to see scientific evidence expressed as numbers. This further demonstrates the importance of learning as much as possible about specific policymakers in order to tailor messages to them,[9] as well as the need to consider using both narrative and number-based messages in written materials or in oral presentations to heterogeneous audiences.

Written Materials

Research studies provide guidance about types of written materials to develop for policymakers.[6,8–9,22,25–27,48–49] Brief reports, such as policy briefs focused on the specific issue and policy, are often helpful for policymakers. These should be no longer than 1,500 words (2–4 pages) and should contain timely information and action items such

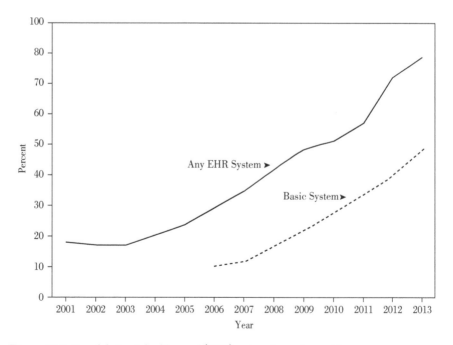

Figure 16.5 Use of electronic health record (EHR) systems is growing rapidly.

Source: Adapted from Hsiao CJ, Hing E. Use and characteristics of electronic health record systems among office-based physician practices: United States, 2001–2013. National Center for Health Statistics Data Brief. 2014;143:1–8. http://www.cdc.gov/nchs/data/databriefs/db143.htm. Accessed March 22, 2015.

> **Box 16.4** Recommendations for Developing Fact Sheets
>
> - Limit to one page
> - Use large enough font and maintain sufficient white space; highlight key points (e.g., through bold font, different colors) so they can be easily read
> - Keep messages simple and tailored to policymakers
> - Summarize the problem in one or two sentences
> - Prominently mention the expected benefits of the policy, including cost savings, if applicable
> - Include local data and consider comparing with other geographic areas (e.g., other counties, states, or national data)
> - Consider adding a professionally produced chart or infographic that clearly highlights one key finding
> - Include name, e-mail address, phone number, and mailing address for the contact person

as specific policy recommendations. Executive summaries should be used if longer reports are provided. Short quotations illustrating key points are helpful because they can be easily remembered and reused by supportive policymakers. Additional materials should be made available through research clearinghouses or some other means, and these should be easily accessible for policymakers or their aides who want more in-depth information. Fact sheets, often referred to as "one pagers," are used to simply and briefly highlight key information, including data.[3,48] Box 16.4 contains recommendations for developing fact sheets to be used in support of a public health policy.[3]

In-person Meetings

In-person meetings with policymakers usually occur in one of two ways: a face-to-face meeting with an individual policymaker (and likely one or more of his or her staff); or a legislative hearing, or other type of committee meeting, in which formal testimony is given or in which experts or other individuals are questioned by policymakers.[3] Box 16.5 contains suggestions for face-to-face communication with an individual policymaker.

Legislative committee hearings about a proposed new public health policy usually involve one or more experts providing short testimonies to policymakers, followed by questions from legislators.[3] Testimony is usually short (a few minutes), and it is sometimes prepared in advance and read to committee members. If data are to be presented, this may be done through the use of posters rather than PowerPoint or some other type of slide presentation software. Information needs to be presented in a direct and nonconfrontational manner to all legislators, regardless of the perception of their voting records or whether they have negative opinions about the policy.[3] Being well-prepared to communicate key messages, and responding appropriately to questions, is crucial because committee hearings can generate a lot of interest from policymakers and media representatives. Spokespeople always need to act professionally, not become defensive, and maintain their composure.[3]

Anticipate Potential Opposition Arguments and Strategies

It is essential to anticipate opposition arguments to the policy and be prepared to address them.[6,12,28,61] Powerful interest groups and individuals with economic interests, for example, may attempt to persuade policymakers to oppose the new public health policy. It is especially important to anticipate what opponents are likely to do in formal testimony settings with policymakers so that one can, if necessary, be able to rebut their arguments with solid scientific evidence. Box 16.6 contains some common arguments and strategies used to oppose public health policies.[12,62-63]

Follow-up

Follow-up is the final aspect of communication planning.[3] If asked by county council members to provide additional information from a scientific study or report to them

after a session is over, get the material to them as soon as possible (ideally within 24
to 48 hours). If working closely with a specific policymaker and his or her staff in a
policy effort, they will appreciate receiving a personalized written note, e-mail, text
message, phone call, or visit thanking them for their support or help regardless of the
outcome of the policy effort. This will help sustain good relationships, which is especially important because many policy efforts take a long time and a lot of effort before
ultimately being successful.

As mentioned in this chapter, the two important aspects to consider when communicating with policymakers are (1) having a good understanding of the environment in
which policymakers operate and (2) engaging in communication planning, which includes
devising a strategy and developing key messages. Box 16.7 presents a case study displaying
some of the key steps involved in advocating for a policy change.

Challenges and Barriers

*It must be a very good and rare day indeed when policymakers take their cues mainly
from scientific knowledge.* Brown[65]

There are many aspects involved in effectively communicating scientific information
to policymakers. It is also important, however, to acknowledge that there are important challenges and barriers (Box 16.8).

Other Factors Influencing Policy Decisions

Policymakers are influenced by many factors.[14–16] Regardless of the quality of studies, consistency of research findings, and level of consensus within the scientific

community regarding the benefits of a policy, scientific evidence is but one of many considerations policymakers weigh when making decisions. There are, unfortunately, many examples from the local to the international level, where policymakers ignored strong scientific evidence. Scientific research findings and recommendations included in policy discussions are viewed as one type of evidence used in debates, not as "absolute truth."[12] Personal anecdotes, and the opinions and beliefs of lay individuals, also may be seen as credible forms of evidence. One need look no further than recent debates, and selected U.S. state and local policies, for example, on childhood immunizations[66–68] and water fluoridation,[69–70] to understand that long "settled science" demonstrating the benefits of these major public health advancements has not resulted in universal adoption because of factors besides science influencing policymakers' decisions.

What are some of these other factors? The following quote from a state legislator nicely highlights three that are especially prominent[71]:

> *"Keep in mind that most of us pay serious attention to three factors: (1) votes, (2) money, and (3) media. To stay in office, we must have votes and must respect the views, interests, and values of those who elected us. We have to run campaigns and we need support for that. Also, we don't easily forget those who provided support for a priority issue we were pushing for—it's called reciprocity. Media is critical because it equals exposure—it helps bring attention to an important issue or debate, and us as well."*

It is not surprising that the views and preferences of constituents (for elected policymakers), or of higher-level officials (for administrative policymakers), are a major factor.[14–16] The effect of money in public policy decision-making is often evidenced through the role of interest groups, especially those likely to experience adverse financial impacts from a proposed policy.[3,12] The presence of "scientific uncertainty" may be used by such groups in arguments to oppose laws or regulations.[62–63]

Cost considerations can be a major deterrent to adopting certain public health policies, especially during tight budgetary times. Ideology and strongly held personal beliefs of policymakers are also influential.[26,72–73] Some individuals strongly oppose governmental interventions regardless of the evidence of their effectiveness. They are concerned about restricting people's personal decision-making (freedom of choice) and the creation of the so-called "nanny state." Furthermore, some policymakers may simply distrust scientists and the scientific process.

Commitment of Time and Energy

Another major barrier is the commitment of time and energy required.[11] Whether at the local, state, or national level, it takes time to understand the policymaking process fully, learn about policymakers and their environments, and cultivate relationships with staffers and policymakers. Educating policymakers or their staff members about public health issues can be time-consuming and may not always be successful. Policy efforts inevitably involve working with individuals and organizations as part of coalitions, and many meetings may be needed. If media advocacy activities are part of the strategy, that requires additional time and effort.

Creating succinct written communication products, such as policy briefs, one-page summaries, or longer reports, as well as visual presentations or materials, which policymakers can readily locate and understand, is not easy. This takes guidance and training from individuals who work in the policy arena, because learning how to translate science to policymakers effectively is not something that scientists are taught in formal schooling. Preparing and providing written or oral testimony, developing potential answers to address opposing arguments, and responding appropriately to potentially challenging or even hostile questioning from policymakers, are all skills that take energy and time to master.

It is important to have a long-term time frame for public health policy efforts.[3,74] This means it may take multiple communication attempts, sometimes over several years, to achieve a public health policy victory. This is especially true when there is powerful and committed opposition.

Ethical Considerations

The purpose of communicating with policymakers is persuasion. Ethical considerations are critical, therefore, when deciding what information to select (or omit) and how to present that information, particularly when it comes to data.[12] One may be tempted to oversimplify or overstate, for example, the projected population impact of enacting a new law or regulation, or to ignore research findings not supportive of the policy. Scientists, in particular, need to be especially careful to maintain their credibility with policymakers by understanding that their role, to the greatest extent possible, is to be perceived as unbiased experts in science who are objective and trustworthy.[19,42]

Unable to Provide Information Desired by Policymakers

The types of information, as well as the communication products and formats, which policymakers and their assistants prefer to receive about scientific topics, are generally well-known. First and foremost, they would like definitive answers to questions such as (1) Will the policy produce its intended effects? and (2) Are the fiscal estimates for the policy correct?

Unfortunately, simple, straightforward, and accurate answers to these and similar questions are often not available. Current scientific and cost-estimate knowledge may not be able to provide an answer. Research results are often in the form of probability estimate (e.g., relative risks) based on study populations that differ from those in a specific county or state, and cost estimates or projections may be inaccurate. Timely research findings, availability of locally relevant data, and an information infrastructure and personnel sufficient to make research products readily available and tailored to the needs of policymakers and their staff members are all desirable. In reality, some of these or even all of them may not be available, or even achievable, with available resources.

Bad Luck

It is possible to do an outstanding job of communicating with policymakers and still be unsuccessful because of unforeseen circumstances.[44] A public health bill may be on track to be approved by a city council or state legislature, only to be delayed or not considered because policymakers are overcome by other issues or events. Legislative sessions are short in some states and other jurisdictions, leading to frustrating postponements and a need to "start all over" in the next session. Compromises and dealmaking may result in adoption of weaker policies than desired.[14-16] Long-term relationships may have been cultivated with key administrative or legislative leaders (political champions) and their aides, but these individuals can lose their leadership positions or their jobs as the result of an election, retirement, or ill health.[11]

Professional Risks

Finally, there can be professional risks involved in actively communicating about efforts to support a public health policy. Government or private organization employees may be officially restricted, or strongly discouraged by higher-level managers, from being involved in policy activities.[3] Harassment by opponents in the form of broad Freedom of Information Act requests and legal action has been used against scientists supporting certain public policies, such as tobacco control and reducing carbon emissions to prevent global warming.[75-76]

Although much less dramatic, there are other potential professional risks. Other scientists may view scientists involved in policy work as advocates who have lost their objectivity.[11] For scientists in universities or other research institutions, considerable time may be devoted to working on policy issues.[11,77] Policy and other service-related activities generally are considered less important than grant writing success, conducting research, and publishing, especially when it comes to decisions about tenure.

CONCLUSION

Well-executed and persistent communication efforts with policymakers are essential for evidence-based scientific knowledge to successfully influence policy decisions and improve the public's health. For many reasons, however, effective communication with key policymakers is complex and challenging. Fortunately, research studies and practice-based experiences of recent years provide insights on how to communicate clearly and concisely with policymakers in ways that are more likely to meet their needs.

There will inevitably always be differences in roles, perspectives, and influential factors between science and policy. And of course, no single communication approach will work with policymakers in every situation or setting. But consistently applying the communication-related suggestions mentioned in this chapter substantially increases the chance of success when working with policymakers on public health policy issues.

REFERENCES

1. Teitlebaum JB, Wilensky S. *Essentials of Health Policy and Law*. 2nd ed. Burlington, MA: Jones & Bartlett; 2012.
2. Brownson RC. Epidemiology and health policy. In: Brownson RC, Pettiti DB (Eds.). *Applied Epidemiology: Theory to Practice*. 2nd ed. New York: Oxford University Press; 2006: 260–288.
3. Brownson RC, Jones E, Parvanta C. Communicating for policy and advocacy. In: Parvanta C, Nelson DE, Parvanta SA, Harner RN (Eds.). *Essentials of Public Health Communication*. Burlington, MA: Jones & Bartlett; 2011: 91–118.
4. Sleet DA, Schieber RA, Gilchrest J. Health promotion policy and politics: lessons from childhood injury prevention. *Health Promot Pract*. 2003;4(2):103–108.
5. Heath GW, Parra DC, Sarmiento OL, Andersen LB, Owen N, Goenka S, et al. Evidence-based intervention in physical activity: lessons from around the world. *Lancet*. 2012;380:272–281.
6. Trostle J, Bronfman M, Langer A. How do researchers influence decision makers? Case studies of Mexican policies. *Health Policy Plan*. 1999;14(2):103–114.
7. Koppaka R. Ten great public health achievements—worldwide, 2001–2010. *MMWR*. 2011;60(24):814–818.
8. Orton L, Lloyd-Williams F, Taylor-Robinson D, O'Flaherty M, Capewell S. The use of research evidence in public health decision making processes: systematic review. *PLoS One*. 2011;6(7):e21704.
9. Brownson RC, Dodson EA, Stamatakis KA, et al. Communicating evidence-based information on cancer prevention to state-level policy makers. *J Natl Cancer Inst*. 2011;103:306–316.
10. Garvin T. Analytical paradigms: the epistemological distances between scientists, policy makers, and the public. *Risk Analysis*. 2001;21(3):443–445.
11. Brownson RC, Royer C, Ewing R, McBride TD. Researchers and policymakers: travelers in parallel universes. *Am J Prev Med*. 2006;30(2):164–172.
12. Nelson DE, Hesse B, Croyle R. *Making Data Talk: Communicating Public Health Findings to the Public, Policy Makers, and the Press*. New York: Oxford University Press; 2009.
13. Brownson RC, Chriqui JF, Stamatakis KA. Understanding evidence-based public health policy. *Am J Public Health*. 2009;99(9):1576–1583.
14. Stone DA. *Policy Paradox: The Art of Political Decision Making*. 3rd ed. New York: Norton; 2011.
15. Kingdon J. *Agendas, Alternatives, and Public Policies*, 2nd ed. Upper Saddle River, NJ: Pearson; 2010.

16. Birkland TA. *An Introduction to the Policy Process: Theories, Concepts, and Models of Public Policy Making.* 3rd ed. New York: Routledge; 2010.

17. National Cancer Institute. *Making Data Talk. A Workbook.* NIH Pub No. 11–7724. Rockville, MD: Author; 2011.

18. National Conference of State Legislatures. Legislator data. http://www.ncsl.org/research/about-state-legislatures/legislator-data.aspx. Accessed March 22, 2015.

19. Moreland-Russell S, Barbero C, Andersen S, Geary N, Dodson EA, Brownson RC. "Hearing from all sides" How legislative testimony influences state level policy-makers in the United States. *Int J Health Policy Manag.* 2015;4(2):91–98.

20. Brownson RC, Malone BR. Communicating public health information to policy makers. In: Nelson DE, Brownson RC, Remington PL, Parvanta C (Eds). *Communicating Public Health Information Effectively.* Washington, DC: American Public Health Association; 2002: 97–114.

21. Dodson EA, Stamatakis KA, Chalifour S, Haire-Joshu D, McBride T, Brownson RC. State legislators' work on public health-related issues: what influences priorities? *J Public Health Manag Pract.* 2013; 19(1):25–29.

22. Sorian R, Baugh T. Power of information: closing the gap between research and policy. *Health Affairs.* 2002;21(2):264–273.

23. Jones E, Kreuter M, Pritchett S, Matulionis RM, Hann N. State health policy makers: what's the message and who's listening? *Health Promot Pract.* 2006;7(3):280–286.

24. Janse G. Communication between forest scientists and forest policy-makers in Europe—a survey on both sides of the science/policy interface. *Forest Policy Economics.* 2008;10:183–194.

25. Innvaer S, Vist G, Trommald T, Oxman A. Health policy-makers' perceptions of their use of evidence: a systematic review. *J Health Services Res Policy.* 2002;7(4):239–244.

26. Schmidt AM, Ranney LM, Goldstein AO. Communicating program outcomes to encourage policymaker support for evidence-based state tobacco control. *Int J Environ Res Public Health.* 2014;11:12562–12574.

27. McBride T, Coburn A, MacKinney C, Mueller K, Slifkin R, Wakefield M. Bridging health research and policy: effective dissemination strategies. *J Public Health Manag Pract.* 2008;14(2):150–154.

28. Williams-Crowe SM, Aultman TV. State health agencies and the legislative policy process. *Public Health Rep.* 1994;109(3):361–367.

29. Campbell DM, Redman S, Jorm L, Cooke M, Zwi AB, Rychetnik L. Increasing the use of evidence in health policy: practice and views of policy makers and research. *Austral N Zealand Health Policy.* 2009;6:21.

30. Gandy, OH Jr. *Beyond Agenda Setting: Information Subsidies and Public Policy.* Norwood, NJ: Ablex Publishing; 1982.

31. Ragas MW. Agenda building during activist shareholder campaigns. *Public Relations Rev.* 2013;39(3):219–221.

32. Jones E, Eyler AA, Nguyen L, Kong J, Brownson RC, Bailey JH. It's all in the lens: differences in views on obesity prevention between advocates and policy makers. *Childhood Obesity.* 2012;8(3):243–250.

33. Deppen SA, Aldrich MC, Hartge P, Berg CD, Colditz GA, Petitti DB, et al. Cancer screening: the journey from epidemiology to policy. *Ann Epidemiol.* 2012;22:439–435.

34. McCombs M. *Setting the Agenda: Mass Media and Public Opinion.* 2nd ed. Malden, MA: Polity Press; 2014.

35. Rodari P, Bultitude K, Desborough K. Science communication between researchers and policy makers. Reflections from a European project. *J Science Comm*. 2012;11(3): C07.

36. Dorfman L, Krasnow ID. Public health and media advocacy. *Annu Rev Public Health*. 2014;35:293–306.

37. National Physical Activity Plan Alliance. 2014 United States Report Card on Physical Activity for Children and Youth. http://www.physicalactivityplan.org/reportcard/NationalReportCard_longform_final%20for%20web.pdf. Accessed March 22, 2015.

38. United States Department of Health and Human Services. Physical Activity Guidelines. Chapter 3: Active children and adolescents. http://www.health.gov/paguidelines/guidelines/chapter3.aspx#top. Accessed March 22, 2015.

39. Eyler AA, Brownson RC, Evenson KR, Levinger D, Maddock JE, Pluto D, et al. Policy influences on community trail development. *J Health Politics Policy Law*. 2008;33(3): 407–424.

40. Dodson EA, Fleming C, Boehmer TK, Haire-Joshu D, Luke DA, Brownson RC. Preventing childhood obesity through state policy: qualitative assessment of enablers and barriers. *J Public Health Policy*. 2009;30:S161–S176.

41. Brownson RC, Chriqui JF, Burgeson CR, Fisher MC, Ness RA. Translating epidemiology into policy to prevent childhood obesity: the case for promoting physical activity in school settings. *Ann Epidemiol*. 2010;20:436–444.

42. Brownson RC, Hartge P, Samet JM, Ness RB. From epidemiology to policy: toward more effective practice. *Ann Epidemiol*. 2010;20(6):409–411.

43. Davis FG, Peterson CE, Bandiera F, Carter-Pokras O, Brownson RC. How do we more effectively move epidemiology into policy action? *Ann Epidemiol*. 2012;22:413–416.

44. McDonough JE. *Experiencing Politics: A Legislator's Stories of Government and Health Care*. Berkeley, CA: University of California Press; 2000.

45. Warner KE. Bags, buckles, and belts: the debate over mandatory passive restraints in automobiles. *J Health Politics Policy Law*. 1983;8(1):44–75.

46. Pornpitkakpan C. The persuasiveness of source credibility: a critical review of five decades' evidence. *J Appl Social Psychol*. 2004;34(2):243–281.

47. Rother H-A. Communicating pesticide neurotoxicity research findings and risks to decision-makers and the public. *NeuroToxicology*. 2014;45:327–337.

48. Izumi BT, Schulz AJ, Israel BA, Reyes AG, Martin J, Lichtenstein RL, et al. The one-pager: a practical policy advocacy tool for translating community-based participatory research into action. *Prog Community Health Partnersh*. 2010;4(2):141–147.

49. Hyder AA, Corluka A, Winch PJ, El-Shinnawy A, Ghassany H, Malekafzali H, et al. National policy-makers speak out: are researchers giving them what they need? *Health Policy Planning*. 2011;26:73–82.

50. Wallack L, Winett L, Lee A. Successful public policy change in California: firearms and youth resources. *J Public Health Policy*. 2005;26:206–226.

51. Association of Asian Pacific Community Health Organizations. Hepatitis B. Policy Brief 2009. http://www.aapcho.org/wp/wp-content/uploads/2012/12/hep_policy_brief_2009_final_2.pdf. Accessed April 30, 2015.

52. Parvanta C, Nelson DE, Parvanta SA, Harner RN. *Essentials of Public Health Communication*. Sudbury, MA: Jones & Bartlett Learning; 2011.

53. Thompson T, Kreuter MW. Using written narratives in public health practice: A creative writing perspective. *Prev Chronic Dis*. 2014;11:130402.

54. Kreuter MW, Green MC, Cappella JN, et al. Narrative communication in cancer prevention and control: a framework to guide research and application. *Ann Behav Med.* 2007;33(3):221–235.
55. Kopfman JE, Smith SW, Ah Yun JK, Hodges A. Affective and cognitive reactions to narrative versus statistical evidence organ donation messages. *Journal of Applied Communications Research.* 1998;26:279–300.
56. Stamatakis KA, McBride TD, Brownson RC. Communicating prevention messages to policy makers: The role of stories in promoting physical activity. *J Phys Act Health.* 2010;7(1):S99–107.
57. Centers for Disease Control and Prevention. "Colorectal Cancer Personal Screening Stories." http://www.cdc.gov/cancer/colorectal/basic_info/stories.htm. Accessed March 22, 2015.
58. Centers for Disease Control and Prevention. Policy Impact: Prescription Painkiller Overdoses. http://www.cdc.gov/HomeandRecreationalSafety/pdf/PolicyImpact-Prescription PainkillerOD.pdf. Accessed March 14, 2015.
59. Centers for Disease Control and Prevention. Policy Impact: Teen Driver Safety. http://www.cdc.gov/motorvehiclesafety/pdf/policyimpact-teendriversafety-a.pdf. Accessed March 14, 2015.
60. Hsiao CJ, Hing E. Use and Characteristics of Electronic Health Record Systems among Office-based Physician Practices: United States, 2001–2013. National Center for Health Statistics Data Brief No. 143. 2014;143:1–8. http://www.cdc.gov/nchs/data/databriefs/db143.htm. Accessed March 22, 2015.
61. Widome R, Samet JM, Hiatt RA, Luke DA, Orleans T, Ponkshe P, et al. Science, prudence, and politics: the case of smoke-free indoor spaces. *Ann Epidemiol.* 2010;20:428–435.
62. Michaels, D. *Doubt Is Their Product: How Industry's Assault on Science Threatens your Health.* New York: Oxford University Press; 2008.
63. McGarrity TO, Wagner WE. *Bending Science: How Special Interests Corrupt Public Health.* Cambridge, MA: Harvard University Press; 2012.
64. Association of State and Territorial Health Officials. State Story. Minnesota increases tobacco taxes to reduce smoking. http://www.astho.org/Prevention/Tobacco/Case-Study/Minnesota/. Accessed March 23, 2015.
65. Brown LD. Knowledge and power: health services research as a political resource. In: Ginzberg E (Ed.). *Health Services Research: Key to Health Policy.* Cambridge, MA: Harvard University Press; 1991: 20–45.
66. Gostin LO. Law, ethics, and public health in the vaccination debates: politics of the measles outbreak. *JAMA: The Journal of the American Medical Association.* 2015;313(11):1099–100.
67. Constable C, Blank NR, Kaplan A. Rising rates of vaccine exemptions: problems with current policy and more promising remedies. *Vaccine.* 2014;32(16):1793–1797.
68. Abiola SE, Colgrove J, Mello M. The politics of HPV vaccination policy formation in the United States. *J Health Polit Policy Law.* 2013;38(4):645–681.
69. Pratt E Jr., Rawson RD, Rubin M. Fluoridation at fifty: what have we learned? *J Law Med Ethics.* 2002;30(Suppl 3):117–121.
70. Mertz A, Allukian M. Community water fluoridation on the Internet and social media. *J Mass Dental Soc.* Summer 2014. http://mydigimag.rrd.com/article/Community+Water+Fluoridation+on+the+Internet+and+Social+Media/1782859/0/article.html. Accessed February 17, 2015.

71. Kreuter M, Jones E, Pritchett S. Communicating effectiveness of health promotion to state-level decisionmakers and legislators. Directors of Health Promotion and Education. http://c.ymcdn.com/sites/www.dhpe.org/resource/resmgr/Docs/Communicating HealthPromotion.pdf?hhSearchTerms=%22white+and+paper%22. Accessed February 16, 2015.

72. Bogenschneider K, Corbett TJ. *Evidence-Based Policymaking: Insights from Policy-Minded Researchers and Research-Minded Policymakers*. New York: Routledge; 2010.

73. Cook C, Lane J. Legislator ideology and corrections and sentencing policy in Florida: a research note. *Criminal Justice Policy Rev.* 2009;20(2):209–235.

74. Likens GE. The role of science in decision making: Does evidence-based science drive environmental policy? *Front Ecol Environ.* 2010;8(6):e1–e9.

75. Swerda EL, Daynard R. Tobacco industry tactics. *Br Med J.* 1996;52(1):183–192.

76. Schiffman R. Harassment of climate scientists needs to stop. *The Guardian.* January 9, 2014. http://www.theguardian.com/commentisfree/2014/jan/09/denialist-harassment-of-climate-scientists-needs-to-stop. Accessed February 17, 2015.

77. Appel LJ, Angell SY, Cobb L, et al. Population-wide sodium reduction: the bumpy road from evidence to policy. *Ann Epidemiol.* 2012;22(6):417–425.

17

Advocacy and Public Health Policy

Roberta R. Friedman and Marlene B. Schwartz

The business of improving population health has always been linked to action. First document, then analyze, then act, then document the effect. Public health takes place in boardrooms, on street corners, in our homes, and in the legislature. So, too, does public health advocacy.
Mary T. Bassett[1]

LEARNING OBJECTIVES

1. Define advocacy as it relates to public health policy.
2. Explain how advocacy fits within the policy process.
3. Describe the importance of coalitions in advocacy efforts.
4. Describe steps in the advocacy process.

INTRODUCTION

Public health is the "the science and art of preventing disease, prolonging life and promoting health through organized efforts and informed choices of society, organizations, public and private, communities and individuals."[2] Public health research builds the knowledge base and identifies strategies to achieve health promotion and disease reduction. Advocacy uses these research findings to create new public policies to improve health outcomes. Many examples illustrate the critical role advocacy played in passing policies that have had a profound and positive impact on health in the United States. Among the best-known policies are tobacco taxes, seatbelt and recycling laws, and baby-friendly hospital initiatives to encourage breastfeeding.[3]

In this chapter, we define the term advocacy and describe the process of promoting policy change (see Chapter 3). We provide examples from the field of nutrition and childhood obesity to illustrate how advocates work to accomplish their goals. We also highlight the challenges encountered in changing policies, and the importance of understanding the larger political environment.

WHAT IS ADVOCACY?

Advocacy is "the act or process of supporting a cause or proposal."[4] Public health advocacy typically involves influencing legislative or regulatory decision-makers who have the power to change public policy. A successful advocate uses a range of tools and strategies to achieve the desired action. Typical strategies include the following:

- Explaining the benefits of the desired action (in person, in writing, or both), especially in terms of the problem(s) it will solve
- Anticipating objections and preparing responses to them
- Appealing to the emotions of the decision-makers or their constituents
- Forming coalitions
- Pointing to other decision-makers who have taken the requested action
- Negotiating

Not every strategy may fit the situation. The advocate must know enough about the key policymakers to choose the strategies that will have the most impact on their decisions.

Although many public health researchers and practitioners may not have thought about prevention in terms of "strategies" or "advocacy," they may have employed the skills of a successful advocate on a day-to-day basis. As conveyed in the case study below (see Table 17.1), advocacy is often used for something as simple as trying to convince someone to do something, the way Anna, a teenager, seeks to convince the decision-makers in her home (i.e., her parents) to help her reach her goal (getting a dog).

The goal of a public health advocate is to promote public policies that will create healthier environments. The term "environment" is extremely broad, and in this context can include nearly every place and situation a person encounters on a daily basis. To name a few examples, public policies have been proposed to influence a city's built environment (e.g., zoning laws that require new roads to include bike paths and sidewalks); the work environment (e.g., laws that make it illegal to not hire someone because he is obese); the retail environment (e.g., a law that requires only healthy snacks in the checkout lines at grocery stores); the restaurant environment (e.g., a law that requires calorie labeling on menus) and the media environment (e.g., a law that requires food items advertised during children's programming to meet certain nutritional standards).

KEY ELEMENTS IN POLICY

Public Health Policy Should Create Optimal Defaults

People make hundreds of choices every day that influence their health. Some of these choices are conscious and intentional decisions, but many are not. Because every decision requires time and consideration, most people make certain choices by simply following the default option (i.e., what will happen automatically if they do not take

Table 17.1 Case Study: Anna Wants a Dog

Describe the benefits of the desired action; explain the problem it will solve	Anna creates a list of reasons why having a dog will benefit the family, including the ways in which having a dog will mitigate other problems.	"I get lonely when I am home after school by myself and a dog will keep me company." "I'll feel safer with a dog." "It's important to get exercise and I've read that people who have dogs get more exercise."
Anticipate objections and prepare responses	Anna anticipates that her parents will think that a dog will mean more work for them. She knows she needs to convince them that this will not be the case.	"You won't have to do anything because I'll be responsible for feeding him and walking him when I get home from school every day."
Reinforce points with written materials	Anna knows that her parents may not believe she really will walk the dog every day because she does so many other activities.	"Here's a schedule to show you exactly when I will feed and walk the dog every school day and on the weekends."
Make emotional appeals	Anna's experience is that her parents really want her to be happy.	"I've been really sad lately. Having a dog will make me so happy."
Form a coalition	Anna has an older sibling who also wants a dog. They join forces to persuade their parents.	"We both want a dog and we'll work together to take care of the dog."
Point to other decision-makers who have done the requested action	Anna finds examples of other families who have dogs.	"Susie's parents got her a dog and now everyone loves the dog and says he is like a member of the family."
Negotiate	Anna thinks of what her parents really want her to do for them.	"I'll keep my grades up to prove I'm responsible. Then can we get a dog?"

active steps to opt out). Default choices are very influential, even though they may not be experienced as choices at all. For example, restaurant menus may offer meals that automatically come with French fries on the side (the default side dish). It is possible for the customer to substitute another option, such as a garden salad; however, in practice, most people simply accept the default choice rather than make the effort to ask for another option, and some of them may not even be aware that there is a choice.

But consider what would happen if the default side dish was a garden salad (the optimal default in terms of health promotion) and customers needed to specifically ask to substitute fries. Research suggests that salad consumption would increase and French fry consumption would decrease.[5] Based on this concept, advocates look for solutions in the form of policy to displace the unhealthful defaults in the environment with optimal defaults. (See Box 17.1.) The idea is to make the healthy choice the easy choice, or more accurately, the choice that one does not even have to make.

Policies that create optimal defaults usually focus on changing the environment rather than individual behavior. Opponents of these policies often invoke "personal responsibility" to shift attention away from the role of the environment and onto the individual.[6] Advocates need to anticipate this objection, which we discuss in the "solutions" section below.

Public Policy Should Be Effective and Based on Sound Science

The possibilities for new policies are endless. However, not all proposed solutions will be effective; some may lack scientific evidence to support them, and some may even have unintended consequences. This is why public health advocacy is important. Effective advocacy includes providing policymakers with data and other scientific evidence that document the problem in depth, offers solutions based on best practices, and, if possible, provides an analysis of the consequences, both intended and unintended, of the proposed policy. Many policymakers have come to rely on public health professionals for this information.

Public Policy Should Create Health Equity

All Americans do not have the same opportunities to be healthy and to make healthy choices. Sometimes, barriers to health and to healthier decisions are too high for individuals to overcome, even with great motivation.
Braveman and Egerter[7]

Box 17.1 Case Study: Changing the Default in Kids' Meals

Kids' meals at fast food restaurants were designed to default automatically to French fries as a side dish and soda as a beverage, even though other options were available by request. A Rudd Center study documented that McDonald's, Burger King, Wendy's, and KFC were all more likely to provide the less healthy options with kids' meals when the consumer did not specify a choice. As a result of public health advocacy, in 2011, McDonald's changed its default side dish to a serving of both apple slices and French fries, instead of only fries.[26] In 2015, Burger King announced that it would default to water or low-fat milk as a beverage, rather than soda.[27] If a parent prefers to give her child a soda, she must request one to substitute for the water or milk. These new practices help create an optimal default for kids' meals, and make it easier for parents to feed their children a more healthful diet.

Health disparities (defined as "types of unfair health differences closely linked with social, economic or environmental disadvantages that adversely affect groups of color"[8]) are a considerable problem in the United States. Public health policy work should also address health disparities and seek to promote health *equity*. (See Figure 17.1.) Health equity is achieved when every person is given the opportunity to "attain his or her full health potential" and no one is "disadvantaged from achieving this potential because of social position or other socially determined circumstances."[9] Achieving health equity in the United States requires, among other things, steps to mitigate the impact of chronic diseases on disparately affected populations. Creating optimal defaults can promote health *equality*, but that is often not enough. As the cartoon illustrates, with health equality, everyone gets a box to stand on to watch the game. But the "give everyone one box" strategy has not taken into account the differences in height of the target population, and, therefore, the goal of seeing the field to watch the game has not been *equitably* addressed. An advocate should analyze proposed policies for all intended and unintended outcomes in terms of both equality and equity, and support policy language that ensures that the populations that need an extra boost will get it.

LOBBYING

Lobbying can be an important tool for advocacy, but advocacy and lobbying are two different processes. Lobbying involves communicating with a legislator to intentionally influence the way he or she will support or vote for a specific piece of legislation.

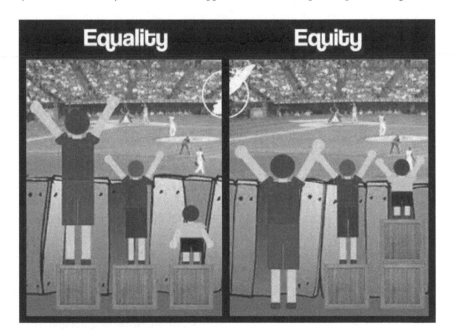

Figure 17.1 Policies should create equity.
Source: http://themetapicture.com/equality-vs-equity/ Accessed March 24, 2015.

Lobbying can be *direct* or *grassroots*. Direct lobbying includes a communication (e.g., a visit, call, or letter) directly to a legislator that reflects a view on a particular piece of legislation. For example, if one writes a letter to one's state representative requesting that she vote in favor of Senate Bill Number 123 that proposes banning smoking from public parks, that is lobbying.[10]

Grassroots lobbying is the process of expressing a view to the public on a certain piece of legislation and including a "call to action." Specifically, this involves asking members of the public to contact their legislators, and providing the public with information on who their legislators are, along with contact information and a way to contact them (e.g., through a petition or a form e-mail). The communication also identifies the legislator's position on a specific bill or notifies the public that the legislator sits on a committee that will vote on the bill. The fictional e-mail below is an example of grassroots lobbying.

Subject: Support House Bill 632
From: Sugar Action Coalition
To: Charlotte Babbin

Dear Charlotte:
Congresswoman Sweeten from your district has said that she will not support House Bill 632, "An act to remove sugar-sweetened beverages from schools." Sugar-sweetened beverages are the single largest source of added sugar in children's diets and have been linked to increases in obesity and type II diabetes. We know you care about the health of the children in your state. Please show your support for this legislation by clicking the link below to send Congresswoman Sweeten an e-mail asking her to support House Bill 632.

For many advocates, lobbying is an intrinsic part of policy advocacy. But for others, lobbying may be restricted or prohibited altogether depending on the tax status of the organization, agency, or academic institution that the advocate represents. For instance, employees of a charitable organization with 501(c)(3) status can legally conduct a limited amount of lobbying, but may have to receive permission to engage in lobbying activity. On the other hand, employees of a private university may be asked by the university's Office of Federal Relations to restrict lobbying activity or to limit and track lobbying hours. Before beginning advocacy work, public health practitioners should find out the tax status of their organization and whether or not lobbying is permitted; they should also learn the definition of lobbying under the governing state's laws.

There are many ways to advocate on behalf of a public health issue without crossing the line into lobbying. For example, submission of a public comment on a proposed regulation, or completion of objective research and analysis on an issue can be used to communicate findings to policymakers. If invited by a legislative committee to testify, this activity would include providing perspective on the issue before the legislature. Perhaps the most common nonlobbying way to deliver public health messages to policymakers and the public is to educate them about the issue before legislation is introduced. To return to our example above, a student advocate could have sent the following e-mail to Congresswoman Sweeten before the sugar-sweetened beverage bill was introduced. Such a message would not be considered lobbying because it does not refer to a specific piece of active legislation.

Subject: Soda machines don't belong in high schools
From: Molly Babbin
To: Congresswoman Sweeten

Dear Congresswoman Sweeten:
My high school has six vending machines filled with soda, sports drinks, and sweetened teas. I see students drinking these beverages every day in my school. I do not think that schools should be selling sugary drinks to students. I learned in health class that these beverages are the single largest source of added sugar in children's diets and have been linked to increases in obesity and type II diabetes. I also learned that some beverage companies pay schools to sell only their brands. I think this is wrong. Why is my school taking money from companies to sell soda when we are taught in class that soda is not healthy? I think this is a big problem.

WHO CAN ADVOCATE?

Individuals, organizations, and coalitions can all advocate. As seen in the above example, an individual high school student can be an advocate. In fact, individuals can be remarkably influential advocates if they have a powerful personal story to tell. One of the largest and most successful advocacy groups in the world, Mothers Against Drunk Driving, was founded by an individual, Candy Lightner, whose daughter was killed by a drunk driver in 1980.[11] More recently, former Congresswoman Gabrielle Giffords became an advocate for gun control laws following the attempt on her life in January 2011.[12] She and her husband began an organization called Americans For Responsible Solutions, which seeks to require background checks before gun purchases and to keep guns out of the hands of people who are mentally ill.[13]

Although individuals and organizations can advocate on their own, coalitions are particularly effective for public health advocacy. A coalition is a group of organizations that come together to achieve a goal on a shared interest. A coalition can include for-profit companies, nonprofit organizations, grassroots groups, state and local health departments, academics and researchers, faith-based organizations, and health and social justice organizations. The individual organizations may have differing, or even conflicting, missions, but they come together to agree on a solution to a particular problem that affects their collective constituencies. It is important to form coalitions early in the advocacy process. The coalition should include, if not be led by, organizations that represent those most adversely affected by the problem all are trying to prevent.

STEPS IN THE ADVOCACY PROCESS

There are a number of steps in the advocacy process, and the process is not always linear. The sections below identify some key parts of the process, although not every advocacy effort will include all parts or occur in this order. These steps complement the guidance on communicating with policymakers in Chapter 16.

1. Define the problem and outline possible solutions

After the general issue for advocacy attention has been identified, it is important to begin to collect information that is directly and indirectly related to it. A list of questions about the issue is a good place to start. Examples might include:

- What national, state, regional, or local data are available to document the scope of the problem?
- Who is affected by the problem? Identify:

  - Percentage of the population affected
  - Percentage of low-income or vulnerable populations affected relative to others
  - Regional differences in impact

- What has been written on the issue? Collect:

  - Studies and commentaries published in peer-reviewed journals that are directly or indirectly related
  - Media coverage: editorials, opinion pieces, investigative journalism
  - Blogs

- What is the economic impact of the problem?

  - Identify the healthcare costs associated with the problem
  - Document if the problem has an impact on employee absenteeism or presenteeism (i.e., attending work while ill)

- What work is presently being done on it by governmental and nongovernmental (national, state, local) agencies?
- What are some possible solutions?

  - Are they "reasonable and justifiable?"[14]
  - Have they been evaluated? If so, are they scientifically based and likely to be effective?
  - What are the costs?

Although defining the problem may seem like a straightforward process, some problems are so large that the field must revisit these questions repeatedly throughout the advocacy effort. For example, childhood obesity is an extremely complicated problem, with hundreds of studies and reports that attempt to identify the extent of it, its causes, and what to do about it. The first Institute of Medicine (IOM) report on childhood obesity, titled *Preventing Childhood Obesity: Health in the Balance,* was published in 2004.[15] Over the subsequent decade, dozens of additional IOM workshops have been held and reports written; each revisits a particular aspect of the problem and looks at new possibilities for prevention and evaluation, such as improving school meals, increasing physical activity, engaging local governments, and measuring progress.

2. Form a Coalition

As we noted above, individuals certainly can advocate on their own, but coalitions can be particularly powerful and effective in public health advocacy. One key to forming an effective coalition is to include a variety of members, including ones who might not be immediately obvious as advocates on your issue. To help identify potential coalition members, create an "asset map." (See Table 17.2.) Such a map lists the skills, knowledge, representation, and resources needed in order to achieve the policy change sought. By plugging in the existing members' assets, gaps can be identified and filled by inviting other members to join. Once a member list is established, it is important to convene the group to begin the process of agreeing on a solution or solutions and drafting the appropriate policy language to achieve them.

Asset-mapping example: The Food Marketing Workgroup[16]

In 2007, the first meeting of the Food Marketing Workgroup was convened in Washington DC to establish a policy agenda for food and beverage marketing to children. As its statement of purpose explains:

The need to limit marketing of unhealthy food to children has never been more urgent. According to the Institute of Medicine, most foods marketed to children are high in sugars, saturated fat, and salt—and marketing influences what children and adolescents eat. Aggressive, widespread food marketing undermines parents' attempts to feed their children healthfully. Food companies spend $2 billion annually to reach children through television, the Internet, mobile phones, magazines, product placement in movies and television, product packages, toys, and anywhere else a logo or product image can be shown. The Food Marketing Workgroup (FMW) believes we can and must do better.

Today, the coalition consists of more than 200 members, with a steering committee of 13 organizations and individuals. The organizations bring a wealth of assets to the workgroup. For example (a partial list):

Table 17.2 Asset-mapping

Asset Needed	Representation
Media expertise and advocacy	Berkeley Media Studies Group
	Center for Digital Democracy
	Common Sense Media
	Campaign for a Commercial-Free Childhood
Target population expertise	Praxis Project
	Black Women's Health Imperative
	California Pan-Ethnic Health Network
	Hispanic Dental Association
	League of United Latin American Citizens
	NAACP
Research expertise	UConn Rudd Center for Food Policy and Obesity
	African American Collaborative Obesity Research Network
	Commercialism in Education Research Unit, National Education Policy Center
Issue-focused public health	Academy of General Dentistry
	American College of Preventive Medicine
	American Diabetes Association
	American Heart Association
	National Action Against Obesity
Education	National Association of State Boards of Education
	American School Health Association
Nutrition expertise	American Academy of Sports Dietitians and Nutritionists
	Gretchen Swanson Center for Nutrition
Legal expertise	ChangeLab Solutions
	Public Health Law Center
Youth	Youth Empowered Solutions (YES!)
	Youth Leadership Institute

3. Begin "Ground Softening"

Once a coalition has identified the specific aspect of the problem to address, they need to raise awareness about the issue among the public and government decision-makers (legislators, agency officials, or both), and explain why it is a public health issue, who is affected, and what policy solutions are warranted. This process, sometimes called "ground softening," is often a necessary first step before viable legislation can be introduced. An advocacy role in this first phase is of an expert and educator who introduces people to the problem and explains why it should be a priority.

In 2009, the New York City Department of Health and Human Hygiene launched its "Pouring on the Pounds"[17] public awareness campaign to educate New Yorkers about the relationship between consumption of sugary beverages and weight gain. A centerpiece of the multifaceted campaign was a short video depicting soda turning to fat as it is poured into a glass, and a man drinking the fat. This was accompanied by posters, brochures, and other educational materials, as well as other videos, and served to raise awareness about the harmful role that sugary drinks play in weight gain and obesity. The campaign served to educate the public (soften the ground) in preparation for proposals designed to help New Yorkers limit the amount of sugary drinks they consume, such as the "portion cap" policy on the size of sugary beverages that could be sold in food service establishments regulated by the Department.[18]

4. Determine Who Has the Power to Make the Change Sought

Public health policy can be accomplished on local, state, and national levels. A coalition may decide that the best initial approach will be to change policy on a local level, before trying for statewide or even national change. This was a successful strategy in the fight to restrict smoking in public places:

> In 1990, the community of San Luis Obispo, California, adopted the first law in the United States eliminating smoking in bars. During the 1990s, smoke-free bar laws were largely limited to communities in California and Massachusetts.... The progress made during the past decade in enacting comprehensive state smoke-free laws is an extraordinary public health achievement. In the span of 10 years, smoke-free workplaces, restaurants, and bars went from being relatively rare to being the norm in half of the states and DC. Several factors appear to have contributed to this outcome . . . as state and local smoke-free laws were enacted across the country, other states and communities learned from the experiences of similar jurisdictions and were able to adapt and implement such laws.[19]

Once the coalition identifies the policy to pursue and the jurisdiction in which to make an impact, the next step is to do the necessary research to determine who has the power to make the desired change. It may be the head of the local town council, the state Speaker of the House or Senate President, a potential sponsor of a future bill, or the chair of a key committee in Congress. Or it may be the director or staff of the municipal, state, or federal agency with the responsibility for relevant regulation.

The coalition members already may have built relationships with the individuals who have the power to make the proposed policy changes. But if not, background research on key people helps to determine how best to approach them. You can accomplish this by conducting "pathways of influence"[20] research to discover answers to the following questions:

- Do they have personal connections to your issue?
- What are their current positions? What are their future ambitions?
- How have they talked about or voted on your issue?
- What is their social media presence?

- What motivates their colleagues?
- What do their constituents care about?
- Who are their financial supporters?
- What are their favorite sources of news and information?
- What are their pet issues?

As this list illustrates, legislators and government officials are *people*, who have personal viewpoints, preferences, histories, and interests that affect how they carry out their work. Learning what key decision-makers care about and are motivated by, who they know and are influenced by, what kinds of arguments are and are not effective with them, and what positions they previously have taken on similar issues, will help determine how to frame the issue in a way that can spark their interest in a particular cause.

5. Translate Research for Decision-makers and the Public

Policymakers have multiple competing demands and priorities and limited time and attention, which can make them particularly challenging to reach. An advocate must be able to quickly convince the policymaker that her issue is important and present a compelling case of why a change in public policy is necessary. Coalition members can identify the key scientific studies related to making the case. Scientific studies are often not user-friendly for nonscientists; they can be difficult to interpret and full of unfamiliar jargon. Therefore, a key part of the advocacy process is to work with coalition partners to translate the studies, data, and tables into easy-to-understand fact sheets, policy briefs, and one-pagers for policymakers and the public. Graphic representations of compelling research findings can communicate the importance of a policy issue or intervention quickly and clearly. All materials should include references to the sources of the data and should be in formats that are easy for the coalition to disseminate.

The example below is taken from a fact sheet written for advocating policies to help Americans decrease their intake of added sugars. (See Figure 17.2.) The data are from a U.S. national survey of dietary intake and the sources of added sugar in people's diets. The graph makes it easy to see that sugary drinks are providing a significant amount of added sugar to the diets of adults and children, and helps policymakers understand why these products are important to address with public policy.

How Much Added Sugar Do Foods And Beverages
Contribute To Our Diets?[21]

Foods and beverages contribute nearly the same percentage of added sugar to the diets of 2- to 19-year-olds (52% and 48% respectively). **Soda is the single largest source of added sugar (22.8%).**

Policymakers, other decision-makers, or members of the coalition may ask questions that require additional research. Coalition members who are researchers should

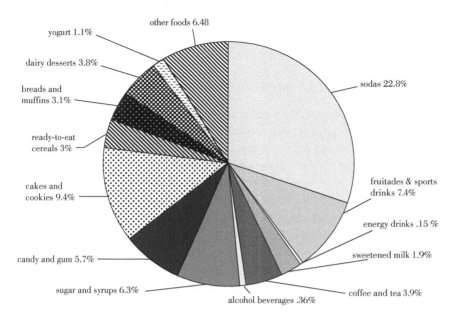

Figure 17.2 Sources of added sugar in the diets of adults and children 2 years and older; NHANES 2007–2008.

Source: Welsh JA, Sharma AJ, Grellinger L, Vos MB. Consumption of added sugars is decreasing in the United States. *Am J Clin Nutr.* 2011;94(3):726–734.

be made aware of research needs, and, if it is not possible for them to conduct the research, should communicate this need to other researchers in the field, so that the policy discussion can move forward. (See Box 17.2.)

As we mentioned above in the "Form a Coalition" section, effective coalitions often include organizations that might not be immediately obvious as advocates on the policy issue. This may prove helpful when it comes time to provide policymakers with analyses of other potential impacts of a policy, beyond those of public health. For example, a state legislator may want to know what the economic impact of a policy solution will be on jobs or the state budget; a local city council person may want to understand how his business district will benefit from a proposed policy. If policy

---

Box 17.2 Case Study: Finances versus Nutrition Standards in Schools

Advocates for better school food have been working for years to improve the nutrition standards of "competitive foods," which are the foods sold or served in vending machines, school stores, and a la carte lines, separately from the National School Lunch Program menu. Opponents of change argued that switching to healthier snacks in middle and high schools would be too expensive, causing the school to suffer serious financial consequences. In order to study this issue, the Centers for Disease Control and Prevention supported a research project to identify and understand the experiences of a sample of school districts around the country that had been able to successfully implement strong competitive food standards without negative financial consequences.[28]

---

sponsors are provided with information about the broader impacts of a proposal, they will be better positioned to gain the support of their colleagues.

6. Understand the Opposition

Whenever policy change is proposed, it inevitably encounters opposition. It may come from industry, or from government entities being lobbied by industry; it may come from grassroots advocacy organizations, or from politicians who are on the other end of the political spectrum from those advocating for it. It may even come from people or organizations who are usually allies on other issues. No matter who the opposition is, what viewpoints they represent, or what the potential solution is, it is critical to a successful advocacy campaign to know as much about the opposition as possible, learn what their arguments will be, and prepare counterarguments in response. It is possible, of course, to work on an issue that has a "win-win" outcome for both sides. Even so, preparing for opposition is critical.

If the issue is one that has already been through a legislative cycle, public testimony from hearings, news articles, the opposition's website, or even social media can be used to find out how the opposition frames their arguments. (See Box 17.3.) Review other public health campaigns, even on different health issues, for patterns in how an affected industry will oppose the policy. Brownell and Warner, for example, illustrate the similarities between the "playbook" that the tobacco industry used to oppose tobacco taxes and the strategies employed by large food companies to oppose sugary-drink taxes. They describe how in both situations the industry in question invoked

---

Box 17.3 Case Study: Opposition to Sugary Drink Taxes

As coalitions in states and localities around the country have prepared campaigns to pass excise taxes on sugary drinks (to reduce consumption and raise revenue for obesity and diabetes prevention) they have had ample opportunity to observe how the beverage industry routinely responds. By analyzing the industry's antitax ads, listening to industry representatives in media interviews, and studying their testimony and that of other opponents, advocates were able to write responses to the arguments against taxes, and prepare their coalitions, policymakers, and other allies to publicly respond to the industry's assertions.

Testimony of Dr. Danielle Greenberg, PepsiCo Inc. before the New York State Joint Legislative Committees on the 2010–2011 Executive Budget, Health/Medicaid Proposals February 9, 2010
. . .*The only way to address the multi-faceted problem of obesity is with comprehensive approaches that address both sides of the energy balance equation: that is the calories we consume in our total diet need to balance with the calories we burn through our daily activities and through planned exercise. Weight management is really very simple—not EASY—but simple. It's all about energy balance and any solution to the obesity challenge must address both sides of the equation—through education, balanced diets, and physical activity.*

---

arguments about personal responsibility; challenged the science that had been done on the issue as biased or inaccurate; funded scientists who did studies that supported industry arguments; vilified critics; and spent tremendous resources lobbying legislators to protect their interests.[22]

7. Understand Public Opinion

Once supporting and opposing parties are defined, it is important to understand the public's opinion on the issue. Are most people aware of the problem? Do people already have strong feelings one way or another about possible solutions? Do attitudes about the issue tend to be associated with particular demographic characteristics, such as sex, age, socioeconomic status, race, ethnicity, political orientation, or geography?

If resources are available, a useful tool to understand the public's opinion regarding an issue is a public opinion survey. Media outlets, universities, and professional organizations that regularly conduct national public opinion polls can be important partners in designing and administering the survey. The goal of a survey is to understand allies and opponents, and identify the biggest obstacles to public acceptance of the policy proposal. Polling also can be used as an advocacy strategy to raise public awareness and gain legislator support. A poll that shows substantial support for a policy near the date of the hearing or vote can reassure the legislators involved that they are reflecting the desires of the people they represent.

8. Outline a Set of Possible Solutions

As we noted above, identifying solutions can be a long and complex process. Begin by working with the coalition to identify a range of possible policy solutions. Formative research, including a literature search for systematic reviews (i.e., syntheses of research studies on a particular topic) and evaluations of experiments and other initiatives that have been tested and found to be successful, can help in identifying possible solutions. This process will help weed out solutions that have no evidence of being effective. Discuss the pros and cons of each strategy with the coalition. Which solutions hold the promise of achieving the maximum impact? Consider health equity—will the proposed solutions reach the populations most affected? Are some solutions good but unrealistic? Or, are they asking for too much? In order to build momentum toward an ultimate goal, advocates sometimes decide to pursue policies with a higher likelihood of success, even if those policies on their own may have limited impact (see Box 17.4).

8. Consider Unintended Consequences

Talking to any and all parties who may be affected by the proposed policy approach, especially those parties who will need to implement the changes, will help to prevent

Box 17.4 Case Study: School Wellness Policies

In the early 2000s advocates were interested in reducing or eliminating unhealthy snacks and beverages from schools. Many wanted federal regulation to require the complete removal of these products, but there was not enough political will or public support to achieve this goal. An interim policy was proposed instead, requiring school districts to write "wellness policies," which would include setting nutritional standards for competitive foods. Although the requirement to have a wellness policy did not guarantee that any districts would remove unhealthy competitive foods, it did increase the public's awareness of the issue and created an opportunity for local school districts to discuss the topic. Eventually, as public support grew, the federal government was able to push forward new regulations for competitive foods through the Healthy, Hunger-Free Kids Act.

unintended consequences (see Box 17.5). Coalition members can help identify these key stakeholders.

9. Plan Your Media Advocacy Strategy

Media advocacy harnesses the power of the news to mobilize advocates and apply pressure for policy change. . . . The public and policymakers do not consider issues seriously unless they are visible, and they are not visible unless the media have brought them to light.
Lori Dorfman and Priscilla Gonzalez[23]

In order to gain public support for a policy, the public must be informed about the issue and made aware of the proposed policy solution. Newspaper and electronic media are

Box 17.5 Case Study of Unintended Consequences: How Sodium Became Chocolate

A Connecticut state legislator wanted to create a policy to reduce the amount of sodium that children were consuming in meals at school. When he learned that there was sodium added to the milk being served, he introduced a policy that would set a sodium limit on the milk purchased by the food service. He did not realize, however, that there were no chocolate milk products on the market that met the proposed sodium limits. His sodium reduction policy quickly became an anti-chocolate milk policy. The advocates representing the state's school nutrition association and the dairy council came out strongly against the policy. The advocates who typically support improvements to the school food environment were caught in a bind because while they wanted to support the sodium reduction, they were not prepared to take on the issue of removing chocolate milk from schools. The bill passed the both houses of the legislature, but was vetoed by the governor.[29] If the legislator who had introduced the bill had met with the school nutrition advocacy groups while crafting the original policy, this situation might have been avoided.

principal forums for educating the public. The traditional, and still useful, approach to generating media attention is the press release, or in some cases, the press conference. Whenever there is an event, a legislative development, or a new poll or research article, a coalition can write a short (one- or two-page) statement about it and send this to media organizations. Press releases also can be posted on coalition websites. A good press release should be brief, clear, and quotable. Not every press release gets journalists' attention, but some serve as the basis for widely read and influential articles.

A media strategy is an important element in every advocacy campaign. Even in the absence of time or resources to support a sophisticated campaign, media can be utilized to draw attention to the issue. Low-cost methods include writing letters to the editor, writing opinion editorials for the newspapers that key decision-makers read, and reaching audiences through social media. Today, advocacy campaigns use blogs, Facebook, Twitter, Instagram, YouTube, and Snapchat, and by the time this book is published, there will no doubt be many more electronic communication platforms from which to choose.

Sometimes earned media can be used to get journalists' attention. For example, in 2007 when the California legislature was considering a bill on restaurant menu labeling, the California Center for Public Health Advocacy (CCPHA) posted an apparently simple quiz on its website.

The 'fast food nutrition quiz' included four seemingly easy questions about items served at fast food restaurants, asking participants to pick the one they thought had the fewest calories, salt, or fat. No one answered all four questions correctly, and 68% were unable to answer even one correctly. These scores were poor regardless of education or income levels. When CCPHA. . . distributed the quiz to the media, their strategy proved to be exceptionally smart and, inadvertently, because became a strategic viral marketing tool. When journalists took the quiz and did as poorly as the average citizen, their amazement at their own ignorance and inability to answer the questions correctly prompted them to send the quiz to other pressrooms around the state. After that the story 'wrote itself,'. . .showing up in editorials, features, and food sections in all the major California newspapers, and many local papers as well.[24]

10. Evaluate Your Advocacy Efforts

Whether or not advocacy work ends successfully with policy change, it is always important to evaluate your efforts. There are several reasons for this. Policy change rarely takes place quickly, and it often requires multiple attempts by advocates. Evaluation helps to document what did and did not work in the advocacy campaign and the lessons learned in the process. Sharing evaluation results also can help others working on the same, or similar, policy goals. Demonstrating to potential funders why your policy solution will be an improvement over what was done previously can help to secure future funding for more policy work on the same issue.

Various aspects of a campaign can be evaluated. For instance, evaluation can include examining organizational capacity, alliances, or strength of support. Other ideas for evaluation include an assessment of improved policies resulting from advocacy efforts, and if implemented, the changes in impact.[25] Even if a formal evaluation is not conducted, informal evaluations and lessons learned in the form of short policy briefs or case studies also can be useful to the field. Interviewing a wide range of people, including representatives of health equity organizations, is needed to gain insight into the extent to which the work was inclusive and focused on the communities most affected by the issue and potential policy solution.

CONCLUSION

Advocacy or the "act of supporting a policy or proposal" is a critical part of public health practice. Sound public health policy creates optimal defaults, promotes health equity, is based on thorough science, and changes the environments in which we live, work, and play to make it easy to practice healthful behavior. Lobbying can be an important tool for advocacy, but significant progress in public health policy can still be achieved without lobbying. Although individuals and organizations can advocate on their own, coalitions are particularly effective for public health advocacy.

We have identified a number of steps in the advocacy process, from defining the problem and outlining possible solutions, to forming a coalition, doing "ground softening" education, and determining who has the power to make changes. Other important steps include translating research for decision-makers and the public, understanding public opinion on the issue and any possible opposition, proposing policy solutions, and creating a media plan. Finally, public health advocates should always evaluate their efforts and share the results.

REFERENCES

1. Bassett MT. Public health advocacy. *Am J Public Health.* 2003;93(8):1204.
2. Winslow CEA. The untilled fields of public health. *Science.*1920;51(1306):23–33.
3. Economos CD, Brownson RC, DeAngelis MA, et al. What lessons have been learned from other attempts to guide social change? *Nutr Rev.* 2001;59(3):S40–S56.
4. Merriam-Webster website. http://www.merriam-webster.com/dictionary/advocacy. Accessed January 28, 2015.
5. Radnitz C, Loeb KL, DiMatteo J, Keller KL, Zucker N, Schwartz MB. Optimal defaults in the prevention of pediatric obesity: from platform to practice. *J Food Nutr Disord.* 2013;2(5):1.
6. Brownell KD, Kersh R, Ludwig DS, et al. Personal responsibility and obesity: a constructive approach to a controversial issue. *Health Aff (Millwood).* 2010;29(3):379–387.
7. Braveman P, Egerter S. Overcoming obstacles to health in 2013 and beyond. *Robert Wood Johnson Foundation Commission to Build a Healthier America.* 2013; http://www.rwjf.org/content/dam/farm/reports/reports/2013/rwjf406474. Accessed March 24, 2015.

8. Brennan Ramirez LK, Baker EA, Metzler M. Promoting health equity: A resource to help communities address social determinants of health. In: *Promoting Health Equity: A Resource to Help Communities Address Social Determinants of Health*. Atlanta, GA: Centers for Disease Control and Prevention; 2008. http://www.cdc.gov/nccdphp/dch/programs/healthycommunitiesprogram/overview/healthequity.htm. Accessed March 22, 2015.

9. Brennan Ramirez LK, Baker EA, Metzler M. Promoting health equity: A resource to help communities address social determinants of health. In: *Promoting Health Equity: A Resource To Help Communities Address Social Determinants of Health*. Atlanta, GA: Centers for Disease Control and Prevention; 2008:111.

10. Federal law defines and regulates lobbying the federal government, and the law of each state defines and regulates lobbying in that state.

11. Candy Lightner. The Biography.com website. 2015; http://www.biography.com/people/candy-lightner-21173669. Accessed March 22, 2015.

12. Gabrielle Giffords. The Biography.com website. 2015; http://www.biography.com/people/gabrielle-giffords-20550593. Accessed March 22, 2015.

13. Newcomb A, Zak L, Giffords, K. Say "Enough" to gun violence on the 2nd anniversary of Tucson shooting. *ABC News*. January 8, 2013. http://abcnews.go.com/US/giffords-kelly-gun-violence-2nd-anniversary-tucson-shooting/story?id=18145328&singlePage=true. Accessed March 21, 2015.

14. Goldstein H. Commentary: translating research into public policy. *J Public Health Policy*. 2009;30(Suppl 1):S16–S20.

15. Kraak VA, Liverman CT, Koplan JP. *Preventing Childhood Obesity: Health in the Balance*. Washington, DC: The National Academies Press; 2005. http://www.iom.edu/Reports/2004/Preventing-Childhood-Obesity-Health-in-the-Balance.aspx. Accessed March 24, 2015.

16. Food Marketing Workgroup. http://www.foodmarketing.org. Accessed March 24, 2015.

17. New York City Department of Health and Mental Hygiene. Pouring on the Pounds Campaign. http://www.nyc.gov/html/doh/html/living/sugarydrink-media-archive.shtml. Accessed March 24, 2015.

18. New York City Department of Health and Mental Hygiene. Your kids could be drinking themselves sick. http://www.nyc.gov/html/doh/html/living/cdp_pan_pop.shtml. Accessed March 24, 2015.

19. Centers for Disease Control and Prevention (CDC). State smoke-free laws for worksites, restaurants, and bars—United States, 2000–2010. *MMWR*. 2011;60(15):472–475. doi: mm6015a2 [pii].

20. Fresina L, Pickles D. PowerPrism: A tool for advocacy, planning, execution and evaluation. http://www.powerprism.org. Accessed March 25, 2015.

21. Rudd Center for Food Policy and Obesity. Added Sugars Fact Sheet. 2014; http://www.uconnruddcenter.org/sugary-drinks-issue-overview-and-fact-sheets. Accessed March 24, 2015.

22. Brownell KD, Warner KE. The perils of ignoring history: Big Tobacco played dirty and millions died. How similar is Big Food? *Milbank Q*. 2009;87(1):259–294.

23. Dorfman L, Gonzalez P. Media advocacy: a strategy for helping communities change policy. In Minkler M. (Ed.), *Community Organizing and Community Building for Health and Welfare*. Rutgers University Press; 2012.

24. Rudd Center for Food Policy and Obesity, Yale University. A case study of California's menu labeling legislation. 2008; http://www.uconnruddcenter.org/resources/upload/

docs/what/policy/CaliforniaSB120MenuLabelCaseStudy.pdf. Accessed March 25, 2015.

25. Reisman J, Gienapp A, Stachowiak S. A guide to measuring policy and advocacy. Organizational Research Services. 2007; http://www.organizationalresearch.com/publicationsandresources/a_guide_to_measuring_advocacy_and_policy.pdf. Accessed April 15, 2015.

26. Baertlein, L. McDonald's Happy Meals get apples, fewer fries. *Reuters.* July 26, 2011. http://www.reuters.com/article/2011/07/26/us-mcdonalds-idUSTRE76P41I20110726. Accessed April 15, 2015.

27. Horovitz B. Burger King drops soft drinks from kids' meals. *USA Today.* March 10, 2015. http://www.usatoday.com/story/money/2015/03/09/burger-king-fast-food-restaurants-soft-drinks-beverages/24661959/. Accessed April 15, 2015

28. Bassler EJ, Chriqui JF, Stagg K, Schneider LM, Infusino K, Asada Y. *Controlling Junk Food and the Bottom Line: Case Studies of Schools Successfully Implementing Strong Nutrition Standards for Competitive Foods and Beverages.* Chicago: Illinois Public Health Institute; 2013; http://iphionline.org/2013/03/controlling-junk-food/. Accessed April 15, 2015.

29. Blad, E. Chocolate milk almost accidentally banned in Connecticut schools. *Education Week.* May 2014. http://blogs.edweek.org/edweek/rulesforengagement/2014/05/chocolate_milk_almost_accidentally_banned_in_connecticut_schools.html. Accessed March 23, 2015.

18

Future Directions for Improving Public Health through Policy

Ross C. Brownson and Amy A. Eyler

"Prediction is very difficult, especially if it's about the future."
Nils Bohr, Nobel laureate in physics

LEARNING OBJECTIVES

1. Describe issues related to advancing practice and research in public health policy.
2. Report emerging trends for policy, prevention, and public health.
3. Recommend new policy-related skills for the public health workforce.

INTRODUCTION

As described in the earlier chapters in this book, health policies (in the form of laws, regulations, organizational practices, and funding priorities) have a substantial impact on the health and well-being of populations. One simple way of measuring policy-related impact is in the life expectancy, which grew very slowly for two millennia. Yet we have had remarkable gains in the past few centuries, particularly in the last century. Since 1900, Americans have gained over 30 years of life[1]; put another way, for every week of time that has elapsed, we have gained an average of two additional days of life. This is remarkable and is due largely to health-related policy measures, such as motor vehicle safety, safer workplaces, family-planning policies, laws regulating tobacco use, and vaccination policies.[2] One of the advantages of policy interventions for population health is that policies often cross-cut numerous risk factors and conditions and reduce the emphasis on a "silo'd" approach to public health (i.e., separate programs/policies for every major risk factor and disease).[3-7]

In this chapter, we highlight several topics that we believe are among the most pressing areas for future policy-related progress. In part, our list was developed from the content of the previous 17 chapters. The issues covered are not meant to be exhaustive; rather, we seek to identify the most promising areas that will move forward practice and research in public health policy.

EVIDENCE OF POLICY INTERVENTION EFFECTIVENESS AND GENERALIZABILITY

An ever-increasing body of evidence is revealing which policies work and which are ineffective; to supplement this evidence on policy effectiveness, a few related topics deserve attention.

Further Develop the Evidence Base on External Validity

As described in this book, there are numerous forms of policy-related evidence. Some types of evidence demonstrate the relative effectiveness of specific policy interventions to address a particular health condition. What is fundamental to policy research, however, and is often missing, is a body of evidence that can help to determine the generalizability of an intervention from one population and/or setting to another (i.e., the core concepts of external validity).[8] There are many remaining research questions related to external validity, including: Which factors need to be taken into account when an internally valid policy is implemented in a different setting or with a different population subgroup? How does one balance the concepts of intervention fidelity and adaptation (reinvention)? If the adaptation process changes the original policy to such an extent that the original efficacy data may no longer apply, then the program may be viewed as a new intervention under very different contextual conditions. How might we efficiently and effectively measure external validity across a wide range of policy-related settings? How can systematic reviews more fully incorporate concepts of external validity?

This greater attention to external validity of policy has many benefits. These include greater relevance and enhanced credibility of findings from research for policymakers and a better understanding of what constitutes an "effective" policy approach (i.e., based solely on whether it worked in a narrowly defined population or a broader understanding of the key factors needed for replication or "scaling-up"[9]).

Apply Concepts from Diffusion Theory

A greater application of diffusion theory will benefit our understanding of the effectiveness and scale-up potential of policy-related interventions. Diffusion theory is a widely used theory designed to understand and predict how innovations (e.g., policies) are adopted by different individuals and organizations. Many of the current properties of diffusion were formalized by the late Everett M. Rogers, who was trained as a rural sociologist, in his classic text, *Diffusion of Innovations*.[10] Diffusion theory has taught us about specific properties of innovations that affect the rate and extent of adoption (as described in Chapter 3, particularly in Table 3.2).[11-15] Although these attributes have been applied to multiple disciplines (e.g., rural sociology, medical sociology, communication, marketing)[16] and some public health programs,[17,18] their use in policy settings is limited. Greater application of the tenets of diffusion theory is likely to enhance policy research and translation of policy into change.

Focus More Strongly on Social Determinants

Public health problems—such as violence, mental illness, and obesity—have complex, underlying direct and indirect causes—the so-called "social determinants of health" (i.e., a group of highly interrelated policy-related factors including poverty, education, housing, and employment)[19,20] (as discussed in Chapter 5). There is now a large body of observational research establishing the links among multiple social determinants and a wide array of health outcomes.[20] Addressing these variables involves aligning structures to optimize health (e.g., improving the built environment), shifting social norms, or developing and assessing evidence to address the well established "causes of causes," including large and powerful industries (e.g., alcohol, tobacco, beverage, and firearms).

Significant challenges to changing the policy environment are often present in low-resource, socially disadvantaged communities—requiring a greater commitment of time and other resources. The greater difficulty and cost may be a deterrent to taking action. On the other hand, any broad policy change undertaken to enable prevention in the society at large will probably yield a greater than average return in high-risk communities. Braverman and colleagues have outlined several priorities for social determinants research, including additional longitudinal research, elucidation of the pathways through which upstream determinants of health operate, understanding political barriers to action, and testing multidimensional interventions that address social determinants.[20]

IMPROVEMENTS IN SURVEILLANCE AND EVALUATION

To increase the scope and frequency of evidence-based policies, practitioners, policymakers, and researchers need an up-to-date list of policy solutions. Long-established principles of surveillance and evaluation are essential for progress.

Enhance Policy Surveillance

Public health surveillance, namely, the ongoing systematic collection, analysis, and interpretation of outcome-specific health data, is a cornerstone of public health[21]—it brings to mind the adage: "What gets measured, gets done."[22] Although we have built many excellent surveillance systems for measuring long-term change (e.g., behavioral risk factors, mortality, cancer incidence), most of these are only partially helpful for policy research, where a greater focus is needed on not only the outcome but on the independent variable (the policy).[23] To supplement existing systems, we need expanded policy surveillance that will enhance our ability to examine time trends in policies and to conduct more sophisticated research on the determinants, implementation, and effectiveness of prevention policies. In addition, by triangulating various surveillance data, hypotheses can be developed (e.g., examining whether state-level policy influences risk factors), which can, in turn, be tested in intervention studies. Importantly, resources are needed to support the continued maintenance and development of policy surveillance systems over time. Many systems initially are funded to create such systems, but unless they continue to be supported over time, it will be difficult to truly measure the long-term impact of policies on key public health outcomes. A few notable efforts are underway to develop public health policy surveillance systems. For example, a group of federal and voluntary agencies have developed policy surveillance systems for tobacco, alcohol, and more recently, school-based nutrition and physical education (see Chapter 15, particularly Table 15.2).[24-27]

Develop Better Measures for "Upstream" Determinants

Successful progress of policy science will require the development of practical measures of outcomes that are both reliable and valid. These enable empirical testing of the success of policy efforts. Related to the previous discussion of social determinants of health, much more emphasis has been placed on measuring the distal results of policies (risk factors, diseases), rather than the "midstream" and "upstream" factors.[28,29]

As new measures are developed (or existing metrics adapted), some key considerations include: which outcomes should be tracked and how long it will take to show progress; how policy fidelity and adaptation can best be measured across a broad range of circumstances; how to best determine criterion validity (how a measure compares with a "gold standard"); how to best measure moderating factors across a range of settings (e.g., schools, worksites); and how common, practical, measures can be developed and shared so researchers are not constantly reinventing measures.

Increase the Volume of Natural Experiments

There is great demand for increased quantity and quality of evidence related to health outcomes of policy interventions. Unfortunately, many aspects of policy change are not applicable for randomization, thus eliminating the use of the strongest experimental design—the randomized controlled trial.[30,31] Practical, political, and ethical reasons inhibit randomization related to, for example, new roads, urban development, or zoning changes. An alternative to randomized controlled trials for evaluating population-level policy and environmental interventions is the "natural experiment." A natural experiment can be defined as a study where the exposure to the event or intervention of interest has not been manipulated by the researcher, but is the result of policy or program change with varied implementation along a number of possible dimensions, such as time, geography, or content.[32] Natural experimental approaches work best when the effects of the intervention are large and rapid, and quality data on exposure and outcomes in a large population are available.[32] By nature, these studies are more susceptible to bias and confounding, but hold promise in building the evidence base for health impact from policy change.

Because natural experiments are different from more traditional experimental designs, flexible forms of research funding are needed. Several institutes and centers at the National Institutes of Health have jointly issued funding opportunity announcements intended to support rigorous evaluation of natural experiments related to obesity and/or diabetes outcomes.[33] The National Institute of Mental Health also offers opportunities for study natural experiments related to mental illness. Despite the availability of funding, applications often are disadvantaged by being judged against the rigor of standard experiments. As policy change continues to be a lever for health impact, more long-term evaluations are needed. These will require appropriate methodology and rapid response funding.

EMERGING TRENDS IN PUBLIC HEALTH

The landscape for prevention and public health is changing constantly due to a variety of inputs (e.g., new diseases/treatments, new information technologies, changing social conditions). These macro-level changes have significant implications for policy-related intervention and research.

Address Climate Change

A wide range of policy issues are connected with climate change, which is increasingly becoming a front-burner issue for public health.[34,35] The range of issues impacted by climate change is diverse, changing, and crosses multiple sectors. Climate change is affecting the following: (1) the ecology of infectious diseases (e.g., increasing the range or abundance of animal reservoirs or insect vectors), (2) catastrophic weather or weather-related events (e.g., flooding, tornadoes, drought, heat waves), (3) rising sea levels, which, in turn, affect the movements of populations, (4) food production changes in relation to weather extremes, and (5) health effects of temperature extremes or air pollution.[36]

Helpful policy-related recommendations have come from the United Kingdom suggesting the need for more research on the most effective policies to address climate change, development of coalitions between policy advocates and health professionals (especially those bridging diverse sectors such as economic development, housing, transportation), and developing policy statements to encourage health professionals to address climate changes.[35,37]

Respond to Emerging Infections

An emerging infectious disease is an infectious disease that has newly appeared in a population (e.g., Severe Acute Respiratory Syndrome [SARS]), has undergone ecologic transformation (e.g., West Nile virus), or has been known for some time but has re-emerged and is increasing rapidly in incidence and/or geographic spread (e.g., influenza). As with many other diseases, emerging infectious diseases occur due to a complex array of variables, including microbial adaptation, climate change, population growth, globalized travel, poverty, and changing human susceptibility.

Emerging infectious diseases can be addressed via a range of policy actions, including: (1) strengthening global surveillance efforts; (2) stronger international standards for control; and (3) capacity building to support the physical infrastructure (e.g., laboratories, research facilities) and personnel for outbreak investigation and medical follow-up.[38,39]

Control Chronic Diseases in a Global Context

Chronic diseases (e.g., heart disease, cancer, stroke, diabetes) now affect all countries across all income groups with almost 80% of chronic diseases occurring in low- and middle-income countries.[40] These chronic diseases are an enormous and growing strain on health systems worldwide and are the source of social and economic costs at national and household levels.

Despite the burden they present in terms of mortality, morbidity, and economic costs, chronic diseases remain neglected, particularly in low- and middle-income countries.[41-43] Because there are many effective and cost-effective methods for controlling chronic diseases, the relative lack of action is more a political than a technological failure.[42] Too often, economic and political incentives favor industry over health-related interests (e.g., subsidies for mass-produced processed foods, or tobacco revenue generated by a government-owned tobacco industry).[43] Additional challenges include the need to bridge diverse disciplines, build the evidence base across countries, and support formal training in public health sciences.[44]

Increase Use of Social Media/Informatics

Emerging technology is changing many aspects of public health. For decades, landline telephone surveys were standard for collecting data, but with the uptake of cell phone usage this method has almost become obsolete. The use of online surveys, text message surveys, or surveying through cell phones are now commonplace. Implementing these new methods will enhance evaluations and help build the evidence base for policy outcomes. Also, learning new technological skills, such as how to use geographic information system, can facilitate both research and dissemination. Maps and graphics can be especially important for identifying specific regions or jurisdictions affected by public policies. Another important technological skill is competence in creating infographics (visual depictions of information or data). Programs and software to develop these innovative ways of presenting information exist. These vary in price (some are free) and skill required (some are simple). Increased use of infographics across all disciplines is making this a necessary skill for successful dissemination.

The use of social media (e.g., Facebook, Twitter, Instagram, YouTube) is increasingly seen as a tool for health promotion and disease prevention intervention and communication. International organizations, federal agencies, state and local health departments, and advocacy groups use social media to provide information and garner support for policies, programs, and initiatives. Researchers are beginning to study the effectiveness of these strategies,[45] along with the growth of their use in public health practice. Keeping up to date on the latest research and trends in the use of social media is recommended.

Continue Implementation of the Affordable Care Act

As highlighted in Chapter 1, the Affordable Care Act (ACA) is a landmark federal policy with many provisions for disease prevention and health promotion. Since it was enacted in 2010, critics have continuously attempted to impede part or all of the legislation, including important public health aspects such as disease screenings or access to birth control. Researchers and practitioners need to become advocates and active voices for the continuation of ACA. The first step is to be familiar with the existing law. Useful summaries and fact sheets for basic information and advocacy are available from the American Public Health Association,[46] the Kaiser Family Foundation,[47] and the U.S. Department of Health and Human Services.[48]

NEW SKILLS FOR THE PUBLIC HEALTH WORKFORCE

Priorities for education of the public health workforce have focused largely on the traditional disciplines of epidemiology, biostatistics, health education, environmental health, and health management/policy. For more rapid future progress, some new and related skills are needed.

Communicate Policy Information More Effectively

The former Speaker of the U.S. House of Representatives, Thomas ("Tip") O'Neill, made famous the phrase, "All politics is local." Evidence becomes more relevant to policymakers when it involves a local example (a story), often describing some type of direct impact on one's local community, family, or constituents.[49] For example, when sample sizes permit, it is probably more policy-relevant to calculate statistics at the voting district or even precinct level than at the city or state level. Research on contextual issues and the importance of narrative communication is beginning to present data in the form of a story that helps to personalize an issue. The premise for this line of research is that storytelling makes messages personally relevant, motivation is gauged by personal susceptibility, and practical information is provided. Policymakers cite the impact on "real people" as one of the most important factors in increasing the coverage and relevance of research.[50]

Fortunately, previous work in the areas of policy development and health communication offer some direction to guide a more systematic approach to using stories (Table 18.1).[51–53] These elements complement the approaches described in

Table 18.1 Attributes of Evidence-based Stories for Policy Advocacy

Attribute	Description of Example Story Element(S)
Expresses an important theme	Revolves around a person (or group of people) at risk for the negative consequences resulting from the risk factor/ absence of policy
Located on underlying distribution of stories	Based on a common case, with respect to risk factor, barriers, and potential impact of a policy intervention
Verifiable	Based on a real-life example (or is at least representative of real-life)
Acknowledges uncertainties in research	Policy interventions described in the story acknowledge the strength of the level
Based on compelling narrative*	Narrative is designed so that intended audience (policymaker) is compelled to share the story with others

Adapted from Steiner[51] and Stamatakis.[52]

*Kreuter and colleagues[53] describe attributes of quality narrative in terms of elements such as coherence of story sequence, character development, story structure, emotional intensity, cultural appropriateness, and production value.

Chapters 16 and 17. Related to narrative communication, there is a need to convert longer research reports into shorter policy "briefs" because policymakers are more likely to read material that is broken into bullets and accompanied by charts or graphs illustrating key points. New skills in this area can build on advice from several teams on how to construct an effective policy brief.[52,54]

Improve Skills in Transdisciplinary Practice

In nearly all cases, policy progress will require new skills and "nontraditional" partnerships with people and organizations not working directly in public health. For example, to address the major physical barriers to physical activity in cities, urban planners, transportation experts, and persons working in parks and recreation are essential in developing an environment and the political will that is physical-activityfriendly. Each of these disciplines has its own priorities, language, acronyms, and assumptions about the role of government. Learning from one another and developing ways to accommodate for differences is essential for the success of transdisciplinary teams. Public health researchers and practitioners can serve as key players on these teams and should enhance leadership, facilitation, and communication skills.

Conduct and Apply Tools from Economic Evaluation

As noted in Chapter 4, economic evaluation is an important tool for policy intervention and research. It can provide information to help assess the relative value of alternative expenditures on policy measures to support health services and public health programs. For example, cost-effectiveness analysis can suggest the relative value of alternative policy interventions (i.e., health return on dollars invested) and can play a key role in a whole range of policy studies. Although cost-effectiveness analysis has been increasingly applied to medical and behavioral health interventions, it could be more widely applied for policy evaluation. In numerous surveys, skills in economic evaluation are among those highly valued by policymakers[55,56] yet most lacking among public health practitioners.[57,58]

CONCLUSION

Predicting the future is a task fraught with challenges and uncertainties. But despite the difficulty of predictions, it is clear that closer linkages between the science of public health and policy audiences are essential if we are to address issues of societal importance and thereby enhance the health of populations.

Policy measures are sometimes (falsely) portrayed as a choice between responsibility of individuals and restriction of freedom by the government.[59] There is a need for strong leadership and new policies, practices, and participation beyond the confines of traditional public health agencies and services.[59] To achieve this progress by furthering evidence-based policy, researchers need to use the best available evidence and expand the role of researchers and practitioners to communicate evidence packaged appropriately for various policy audiences. They also need to understand and engage all three streams[60] (problem, policy, politics) to implement an evidence-based policy process; to develop content based on specific policy elements that are most likely to be effective; and to document outcomes to improve, expand, or terminate policy.

REFERENCES

1. Centers for Disease Control and Prevention (CDC). Ten great public health achievements—United States, 1900–1999. *MMWR.* Apr 1999;48(12):241–243.
2. Centers for Disease Control and Prevention (CDC). Ten great public health achievements—United States, 2001–2010. *MMWR.* May 2011;60(19):619–623.
3. Brownson RC, Haire-Joshu D, Luke DA. Shaping the context of health: a review of environmental and policy approaches in the prevention of chronic diseases. *Annu Rev Public Health.* 2006;27:341–370.
4. Salinsky E, Gursky EA. The case for transforming governmental public health. *Health Aff (Millwood).* Jul–Aug 2006;25(4):1017–1028.
5. Slonim AB, Callaghan C, Daily L, et al. Recommendations for integration of chronic disease programs: are your programs linked? *Prev Chronic Dis.* Apr 2007;4(2):A34.
6. Wiesner PJ. Four diseases of disarray in public health. *Ann Epidemiol.* Mar 1993;3(2):196–198.
7. Allen P, Sequeira S, Best L, Jones E, Baker EA, Brownson RC. Perceived benefits and challenges of coordinated approaches to chronic disease prevention in state health departments. *Prev Chronic Dis.* 2014;11:E76.
8. Green LW, Glasgow RE. Evaluating the relevance, generalization, and applicability of research: issues in external validation and translation methodology. *Eval Health Prof.* Mar 2006;29(1):126–153.

9. Norton W, Mittman B. *Scaling Up Health Promotion/Disease Prevention Programs in Community Settings: Barriers, Facilitators, and Initial Recommendations.* Hartford, CT: Patrick and Catherine Weldon Donaghue Medical Research Foundation; 2010.

10. Rogers EM. *Diffusion of Innovations.* New York: Free Press; 1962.

11. Dearing J, Kee K. Historical roots of dissemination and implementation science. In: Brownson R, Colditz G, Proctor E (Eds.). *Dissemination and Implementation Research in Health: Translating Science to Practice.* New York: Oxford University Press; 2012: 55–71.

12. Oldenburg B, Glanz K. Diffusion of innovations. In: Glanz K, Rimer B, Vishwanath K (Eds.). *Health Behavior and Health Education: Theory, Research and Practice.* 4th ed. San Francisco, CA: Jossey-Bass; 2008: 313–334.

13. Dodson E, Brownson R, Weiss S. Policy dissemination research. In: Brownson R, Colditz G, Proctor E (Eds.). *Dissemination and Implementation Research in Health: Translating Science to Practice.* New York: Oxford University Press; 2012: 437–458.

14. Brownson R, Tabak R, Stamatakis K, Glanz K. Implementation, dissemination and diffusion of public health interventions. In: Glanz K, Rimer B, Viswanath K, (Eds.). *Health Behavior and Health Education.* 5th ed. San Francisco, CA: Jossey-Bass Publishers; 2015: 301–326.

15. Rogers EM. *Diffusion of Innovations.* 5th ed. New York: Free Press; 2003.

16. Dearing JW. Evolution of diffusion and dissemination theory. *J Public Health Manag Pract.* Mar–Apr 2008;14(2):99–108.

17. Dearing JW. Improving the state of health programming by using diffusion theory. *J Health Commun.* 2004;9(Suppl 1):21–36.

18. King L, Hawe P, Wise M. Making dissemination a two-way process. *Health Promotion International.* 1998;13(3):237–244.

19. McKinlay JB, Marceau LD. Upstream healthy public policy: lessons from the battle of tobacco. *Int J Health Serv.* 2000;30(1):49–69.

20. Braveman P, Egerter S, Williams DR. The social determinants of health: coming of age. *Annu Rev Public Health.* 2011;32:381–398.

21. Thacker SB, Berkelman RL. Public health surveillance in the United States. *Epidemiol Rev.* 1988;10:164–190.

22. Thacker SB. Public health surveillance and the prevention of injuries in sports: what gets measured gets done. *J Athl Train.* Apr–Jun 2007;42(2):171–172.

23. Chriqui JF, O'Connor JC, Chaloupka FJ. What gets measured, gets changed: evaluating law and policy for maximum impact. *J Law Med Ethics.* Mar 2011;39(Suppl 1):21–26.

24. Chriqui JF, Frosh MM, Brownson RC, et al. Measuring policy and legislative change. *Evaluating ASSIST: A Blueprint for Understanding State-Level Tobacco Control.* Bethesda, MD: National Cancer Institute; 2006.

25. Masse LC, Chriqui JF, Igoe JF, et al. Development of a Physical Education-Related State Policy Classification System (PERSPCS). *Am J Prev Med.* Oct 2007;33(4 Suppl):S264–276.

26. Masse LC, Frosh MM, Chriqui JF, et al. Development of a School Nutrition-Environment State Policy Classification System (SNESPCS). *Am J Prev Med.* Oct 2007;33(4 Suppl):S277–S291.

27. National Institute on Alcohol Abuse and Alcoholism. Alcohol Policy Information System. http://alcoholpolicy.niaaa.nih.gov/. Accessed May 10, 2015.

28. Brownson RC, Jones E. Bridging the gap: translating research into policy and practice. *Prev Med.* Oct 2009;49(4):313–315.

29. McKinlay JB. Paradigmatic obstacles to improving the health of populations—implications for health policy. *Salud Publica Mex.* Jul–Aug 1998;40(4):369–379.

30. Brownson RC, Diez Roux AV, Swartz K. Commentary: Generating rigorous evidence for public health: the need for new thinking to improve research and practice. *Annu Rev Public Health*. 2014;35:1–7.

31. Mercer SL, Devinney BJ, Fine LJ, Green LW, Dougherty D. Study designs for effectiveness and translation research identifying trade-offs. *Am J Prev Med*. Aug 2007;33(2):139–154.

32. Craig P, Cooper C, Gunnell D, et al. Using natural experiments to evaluate population health interventions: new Medical Research Council guidance. *J Epidemiol Community Health*. Dec 2012;66(12):1182–1186.

33. Hunter CM, McKinnon RA, Esposito L. News from the NIH: research to evaluate "natural experiments" related to obesity and diabetes. *Transl Behav Med*. Jun 2014;4(2):127–129.

34. Fielding JE. Preface: changing climate changing public health. *Annu Rev Public Health*. 2008;29:v–vi.

35. Jackson R, Shields KN. Preparing the U.S. health community for climate change. *Annu Rev Public Health*. 2008;29:57–73.

36. Erwin P, Brownson R. The future of public health practice. In: Erwin P, Brownson R (Eds.). *Scutchfield and Keck's Principles of Public Health Practice*. 4th ed. Clifton Park, NY: Cengage Learning; 2015: In press.

37. Stott R, Godlee F. What should we do about climate change? Health professionals need to act now, collectively and individually. *BMJ*. Nov 2006;333(7576):983–984.

38. Fidler DP. Globalization, international law, and emerging infectious diseases. *Emerg Infect Dis*. Apr Jun 1996;2(2):77 84.

39. Coker RJ, Hunter BM, Rudge JW, Liverani M, Hanvoravongchai P. Emerging infectious diseases in Southeast Asia: regional challenges to control. *Lancet*. Feb 2011;377(9765): 599–609.

40. World Health Organization. *Noncommunicable Diseases—Country Profiles*. Geneva, Switzerland: Author; 2011.

41. Daar AS, Singer PA, Persad DL, et al. Grand challenges in chronic non-communicable diseases. *Nature*. Nov 2007;450(7169):494–496.

42. Geneau R, Stuckler D, Stachenko S, et al. Raising the priority of preventing chronic diseases: a political process. *Lancet*. Nov 2010;376(9753):1689–1698.

43. Narayan KM, Ali MK, Koplan JP. Global noncommunicable diseases—where worlds meet. *N Engl J Med*. Sep 2010;363(13):1196–1198.

44. Diem G, Brownson RC, Grabauskas V, Shatchkute A, Stachenko S. Prevention and control of noncommunicable diseases through evidence-based public health: implementing the NCD 2020 action plan. *Glob Health Promot*. March 10, 2015.

45. Capurro D, Cole K, Echavarria MI, Joe J, Neogi T, Turner AM. The use of social networking sites for public health practice and research: a systematic review. *J Med Internet Res*. 2014;16(3):e79.

46. American Public Health Association. Policy Statements and Advocacy. https://www.apha.org/policies-and-advocacy. Accessed May 16, 2015.

47. The Henry J. Kaiser Family Foundation. http://kff.org/. Accessed May 16, 2015.

48. U.S. Department of Health and Human Services. About the Law. http://www.hhs.gov/healthcare/rights/. Accessed May 16, 2015.

49. Jones E, Kreuter M, Pritchett S, Matulionis RM, Hann N. State health policy makers: what's the message and who's listening? *Health Promot Pract*. Jul 2006;7(3):280–286.

50. Sorian R, Baugh T. Power of information: closing the gap between research and policy. When it comes to conveying complex information to busy policy-makers, a picture is truly worth a thousand words. *Health Aff (Millwood)*. Mar–Apr 2002;21(2):264–273.

51. Steiner JF. Using stories to disseminate research: the attributes of representative stories. *J Gen Intern Med.* Nov 2007;22(11):1603–1607.

52. Stamatakis K, McBride T, Brownson R. Communicating prevention messages to policy makers: The role of stories in promoting physical activity. *J Phys Act Health.* 2010;7(Suppl 1):S00–S107.

53. Kreuter MW, Green MC, Cappella JN, et al. Narrative communication in cancer prevention and control: a framework to guide research and application. *Ann Behav Med.* May–Jun 2007;33(3):221–235.

54. Dodson EA, Eyler AA, Chalifour S, Wintrode CG. A review of obesity-themed policy briefs. *Am J Prev Med.* Sep 2012;43(3 Suppl 2):S143–S148.

55. Haines A, Kuruvilla S, Borchert M. Bridging the implementation gap between knowledge and action for health. *Bull World Health Organ.* Oct 2004;82(10):724–731; discussion 732.

56. Sanderson I. Evaluation, policy learning and evidence-based policy making. *Public Admin.* 2002;80(1):1–22.

57. Jacob RR, Baker EA, Allen P, et al. Training needs and supports for evidence-based decision making among the public health workforce in the United States. *BMC Health Serv Res.* Nov 2014;14(1):564.

58. Jacobs JA, Clayton PF, Dove C, et al. A survey tool for measuring evidence-based decision making capacity in public health agencies. *BMC Health Serv Res.* 2012;12:57.

59. Chokshi DA, Stine NW. Reconsidering the politics of public health. *JAMA: The Journal of the American Medical Association.* Sep 2013;310(10):1025–1026.

60. Kingdon JW. *Agendas, Alternatives, and Public Policies.* Updated 2nd ed. Boston, MA: Longman; 2010.

Index

Arkansas Medicaid Trust Fund, 155
ASPPH. *see* Association of Schools and
      Programs of Public Health (ASPPH)
ASR. *see* Annual Security Report (ASR)
asset building
   preventive health through
      social and economic policy and, 97–98
Association of Schools and Programs of
      Public Health (ASPPH), 12
availability
   in alcohol control policy, 184

BAC. *see* blood alcohol concentration (BAC)
background section
   in public health policy analysis process,
      72–73, 69*f*
ballot initiatives, 269
   in tax-based pricing policies, 122, 122*b*
ballot measures
   general legislative policymaking *vs.*, 28
   in policy enactment, 28
bar charts
   in communicating with policymakers,
      314–315, 315*f*
behavior(s). *see also specific types, e.g.,* sexual
      behavior
   changing of
      injury prevention policies in, 218–220
   risk
      changing social meaning of, 218–219
   sedentary
      prevalence of, 164
   sexual (*see* sexual behavior)
Berkeley SSB-tax initiative (2014), 157
*Best Practices for Comprehensive Tobacco
      Control*
   of CDC, 120
beverage labels
   revision of
      FDA on, 33
bicycle helmet requirements, 221
bill(s)
   amendment to, 25
   budget
      policy implementation related to, 29*b*
   drafting of
      in policy enactment, 25–26, 26*f*, 22*f*

bite(s)
   tick
      prevention of, 202
blood alcohol concentration (BAC)
   in alcohol control policy, 184–185
blood donation
   American Medical Association on, 258
   FDA on, 255, 258
   from MSM, 255, 258
blood donation policy, 255, 258
Bloomberg, M., 33
BMI. *see* body mass index (BMI)
body mass index (BMI), 141
Brazilian Ministry of Health, 169
breastfeeding
   HIV transmission via, 209
Brownell, K.D., 342
Brown, M., 109
Brownson, R.C., 3, 349, x
Buckyballs
   lawsuits related to, 221–222
budget bills
   policy implementation related to, 29*b*
Buggery Act of 1533, 251
Bush, G.W., Pres., 168

California Center for Public Health
   Advocacy (CCPHA), 345
California Evidence-based
      Clearinghouse, Domestic
      Violence Home Visitation
      Intervention, 241
California Lesbian Gay Bisexual Transgender
      (LGBT) Tobacco Education
      Partnership
   case study, 131–133
Camberos, G.J., 93
Campus SaVE. *see* Campus Sexual
      Elimination Act (Campus SaVE)
Campus Sexual Violence Elimination Act
      (Campus SaVE), 234–237
cancer(s)
   lung
      tobacco use and, 117
CARDIA study. *see* Coronary Artery Risk
      Development in Young Adults
      (CARDIA) study

climate change
  addressing
    public health policy in, 353
Clostridium difficile infection
  prevalence of, 208
club drug GHB
    (gamma-hydroxybutyrate), 267
CMS. *see* Centers for Medicare and Medicaid
    Services (CMS)
coalition
  in advocacy process
    formation of, 337, 338t
coal mine explosions
  government interventions in, 19–20
Cochrane Collaboration, 223
Cohen, M.D., 50
collective choice tier
  of IAD Framework, 48, 49
CollegeBound*baby* program, 97
College Kick Start program, 97
colorectal cancer screening
  narrative to encourage, 314b
commercial sexual behavior
  public policy strategies related to, 251–253
Committee on Tobacco Use
  of IOM, 123
common administrative law, 20
common law
  in policy enactment, 27–28
  in public health policy, 31
communal resources
  allocation of
    public policy in, 18
communication
  in Diffusion of Innovation theory, 58
  importance of, 303
  in influencing policy and practice,
    303–327 (*see also* policymaker(s),
    communicating with)
  interpersonal
    in agenda-setting process, 46
  by public health workforce
    policy information–related,
      355–356, 356t
  strategic
    in EHI, 99f, 102–103
communication planning

in communicating with policymakers,
    304b, 308–319
  anticipate potential opposition
    arguments and strategies, 318, 318b
  develop and deliver messages, 304b,
    311–318, 313f, 314b, 315f, 316f,
    317b, 318b
  develop storyline (meta-message),
    304b, 308–309
  follow-up, 318–319, 319b
  select messenger (source) in, 304b,
    310–311, 310f
  timing in, 304b, 309–310
Communities Putting Prevention to Work
    (CPPW) program, 8, 8b
  as example of broad reach of policy, 10
community(ies)
  LGBT
    provisions for VAWRA in, 232, 232f
    tobacco use in, 131–133
  policy, 44
  preventive health in
    social and economic policy and, 98
"Community Action Forums," 110
Community Feedback Forum
  of *For the Sake of All* project, 105f, 106
Community Partner Group (CPG), 103–
    110. *see also For the Sake of All* project
Community Preventive Services Task
    Force, 223
Community Trials Project, 47
Complete Streets
  terminology related to, 172–173
Complete Streets policies
  across U.S.
    diffusion of, 59–60
  case of, 172–173
  described, 60
concussion management
  in youth athletics
    law related to, 32
conditional use permits (CUPs)
  in regulating tobacco retailers, 125, 126b
condom use
  in HIV prevention, 210–211
  in STI/HIV prevention, 254–255,
    256t–257t

1861 Offenses Against the Person Act, 251
Electronic Nicotine Delivery Systems
    (ENDS), 296
emerging infectious disease
  responding to
    public health policy in, 353–354
*Ending the Tobacco Problem: A Blueprint for
    the Nation*
  of IOM, 120
ENDS. *see* Electronic Nicotine Delivery
    Systems (ENDS)
energy balance
  obesity related to factors affecting,
    143–145, 145f
energy commitment
  in communicating with policymakers,
    321, 320b
enforcement
  of injury prevention policies, 220–221
"Engaging Richmond" community–
    university partnership, 100
entrepreneur
  policy
    described, 51
environment(s)
  obesogenic, 143–145, 145f
  physical
    safety modifications of, 218
  policymaking
    in communicating with policymakers,
      304–319, 304b (*see also*
      policymaking environment, in
      communicating with policymakers)
  smoke-free
    creating, 120–121, 121f
  social
    safety modifications of, 218
  types of, 330
Equal Protection Clause of the Fourteenth
    Amendment, 133
equity
  in evaluation criteria, 81b
ethical considerations
  in communicating with policymakers,
    321, 320b
evaluation criteria
  identification of, 80, 81b

in improving public health, 352–354
in public health policy analysis process, 80,
    81b, 69f
Event History Analysis, 60
evidence base
  in evaluation criteria, 81b
  external validity in developing, 350
  in policy analysis, 83, 85
executive branch of government, 20, 21f
  policy implementation by, 29–30
executive orders, 20
  defined, 27
  in policy enactment, 27
experiment(s)
  natural (*see* natural experiment(s))
externalities
  defined, 19
external validity
  develop evidence base on, 350
Eyler, A.A., ix, 3, 163, 291, 349

face-to-face meetings
  with individual policymakers
    recommendations for, 317–318, 318b
FAFH. *see* food consumed away from
    home (FAFH)
fairness
  in evaluation criteria, 81b
Fallin, A., 49
false identification documents (IDs)
  laws prohibiting use or sale of, 185–186
Family Educational Rights and Privacy Act, 236
Family Smoking Prevention and Tobacco
    Control Act, 31
family violence. *see also* intimate partner
    violence (IPV)
  mental health problems related to, 242
FDA. *see* Food and Drug
    Administration (FDA)
FDA v. Brown & Williamson Tobacco Corp, 31
federal agencies with health-related data
  examples of, 71t–72t
federal food and nutrition programs,
    146–147, 146t
federal government
  state government *vs.*
    tasks of, 20–22

federal prevention policy
  ACA on, 7b–8b
Federal Register, 76
"feedback loop," 23, 31, 67
Ferguson, Missouri
  fatal shooting of unarmed teenager in, 109
Fields, R., 93
Fifth Amendment Takings Clause
  in tobacco control, 130–131, 130b
First Amendment commercial speech
  in tobacco control, 130–131, 130b
First Amendment compelled speech
  in tobacco control, 130–131, 130b
focusing events
  in agenda-setting process, 46
FOCUS St. Louis, 109
food, nutrition, and obesity policy, 141–162.
    see also obesity; obesity epidemic
Food and Drug Administration (FDA)
  on blood donation, 255, 258
  on nutritional labeling for vending
      machines and chain restaurants, 7b
  on revising food and beverage labels, 33
  tobacco industry *vs.*, 31
  on tobacco products regulation,
      123–125, 124t
food-borne infections
  mortality data, 197–198
  transmission of
      prevention of, 202–203
food consumed away from home (FAFH)
  as factor in obesity, 145
food labels
  revising
      FDA on, 33
Food Stamp Program, 147
food system
  of U.S., 145
formal policymaking process, 305, 304b
forthesakeofall.org, 105
For the Sake of All project, 98, 103–110
  alignment with City of St. Louis
      Sustainability Plan, 106
  Community Feedback Forum of, 106, 105f
  described, 103
  dissemination of information in, 104–108,
      107f, 108f, 105f

engagement in, 104–108, 107f, 108f, 105f
  goals of, 103
  partnerships in, 104
  response to, 108–109
  second phase of, 109–110
Framework Convention on Tobacco Control
  of WHO, 118
free media
  defined, 34
Freudenberg, N., 96
Frieden, T., 42, 94
Friedman, R.R., 329
"fundamental causes" of health, 93
Futures Without Violence, 241

Galea, S., 105
gamma-hydroxybutyrate (GHB), 267
"Garbage Can" model, 50
gas prices
  physical activity effects of, 173–174
gatekeepers (aides)
  in agenda-setting process, 46
  build relationships with, 306–307, 304b
Gateway Center for Giving, 109
gender
  as factor in obesity, 142
general legislative policymaking
  ballot measures *vs.*, 28
GHB (gamma-hydroxybutyrate), 267
Giffords, G., 335
Gilsinan, J., 41
global connectivity
  as factor in infectious diseases, 198
Global Polio Eradication Initiative, 18
global premature death
  causes of, 197–198, 198t
Golden, S.D., 17, 117
Gordon, B., 131
government(s)
  branches of, 20, 21f
  interventions by (*see* government
      interventions)
  policymaking and rulemaking through, 17
  state *vs.* federal
      tasks of, 20–22
governmental policy systems
  described, 9

Healthy People 2020, 118, 292
hepatitis A vaccination
  occupations requiring, 204
"herd immunity," 205
herpes zoster virus
  vaccine against, 204
HIA. *see* Health Impact Assessment (HIA)
HiAP. *see* "health in all policies" (HiAP)
Higher Education Act of 1965, 236
HITECH Act of 2009. *see* Health
    Information Technology for
    Economic and Clinical Health
    (HITECH) Act of 2009
HIV/AIDS
  in inmates
    Social Construction Framework in
    prevention of, 54
HIV infection
  mandates in U.S. related to
    sex education and, 256t–257t
  mortality data, 208 209
  new cases, 211
  policies related to
    case study, 208–211
  prevention and control of, 208–211
    CDC on, 260
    condom use in, 210–211, 254–255,
    256t–257t
    PrEP in, 210–211
    treatment of infected individuals
    in, 210
  testing for
    CDC on, 210–211
  transmission of, 209
    mother-to-child, 209
Holder, H.D., 47
home visitations
  in violence against women prevention,
    241–242
Hou, N., 174
household-income poverty
  negative outcomes for children and youth
    related to, 97
"How can we save lives–and save money–in
    St. Louis? Invest in economic and
    educational opportunity," 105
HUD. *see* U.S. Department of Housing and
    Urban Development (HUD)

IAD Framework. *see* Institutional Analysis
    and Development (IAD) Framework
identification documents (IDs)
  false
    laws prohibiting use or sale of, 185–186
IDs. *see* identification documents (IDs)
"I Have a Dream" speech, 104
illicit drug(s)
  costs and nature of, 264
  public policy related to, 263–287
    (*see also* illicit drug use)
  types of, 264
illicit drug use
  described, 263–264, 265f
  epidemic of, 220
  fatal, 220
  prevalence of, 264, 265f
  public health risks of, 263–264, 265f
  public policy and, 263–287
  U.S. policy strategies for addressing, 264–
    271, 265f, 266f (*see also* U.S. illicit
    drug policy)
immunity
  "herd," 205
immunization(s). *see* vaccination(s);
    vaccine(s)
improving conditions
  public policy in, 18
inactivity
  physical, 163–165, 164f (*see also* physical
    activity)
individually focused effort
  policy interventions *vs.*, 10
infection(s). *see* specific types
infectious disease(s)
  consequences of, 197–199, 198t
  emerging
    public health in responding
    to, 353–354
  global connectivity and, 198
  human-to-human transmission of
    prevention of, 203–204
  mortality data, 197–198, 198t
  prevention and control of
    case study, 207–211
    contact tracing in, 203
    HCAIs, 207–211
    history of, 197–199

IPV. *see* intimate partner violence (IPV)
issue framing, 24

Jacobson v. Massachusetts, 223
JCAHO standards. *see* Joint Commission
    on Accreditation of Hospital
    Organizations (JCAHO) standards
Jeanne Clery Disclosure of Campus Security
    Policy and Campus Crime Statistics
    Act, 236
Jenner, E., 5
Joint Commission on Accreditation of
    Hospital Organizations (JCAHO)
    standards, 242–243
Jonson-Reid, M., 229
judicial branch of government, 20, 21f
    policy implementation related to, 31

Kennedy, D., 239
Kerlinger, F.N., 41
Kingdon, J.W., 50
King, M.L., Jr., 104
Koop, C.E., 254
Kopfman, J.E., 313
Krebs, C., 234
Kwon, H.T., 303

label(s)
    food and beverage
        FDA on revising, 33
labeling
    nutritional
        for vending machines and chain
            restaurants, 7b
Langhinrichsen-Rohling, J., 241
Lauritsen, J.L., 229
law(s). *see also specific types*
    administrative, 27
    case, 27–28
    in changing behaviors, 219–220
    common, 27–28
        in public health policy, 31
    common administrative, 20
    concussion management in youth
        athletics–related, 32
    consumer products safety–related,
        221–222
    in creating safer consumer products, 222–223

legislative, 20
MLDA
    case study, 189–190
    in prohibiting use or sale of false IDs, 185–186
    in regulating tobacco retailers, 125, 126b
    regulatory, 27
    "Return to Play," 32
    smoke-free, 120–121, 121f
        public support for, 129
    tort, 222
Lawrence v. Texas, 251
lawsuit(s)
    product liability, 222–223
legal issues
    tobacco control policies–related,
        129–131, 130b
legality
    in evaluation criteria, 81b
legalization/regulation
    in illicit drug policy, 270–271, 269f
legislative branch
    of government, 20, 21f
    policy implementation related to, 30
legislative law, 20
legislative policies
    in injury prevention, 217–218
legislative process
    in policy enactment, 25–26, 26f, 22f
lesbian gay bisexual transgender (LGBT)
        community
    provisions for VAWRA in, 232, 232f
    tobacco use in, 131–133
Lesbian Gay Bisexual Transgender (LGBT)
        Tobacco Education Partnership
    case study, 131–133
LGBT community. *see* lesbian gay bisexual
        transgender (LGBT) community
liability
    product
        injury prevention policies related to,
            222–223
licensing laws
    in regulating tobacco retailers, 125, 126b
Lightner, C., 335
line graphs
    in communicating with policymakers,
        315–316, 316f

on sexual violence on college campuses,
235–237

on unwanted sexual behavior, 253

Office of Head Start, Administration for
Children and Families
within Department of Health and Human
Services, 95

O'Neill, T., 355

operational tier
of IAD Framework, 48, 49

opposition arguments and strategies
anticipation of
in communicating with policymakers,
318, 318b

ordinance(s), 26

organizational policies, 217

packaging restrictions
for tobacco products, 123–125, 126b, 124t

paid media
defined, 34

PAPRN. *see* Physical Activity Policy Research
Network (PAPRN)

Patient Protection and Affordable Care Act of
2010, 233

PDMPs. *see* prescription drug monitoring
programs (PDMPs)

PDO. *see* prescription drug overdose (PDO)

PE. *see* physical education (PE)

pertussis
steady rise in cases of, 206–207

Philip Morris USA, 133

physical activity
epidemiology of, 164–165, 164f
gas prices effects on, 173–174
guidelines for, 163
health benefits of, 163
importance of, 163
IOM on, 165
motivation for, 165
prevalence of, 164
public policy and, 163–178 (*see also*
physical activity policy)

physical activity policy, 163–178
advocacy for, 169–170, 171t–172t
case examples, 170, 172–174
framework on, 165–166, 166f

global examples of, 168–169
strategies, 165–169, 167t, 164f

Physical Activity Policy Research Network
(PAPRN), ix

physical education (PE) policies
case for, 170, 172

physical environment
safety modifications of
policies in, 218

physical inactivity
consequences of, 163–165, 164f
geographic predilection for, 164, 164f
prevalence of, 164

pie charts
in communicating with policymakers,
314, 315f

Pigou, A., 188

"Pigovian" taxation, 188

Plunk, A.D., 179

policy(ies). *see also specific types, e.g.,*
immunization policies
adoption of
assessment of, 289–299
alcohol misuse–related, 179–196
"big P" *vs.* "little p," 17
broad reach of
CPPW program as example of, 8, 10, 8b
changes in (*see* policy change(s))
Complete Streets, 59–60, 172–173
elements in, 330–333, 333f, 332b
evidence-based content in
evaluation for, 294–295
HIV infection–related
case study, 208–211
implementation of (*see* policy
implementation)
in improving health, 3–15
benefits of, 9–10
described, 3
introduction, 3–8, 6f, 4t, 7b–8b
public health achievements of last
century and examples of related
policy strategies, 4t
reasons for, 9–10
tobacco-related, 5, 6f, 4t
typhoid fever–related, 4–5
vaccination-related, 5, 4t

problem stream
  in Multiple Streams Framework, 50, 50f
product liability
  injury prevention policies related to,
    222–223
product liability lawsuits, 222–223
professional risks
  in communicating with policymakers,
    322, 320b
prohibition
  in illicit drug policy, 270, 269f
"Project Connect Texas," 241
prostitution
  public policy strategies related to, 251–253
Protect Students from Sexual Assault
  of White House Task Force, 234–236
public goods
  examples of, 18
  provision of
    government interventions in, 18
public health. *see also* public health policy;
    public health policy analysis
  achievements of last century
    examples of related policy strategies, 4t
  assessment of policy adoption and content
    for use in, 289–290
  described, 329
  emerging trends in, 353–355
    address climate change, 353
    continue implementation of ACA, 355
    control chronic diseases in global
      context, 354
    increased use of social media/
      informatics, 354–355
    respond to emerging infection, 353–354
  in illicit drug policy, 271, 269f
  interventions with greatest potential
    impact on, 42–43
  lobbying prevalence related to, 33
  policy theory applied to, 41–44, 43f,
    45t, 42f
    publications on, 45t
  within socio-ecological framework, 8–9
  workforce in
    new skills for, 355–357, 356t
      (*see also* public health workforce,
      new skills for)

public health advocate
  goal of, 330
Public Health Cigarette Smoking Act of
    1969, 10
Public Health Law Research initiative
  of RWJF, 223
Public Health Law Research Program at
    Temple University
  RWJF–supported, 294
public health partners
  as catalysts for tobacco control
    policies, 134
public health policy
  ACA in, 355
  advocacy and, 329–348
    (*see also* advocacy)
  analysis of, 67–92 (*see also* policy analysis;
    public health policy analysis)
  chronic diseases–related
    global context of, 354
  climate change–related, 353
  common law in, 31
  in creating health equity, 332–333, 333f
  in creating optimal defaults,
    330–332, 332b
  effectiveness of, 332, 350–351
  elements in, 330–333, 333f, 332b
  emerging infectious disease–related,
    353–354
  generalizability of, 350–351
  improving, 349–360
    apply concepts from diffusion theory in,
      350–351
    develop better measures for "upstream"
      determinants in, 352
    develop evidence base on external
      validity, 350
    evaluation-related, 352–354
    focus more strongly on social
      determinants, 351
    future directions in, 349–360
    increase volume of natural experiments
      in, 352–353
    introduction, 349–350
    surveillance-related, 351–352
  lobbying and, 333–335
  sound science as basis of, 332

youth athletics
  concussion management in
    law related to, 32

"Zackery Lystedt Law," 32
Zimmerman, E.B., 93
zoning laws